Diabetes & Women's Health Across the Life Stages

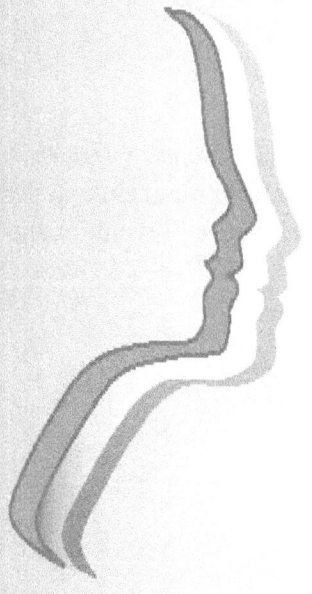

A Public Health Perspective

Gloria L.A. Beckles, MBBS, MSc, and
Patricia E. Thompson-Reid, MAT, MPH
Editors

**U.S. DEPARTMENT OF HEALTH
AND HUMAN SERVICES**
CENTERS FOR DISEASE CONTROL AND PREVENTION

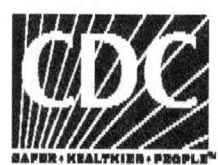

For more information, contact
CDC Division of Diabetes Translation
P. O. Box 8728
Silver Spring, MD 20910

Phone: Toll-free 1-877-CDC-DIAB (232-3422)
Fax: (301) 562-1050
E-Mail: diabetes@cdc.gov
Internet: http://www.cdc.gov/diabetes

Suggested citation:

Beckles GLA, Thompson-Reid PE, editors. *Diabetes and Women's Health Across the Life Stages: A Public Health Perspective.* Atlanta: U.S. Department of Health and Human Services, Centers for Disease Control and Prevention, National Center for Chronic Disease Prevention and Health Promotion, Division of Diabetes Translation, 2001.

Message from Frank Vinicor, MD, MPH
Director, CDC Diabetes Program

Writing this monograph has been important for the diabetes program at the Centers for Disease Control and Prevention (CDC). The monograph has become much more than a "report" by CDC. It has become a model of thought, interaction, and commitment to make a difference in the lives of people—women or men—facing the daily challenges of diabetes.

We have come to better understand the impact of greater societal forces and policies on the lives of people with diabetes, though individuals and health care providers make their own essential contributions. Many cultural, social, organizational, and environmental forces do and will facilitate or limit the impact of our individual decisions, and the need to always coordinate science and clinical medicine with programs and policies has become much more obvious to us.

We (at CDC), along with many partners, have the opportunity to convert the ideas in this monograph into concrete action to assure that efforts to augment programs directed to both the prevention of diabetes and the care of those with the disease will occur. These efforts will synergistically blend clinical and public health strategies. In the next 12 months, CDC and its primary cosponsors, the American Diabetes Association, the Association of State and Territorial Health Officials, and the American Public Health Association, will convene a national call-to-action meeting to develop and then implement the National Public Health Action Plan for Diabetes and Women. Much more effort is required, but with this monograph, the process has begun.

Our clinical care systems have benefited many Americans. Now, with the blending of public health and medical approaches to the prevention of the disease burden associated with diabetes—in this case in women—many more people who face the daily challenges of diabetes can maintain hope.

Foreword

Diabetes has been a serious public health problem for many years. Currently an estimated 16 million Americans have diabetes, more than half of them women. Why, then, has so little progress been made in reducing the burden of this disabling disease? This provocative question is explored by the authors of *Diabetes and Women's Health Across the Life Stages: A Public Health Perspective*. Throughout its pages, editors Gloria L.A. Beckles and Patricia E. Thompson-Reid and their collaborators introduce us to some eye-opening issues and some serious, sobering implications for the health of women.

There is no better time for this in-depth look at diabetes as a women's health issue than now, as we begin a technologically advanced new century. Old or young, one-third of American women are overweight, and more than one-fourth do not participate in any leisure-time physical activity, according to the Third National Health and Nutrition Examination Survey (NHANES III 1988–1994). As a group, American women are aging and growing more obese and less physically active; each of these factors increases their risk for type 2 diabetes. Currently, about 20 million are over age 65. By the year 2030, that number is expected to double to 40 million, or roughly 1 in 4 American women. Astonishingly, more than 7 million women will be past the age of 85, compared with 4 million men.

The face of the American population is also changing: by the year 2050, 1 in 4 American women will be of Hispanic heritage, 1 in 8 African American, 1 in 11 Asian American, and 1 in 100 American Indian. Non-Hispanic whites will represent barely half of the population of women. Currently, the prevalence of diabetes is at least 2–4 times higher among women of color, and if this trend continues, the burden of diabetes could reach unimaginable dimensions.

As the authors point out, the number of persons diagnosed with diabetes increased fivefold between 1958 and 1997, at a direct cost of over $40 billion and an indirect cost of another $50 billion annually from absenteeism, disability, and premature death. These facts carry frustrating, even poignant overtones, because much of the burden of diabetes associated with complications is potentially preventable.

Although we are well aware of the clinical risks and outcomes of diabetes, this monograph adds a new and important public health dimension to diabetes research by looking at the socioeconomic environment that has contributed to the increase of this disease and the challenges we face as we seek to effectively educate women about the behavioral changes necessary for prevention. As this document points out, efforts to reach women with prevention messages will not work if their social environment does not support the messages. The authors conclude that the same social bias that resulted in women's health historically being viewed primarily in the context of their reproductive organs may still influence women's health priorities. The document's uniqueness also lies in its visionary understanding of the changing issues that affect women's health through their life span. Because of this awareness, the document is structured to reflect the different manifestations of diabetes at different stages of a woman's life, including the threat of type 1 and the emergence of type 2 diabetes in youth, gestational diabetes (seen in up to 5% of pregnancies) among women of childbearing age, and type 2 diabetes as a disease of middle-aged and older women.

The authors make a powerful argument that more information is needed on how behavioral and social factors interact with biological factors to affect the health of women, particularly those with diabetes or other chronic illnesses. Until such research gives us a clearer picture of how diabetes develops over time, health care systems should consider custom-designed prevention and control programs tailored for women and based on local and regional attitudes about health care, differing cultural health beliefs, and available social supports. Through the National Diabetes Control Program, the Centers for Disease Control and Prevention collaborates with all 50 states, the District of Columbia, and U.S. territories and jurisdictions to provide a mechanism for implementing such programs.

In the 21st century, the government cannot take on this health care burden alone; diabetes will not receive the concerted effort it deserves without action from both the public and private sectors. This monograph is lush with data and easy to read and reference. It should quickly become a useful tool for health care professionals, advocates, and educators seeking a leadership role in the fight against diabetes.

Wanda K. Jones, DrPH
Deputy Assistant Secretary for Health (Women's Health)
Director, U.S. Department of Health and Human Services
Office on Women's Health

Acknowledgments

This report was prepared by the Centers for Disease Control and Prevention, National Center for Chronic Disease Prevention and Health Promotion, Division of Diabetes Translation.

Jeffrey P. Koplan, MD, MPH, Director, Centers for Disease Control and Prevention, Atlanta, Georgia.

James S. Marks, MD, MPH, Director, National Center for Chronic Disease Prevention and Health Promotion, Centers for Disease Control and Prevention, Atlanta, Georgia.

Frank Vinicor, MD, MPH, Director, Division of Diabetes Translation, National Center for Chronic Disease Prevention and Health Promotion, Centers for Disease Control and Prevention, Atlanta, Georgia.

Kathy Rufo, MPH, Deputy Director, Division of Diabetes Translation, National Center for Chronic Disease Prevention and Health Promotion, Centers for Disease Control and Prevention, Atlanta, Georgia.

Editors

Gloria L.A. Beckles, MBBS, MSc, Scientific Editor, Medical Epidemiologist/Senior Service Fellow, Division of Diabetes Translation, National Center for Chronic Disease Prevention and Health Promotion, Centers for Disease Control and Prevention, Atlanta, Georgia.

Patricia E. Thompson-Reid, MPH, MAT, Managing Editor, Program Development Consultant, Division of Diabetes Translation, National Center for Chronic Disease Prevention and Health Promotion, Centers for Disease Control and Prevention, Atlanta, Georgia.

Contributing Authors

Chapters

Gloria L.A. Beckles, MBBS, MSc, Medical Epidemiologist/Senior Service Fellow, Division of Diabetes Translation, National Center for Chronic Disease Prevention and Health Promotion, Centers for Disease Control and Prevention, Atlanta, Georgia.

Cynthia Berg, MD, MPH, Medical Officer, Division of Reproductive Health, National Center for Chronic Disease Prevention and Health Promotion, Centers for Disease Control and Prevention, Atlanta, Georgia.

Isabella Danel, MD, MPH, Epidemiologist, Division of Reproductive Health, National Center for Chronic Disease Prevention and Health Promotion, Centers for Disease Control and Prevention, Atlanta, Georgia.

Kellie-Ann Ffrench, MA, Department of Psychology, University of Georgia, Athens, Georgia.

Catherine Hennessey, DrPh, Epidemiologist, Division of Adult and Community Health, National Center for Chronic Disease Prevention and Health Promotion, Centers for Disease Control and Prevention, Atlanta, Georgia.

Deanna Hill, MPH, Epidemiologist, Henry Ford Health System, Department of Biostatistics and Research Epidemiology, Detroit, Michigan.

Georgeanna J. Klingensmith, MD, University of Colorado Health Sciences Center, The Barbara Davis Center for Childhood Diabetes, Denver, Colorado.

JoAnn E. Manson, MD, DrPH, Associate Professor, Department of Epidemiology, Harvard School of Public Health, Harvard University, Boston, Massachusetts.

Lily D. McNair, PhD, Assistant Professor, Department of Psychology, University of Georgia, Athens, Georgia.

Jill M. Norris, MPH, PhD, Assistant Professor, Department of Preventive Medicine and Biometrics, University of Colorado School of Medicine, Denver, Colorado.

Diane Rowley, MD, MPH, Associate Director for Science, National Center for Chronic Disease Prevention and Health Promotion, Centers for Disease Control and Prevention, Atlanta, Georgia.

Mary Sabolsi, MD, MPH, Brigham and Women's Hospital, Harvard University, Boston, Massachusetts.

Patricia E. Thompson-Reid, MPH, MAT, Program Development Consultant, Division of Diabetes Translation, National Center for Chronic Disease Prevention and Health Promotion, Centers for Disease Control and Prevention, Atlanta, Georgia.

Frank Vinicor, MD, MPH, Director, Division of Diabetes Translation, National Center for Chronic Disease Prevention and Health Promotion, Centers for Disease Control and Prevention, Atlanta, Georgia.

Case Studies

Ann Albright, PhD, RD, Director, California Diabetes Control Program, California Department of Health, Sacramento, California.

Ann Kollmeyer, RD, MPH, Chief, Office of Policy and Program Information, Wolf Project, Minnesota Department of Health, Minneapolis, Minnesota.

Dawn L. Satterfield, RN, MSN, Health Education Specialist, Division of Diabetes Translation, National Center for Chronic Disease Prevention and Health Promotion, Centers for Disease Control and Prevention, Atlanta, Georgia.

Angela Green-Phillips, MPA, Chief, Office of Policy and Program Information, Division of Diabetes Translation, National Center for Chronic Disease Prevention and Health Promotion, Centers for Disease Control and Prevention, Atlanta, Georgia.

Senior Reviewers

Barbara A. Bowman, PhD, Associate Director for Policy Studies, Division of Diabetes Translation, National Center for Chronic Disease Prevention and Health Promotion, Centers for Disease Control and Prevention, Atlanta, Georgia.

Carl Caspersen, PhD, Associate Director for Science, Division of Diabetes Translation, National Center for Chronic Disease Prevention and Health Promotion, Centers for Disease Control and Prevention, Atlanta, Georgia.

Michael M. Engelgau, MD, Chief, Epidemiology and Statistics Branch, Division of Diabetes Translation, National Center for Chronic Disease Prevention and Health Promotion, Centers for Disease Control and Prevention, Atlanta, Georgia.

Anne Fagot-Campagna, MD, PhD, Visiting Scientist, Division of Diabetes Translation, National Center for Chronic Disease Prevention and Health Promotion, Centers or Disease Control and Prevention, Atlanta, Georgia.

H. Wayne Giles, MD, PhD, Associate Director for Science, Division of Adult and Community Health, National Center for Chronic Disease Prevention and Health Promotion, Centers for Disease Control and Prevention, Atlanta, Georgia.

Nora L. Keenan, PhD, Epidemiologist, Division of Adult and Community Health, National Center for Chronic Disease Prevention and Health Promotion, Centers for Disease Control and Prevention, Atlanta, Georgia.

Juliette Kendrick, MD, Acting Associate Director for Science, Division of Reproductive Health, National Center for Chronic Disease Prevention and Health Promotion, Centers for Disease Control and Prevention, Atlanta, Georgia.

Rodolfo Valdez, PhD, Epidemiologist, Division of Diabetes Translation, National Center for Chronic Disease Prevention and Health Promotion, Centers for Disease Control and Prevention, Atlanta, Georgia.

Other Contributors

Kelly J. Acton, MD, MPH, FACP, Director, National Diabetes Control Program, Indian Health Service, Albuquerque, New Mexico.

Ana Alfaro-Correa, ScD, MA, Program Development Consultant, Division of Diabetes Translation, National Center for Chronic Disease Prevention and Health Promotion, Centers for Disease Control and Prevention, Atlanta, Georgia.

Christopher Benjamin, JD, MPA, Program Development Consultant, Division of Diabetes Translation, National Center for Chronic Disease Prevention and Health Promotion, Centers for Disease Control and Prevention, Atlanta, Georgia.

Donald Betts, MPA, Public Health Analyst, Division of Diabetes Translation, National Center for Chronic Disease Prevention and Health Promotion, Centers for Disease Control and Prevention, Atlanta, Georgia.

Kristen L. Bleau, Research Assistant, Division of Diabetes Translation, National Center for Chronic Disease Prevention and Health Promotion, Centers for Disease Control and Prevention, Atlanta, Georgia.

Diann Braxton, Program Operations Assistant, Division of Diabetes Translation, National Center for Chronic Disease Prevention and Health Promotion, Centers for Disease Control and Prevention, Atlanta, Georgia.

Betty S. Burrier, Center for Beneficiary Services, Centers for Medicare and Medicaid Services, U.S. Department of Health and Human Services, Baltimore, Maryland.

Cynthia K. Clark, MA, Program Development Consultant, Division of Diabetes Translation, National Center for Chronic Disease Prevention and Health Promotion, Centers for Disease Control and Prevention, Atlanta, Georgia

Rita Diaz-Kenney, MPH, Health Education Specialist, Division of Diabetes Translation, National Center for Chronic Disease Prevention and Health Promotion, Centers for Disease Control and Prevention, Atlanta, Georgia.

Van H. Dunn, MD, Senior Vice President, New York City Health and Hospital Corporation, New York, New York.

Linda G. Elsner, Writer-Editor, National Center for Chronic Disease Prevention and Health Promotion, Centers for Disease Control and Prevention, Atlanta, Georgia.

Margaret Fowke, RD, LD, MPA, Presidential Management Intern, Division of Diabetes Translation, National Center for Chronic Disease Prevention and Health Promotion, Centers for Disease Control and Prevention, Atlanta, Georgia.

Christine S. Fralish, MLIS, Chief, Technical Information and Editorial Services Branch, National Center for Chronic Disease Prevention and Health Promotion, Centers for Disease Control and Prevention, Atlanta, Georgia.

Don L. Garcia, MD, Family Practitioner, Medica Health System, Anaheim, California.

Sanford Garfield, PhD, National Institute of Diabetes and Digestive and Kidney Diseases, National Institutes of Health, Bethesda, Maryland.

Julie A. Gothman, RD, South Dakota Department of Health, Pierre, South Dakota.

Yvonne Green, RN, MSN, CNM, Associate Director for Women's Health, Office of the Director, Centers for Disease Control and Prevention, Atlanta, Georgia.

Regina Hardy, MS, Deputy Chief, Epidemiology and Statistics Branch, Division of Diabetes Translation, National Center for Chronic Disease Prevention and Health Promotion, Centers for Disease Control and Prevention, Atlanta, Georgia.

Sabrina M. Harper, MS, Public Health Advisor, Division of Diabetes Translation, National Center for Chronic Disease Prevention and Health Promotion, Centers for Disease Control and Prevention, Atlanta, Georgia.

Nancy Haynie-Mooney, Health Communications Specialist, Division of Diabetes Translation, National Center for Chronic Disease Prevention and Health Promotion, Centers for Disease Control and Prevention, Atlanta, Georgia.

Kathryn Herron, MPH, Presidential Management Intern, Health Resources and Services Administration, U.S. Department of Health and Human Services, Washington, DC.

Rick L. Hull, PhD, Writer-Editor, National Center for Chronic Disease Prevention and Health Promotion, Centers for Disease Control and Prevention, Atlanta, Georgia.

Leonard Jack, Jr. PhD, MS, Acting Chief, Community Intervention Section, Program Development Branch, Division of Diabetes Translation, National Center for Chronic Disease Prevention and Health Promotion, Centers for Disease Control and Prevention, Atlanta, Georgia.

Valerie Johnson, Writer-Editor, National Center for Chronic Disease Prevention and Health Promotion, Centers for Disease Control and Prevention, Atlanta, Georgia.

Wanda K. Jones, DrPH, Deputy Assistant Secretary, Director, Office on Women's Health, U.S. Department of Health and Human Services, Washington, DC.

Lisa M. Kemp, Budget Analyst, Division of Diabetes Translation, National Center for Chronic Disease Prevention and Health Promotion, Centers for Disease Control and Prevention, Atlanta, Georgia.

Carol Krause, MA, Director, Division of Communications, Office on Women's Health, U.S. Department of Health and Human Services, Washington, DC.

Roz D. Lasker, MD, Director, Division of Public Health, The New York Academy of Medicine, New York, New York.

Arlene Lester, DDS, MPH, Program Development Consultant, Division of Diabetes Translation, National Center for Chronic Disease Prevention and Health Promotion, Centers for Disease Control and Prevention, Atlanta, Georgia.

Norma Loner, Committee Management Specialist, Division of Diabetes Translation, National Center for Chronic Disease Prevention and Health Promotion, Centers for Disease Control and Prevention, Atlanta, Georgia.

Ivette A. Lopez, MPH, Health Communications Specialist, Division of Diabetes Translation, National Center for Chronic Disease Prevention and Health Promotion, Centers for Disease Control and Prevention, Atlanta, Georgia.

Mary E. Lowrey, Program Analyst, Division of Diabetes Translation, National Center for Chronic Disease Prevention and Health Promotion, Centers for Disease Control and Prevention, Atlanta, Georgia.

David Marrero, PhD, Associate Professor of Medicine, Indiana University, Indianapolis, Indiana.

Phyllis C. McGuire, Public Health Analyst, Division of Diabetes Translation, National Center for Chronic Disease Prevention and Health Promotion, Centers for Disease Control and Prevention, Atlanta, Georgia.

Phyllis L. Moir, MA, Writer-Editor, National Center for Chronic Disease Prevention and Health Promotion, Centers for Disease Control and Prevention, Atlanta, Georgia.

Kathy Mulcahy, CDE, Liaison, American Association of Diabetes Educators, Chicago, Illinois.

Dara L. Murphy, MPH, Chief, Program Services Branch, Division of Diabetes Translation, National Center for Chronic Disease Prevention and Health Promotion, Centers for Disease Control and Prevention, Atlanta, Georgia.

Venkat Narayan, MD, Chief, Epidemiology Section, Division of Diabetes Translation, National Center for Chronic Disease Prevention and Health Promotion, Centers for Disease Control and Prevention, Atlanta, Georgia.

Carolyn W. Perkins, Administrative Officer, Division of Diabetes Translation, National Center for Chronic Disease Prevention and Health Promotion, Centers for Disease Control and Prevention, Atlanta, Georgia.

Todd W. Pierce, Visual Information Specialist, Division of Diabetes Translation, National Center for Chronic Disease Prevention and Health Promotion, Centers for Disease Control and Prevention, Atlanta, Georgia.

Audrey L. Pinto, Writer-Editor, National Center for Chronic Disease Prevention and Health Promotion, Centers for Disease Control and Prevention, Atlanta, Georgia.

Thomas L. Pitts, MD, Chicago, Illinois.

Robert Pollet, MD, Department of Veterans Affairs, Washington, DC.

Teresa M. Ramsey, MA, Writer-Editor, National Center for Chronic Disease Prevention and Health Promotion, Centers for Disease Control and Prevention, Atlanta, Georgia.

Richard R. Rubin, PhD, Assistant Professor, The Johns Hopkins University School of Medicine, Baltimore, Maryland.

Kathy Rufo, MPH, Deputy Director, Division of Diabetes Translation, National Center for Chronic Disease Prevention and Health Promotion, Centers for Disease Control and Prevention, Atlanta, Georgia.

Marc A. Safran, MD, FACPM, Chief Medical Officer, Division of Diabetes Translation, National Center for Chronic Disease Prevention and Health Promotion, Centers for Disease Control and Prevention, Atlanta, Georgia.

Kathy E. Shaw, RN, Manager, Market Development, Patient Care, Boehringer Mannheim Corporation, Indianapolis, Indiana.

Arlene Sherman, Management Infomation Assistant, Division of Diabetes Translation, National Center for Chronic Disease Prevention and Health Promotion, Centers for Disease Control and Prevention, Atlanta, Georgia.

Russell J. Sniegowski, MPH, Chief, Health Systems Section, Division of Diabetes Translation, National Center for Chronic Disease Prevention and Health Promotion, Centers for Disease Control and Prevention, Atlanta, Georgia.

Mary Kay Sones, Health Communications Specialist, National Center for Chronic Disease Prevention and Health Promotion, Centers for Disease Control and Prevention, Atlanta, Georgia.

Herman L. Surles, Jr., Writer-Editor, National Center for Chronic Disease Prevention and Health Promotion, Centers for Disease Control and Prevention, Atlanta, Georgia.

Darlene Thomas, Secretary, Division of Diabetes Translation, National Center for Chronic Disease Prevention and Health Promotion, Centers for Disease Control and Prevention, Atlanta, Georgia.

Diana J. Toomer, Writer-Editor, National Center for Chronic Disease Prevention and Health Promotion, Centers for Disease Control and Prevention, Atlanta, Georgia.

Galo R. Torres, DDS, Program Consultant for Migrant and Oral Health, Health Resources and Services Administration, U.S. Department of Health and Human Services, Atlanta, Georgia.

Jennifer Tucker, MPA, Program Analyst, National Center for Chronic Disease Prevention and Health Promotion, Centers for Disease Control and Prevention, Atlanta, Georgia.

Michele Whatley, Office Automation Clerk, Division of Diabetes Translation, National Center for Chronic Disease Prevention and Health Promotion, Centers for Disease Control and Prevention, Atlanta, Georgia.

Quion Wilkes, Office Automation Clerk, Division of Diabetes Translation, National Center for Chronic Disease Prevention and Health Promotion, Centers for Disease Control and Prevention, Atlanta, Georgia.

Violet Woo, MS, MPH, Health Policy Analyst, Division of Policy and Data, Office of Minority Health, U.S. Department of Health and Human Services, Rockville, MD.

Publication support was provided by Palladian Partners, Inc., under Contract No. 200-98-0415 for the National Center for Chronic Disease Prevention and Health Promotion, Centers for Disease Control and Prevention, U.S. Department of Health and Human Services.

DIABETES AND WOMEN'S HEALTH ACROSS THE LIFE STAGES: A PUBLIC HEALTH PERSPECTIVE

LIST OF TABLES AND FIGURES

INTRODUCTION

P.E. Thompson-Reid, MAT, MPH, P.C. McGuire, G.L.A. Beckles, MBBS, MSc

Diabetes is a major public health problem that imposes a serious burden on individuals and on society.[1] An estimated 15.7 million Americans have diabetes, and approximately one-third of these persons do not know they have the disease.[2] Even so, the number of persons with diagnosed diabetes increased fivefold between 1958 and 1993.[3] In 1997, the cost of diabetes was estimated to be $98.2 billion, of which $44.1 billion was attributable to direct medical expenditures and $54.1 billion to indirect costs including absenteeism, disability, and premature death.[4] Despite this physical and financial toll, the public generally has not perceived diabetes as a serious disease.[5] As a result, many efficacious and cost-effective preventive practices that can reduce the burden of this disease are not widely used.[6-11]

Diabetes as a Women's Health Issue

In general, American women live complicated and challenging lives. Women with diabetes face the same joys and problems, but with an added element: they battle a chronic disease with various social and personal challenges every hour of the day.

In 1983 the Assistant Secretary for Health established the Public Health Service Task Force on Women's Health Issues.[12] In 1985, this task force published a report that presented health issues across the life stages of women and listed recommendations that encouraged expanded research focusing on conditions and diseases unique to or more prevalent among women.[12] The report also presented criteria for qualifying a health problem as a women's issue. When these criteria are applied to diabetes, this condition can clearly be differentiated

as a women's issue. Diabetes in pregnancy is a serious condition that is unique to women because of its potential to affect the health of both the mother and her unborn child.[13,14] Approximately 2%–5% of all pregnancies in the United States are complicated by gestational diabetes, and this complication is most common among women of racial and ethnic groups at high risk for diabetes (blacks, Hispanics, American Indians, and Asian Americans). Moreover, the burden of diabetes falls disproportionately on women. More than half of all persons with diabetes are women. In addition, among the 8.1 million women aged 20 years or older with diabetes, older women and minority women are disproportionately represented.[2,15] The prevalence of diabetes is at least 2–4 times higher among black, Hispanic, American Indian, and Asian/Pacific Islander women than among white women. This excess of diabetes is even more profound for particular subgroups of women.[16-19] Because of the increasing lifespan of women and the rapid growth of minority populations, the number of women in the United States at high risk for diabetes and its complications is increasing.

The risk for cardiovascular disease, the most common complication attributable to diabetes, is more serious among women than men. Notably, women with diabetes lose their premenopausal protection from ischemic heart disease and have risk for this condition as great as or greater than that of diabetic or nondiabetic men. Furthermore, among people with diabetes who develop ischemic heart disease, women have worse survival and quality of life measures.[20-27] Women are also at greater risk for blindness due to diabetes than men.[28]

Research has shown that many risk factors for diabetes (weight gain, obesity, lack of physical activity) are more common among women than men in all population subgroups.[29] In addition, the natural history of these factors and their relationship to diabetes are quite different among some subgroups of American women. For example, black women retain more weight postpartum than white women with comparable gestational weight gain,[30] increasing their risk for obesity and its sequelae in subsequent pregnancies and at older ages.[31,32] Obesity is associated with the prevalence of type 2 diabetes[29] and is a risk factor for the development of this disease.[33] Among women of minority racial or ethnic origin, there is earlier onset of obesity, and these groups experience disproportionately high levels of excess weight.[18,32,34-36] This variation in risk profiles and cultural norms among the various populations of women with diabetes suggests that the interventions for mediating these risks should also vary accordingly. The results of the primary prevention trials now in progress should provide additional information that may benefit women at risk for type 2 diabetes mellitus.

Challenges and Opportunities

Women have made many strides in promoting equity in their social status; nevertheless, there are entrenched values and structures in our society that continue to negatively affect the health of women in general. The results of the Diabetes Complications and Control Trial and the United Kingdom Prospective Diabetes Study have indicated that most of the complications of type 1 and type 2 diabetes are preventable.[11,37] However, progress in applying this knowledge to reduce the burden of diabetes has been slow. These realities, coupled with gender-related issues, may serve as barriers to the use of this knowledge by health care providers and women with diabetes. The Public Health Service Task Force Report on women's health states that "societal attitudes toward females, the socialization of girls and women, differing economic and occupational status between men and women and among women, as well as changing attitudes toward the family, sexual behavior, and living arrangements all have implications for women's health."[12] More knowledge is required to inform the public health community about how these behavioral and social factors interact with biological factors to affect the health of women, particularly when they are compounded by the existence of a chronic disease such as diabetes.

Historically the concept of women and women's health was defined by the very nature of their biology and social status as compared with those of men. From the times of the Greeks, men and women were seen as having similar biological structures, but women were seen as imperfect because of their differences.[38,39] In addition, until the mid-1900s, the maternal role was thought to require so much energy that other activities such as physical activity and intellectual pursuits were not promoted for women. Implicit in this assumption was the perception that women are inferior to men.[40]

This gender bias created a social environment where women's work and concerns were not taken seriously. Moreover, this perception of women dictated that the primary focus of women's health be on their reproductive function, to the neglect of many other aspects of their general health.[39] Such thinking was also reflected in the types of policies that were directed to women worldwide. For example, many biomedical and public policy studies of the past did not include women.[39-42] As a result, findings of studies on men have been extrapolated to women. Even in conditions specific to women, there are gaps in research and treatment protocols. For example, for women with gestational diabetes, the primary focus is on the clinical management of the mother's glycemic status for positive birth outcomes. After the birth of the child, systematic follow-up of the mother with gestational diabetes has not been uniformly provided to maintain her health and to reduce her risk of developing diabetes immediately postpartum or for several years later.[43] In 1998, the American Diabetes Association Clinical Practice Recommendations for women with gestational diabetes were updated to facilitate a broad-based approach to the follow-up of these women.[44] This has brought renewed attention to the issue; however, there are major systemic and policy barriers that impair the implementation of adequate follow-up for women with gestational diabetes.[45]

As a result of social, political, and economic pressures, the focus of the delivery of services to women is moving from an emphasis on reproductive health and pregnancy to comprehensive services for women throughout their lives.

Notable events have also helped this process along at the federal level:

• Publication of *Women's Health: Report of the Public Health Service Task Force on Women's Health Issues*[12] in 1985.

• Establishment of the Office of Research on Women's Health within the Office of the National Institutes of Health (NIH) Director.

• The NIH Revitalization Act of 1993.

• Establishment of the U.S. Public Health Service's Office of Women's Health in 1994.

• Establishment of the Office of Women's Health at the Centers for Disease Control and Prevention (CDC) in 1994.

• Publication of the *NIH Guidelines on the Inclusion of Women and Minorities as Subjects in Clinical Research* in 1994.

Despite these recent efforts to improve the health status of women, there is still opportunity to examine, modify, and expand this focus as we move forward. An assessment of the health status of women with diabetes in the United States and an examination of the determinants of women's health at the population level, particularly those that cannot be addressed with traditional clinical interventions, could influence changes in policy and the delivery of services and inform the development of appropriate interventions to improve the health of women overall. Many social scientists believe that the interaction of the social and economic environment on the psychological resources and coping

skills of an individual may influence health status much more than was expected.[46-48] It is also likely that these determinants play a role in the health disparities found among women and among racial and ethnic groups at greater risk for diabetes and its complications. As we search for these explanations, we must include a rigorous examination of the economic, social, and environmental factors that affect the health of women and the availability of appropriate curative and preventive services so that the public health community response will be appropriate.

Women's Health at CDC

As the nation's prevention agency, the mission of CDC is to promote health and quality of life by preventing and controlling disease, injury, and disability. The vision of CDC is "Healthy People in a Healthy World—Through Prevention." This is reflected in its 1993 operational priorities:

• To strengthen the core functions of public health.

• To enrich its capacity to respond to urgent threats to health.

• To develop nationwide prevention efforts.

• To promote women's health.

In 1993, in keeping with CDC policy directives, the National Center for Chronic Disease Prevention and Health Promotion established a Women's Health Working Group with representatives from each division to monitor issues related to women's health and to oversee the distribution of resources for activities in this area. As a result of discussions in this broader group, the following questions were presented to each division in the Center:

• From a public health perspective, what are the biggest problems affecting women?

• What is the disease burden for women?

• Can we describe the population at risk?

• What is preventable and what are we doing about it?

Discussions of these questions revealed the lack of a public health perspective on diabetes and women's health issues and formed the seed from which this monograph grew.

Purpose
The intent of this monograph is

- To describe the diversity within the population of American women as a context for the discussion of women's health issues.

- To present a situational analysis of the epidemiological, social, and environmental circumstances in which American women develop and live with diabetes.

- To synthesize and present in a single document the health status of women with diabetes.

- To suggest ways in which public health agencies can contribute to improved access and quality of care for women with diabetes.

- To serve as a general reference document for public health professionals, advocacy groups, and all persons in the diabetes community.

- To increase awareness of the general population that diabetes is a serious health problem.

Conceptual Framework
The monograph is structured to examine the impact of diabetes through the life stages of the woman. The age groups are constrained by standard age structures used in population-based studies and national surveys. In keeping with a public health paradigm, we first examine the sociodemographic characteristics of the population of women in the United States and subsequently look at subgroups of women with diabetes. Chapter 2 of the monograph presents a general profile of women in the United States, looking at population size and growth among various ethnic and racial groups, the psychosocial determinants of health, and the public health implications of these findings. Chapters 3 through 6 begin with case studies that provide a glimpse into the lives of women with diabetes discussed in each specific life stage. In chapters 3

through 6, the authors examine the impact of diabetes on women's health through the life stage of the woman:

- **The Adolescent Years.** The adolescent years are marked by major biological and psychosocial changes that transform the adolescent into an adult. Many adolescents with diabetes face lifestyle choices that can affect their ability to control the disease. Policies—or the lack of appropriate policies—in the wider society may influence the ability of women in this age group and their families to make healthy lifestyle choices.

- **The Reproductive Years.** For women with diabetes, successful passage through this time of greatest personal growth and responsibility (schooling, marriage, career development, and raising children) is enhanced by their ability to control their disease. The development of gestational diabetes during pregnancy puts both the woman and the unborn child at risk for negative health outcomes. For those with few personal resources, this period could place them at higher risk for negative health outcomes and future economic hardship.

- **The Middle Years.** Marked by major physiologic events such as menopause, this is a time when other chronic diseases or complications of diabetes most often first appear, along with many other social and psychological changes (e.g., death, divorce, retirement, poverty).

- **The Older Years.** During this time, women with diabetes become even more vulnerable to other chronic illnesses, disability, poverty, and loss of social support systems. The number of women in this age group is growing exponentially as the American population ages.

Within each chapter, authors discuss the prevalence of diabetes, the sociodemographic characteristics of women with diabetes in the age group, the impact of diabetes on women's health status, health-related behaviors, access to care, the psychosocial determinants of health-related behaviors and health outcomes, comorbid conditions as determinants of health behaviors and health outcomes, and the public health implications of pertinent findings for each life stage described above. Chapter 7 summarizes the findings in chapters 3 through 6 and presents their public health implications.

Audience and Scope

This document is intended for public health professionals, policy makers, staff of community-based organizations and voluntary organizations, researchers, and advocates for women's health, as well as persons interested in issues related to women and diabetes. In particular, this document seeks to provide essential information for persons charged with making decisions and setting policies related to diabetes and women's health.

In addition to the seven chapters, including four on the different life stages of women, several tools have been added to enhance the reader's use of the monograph and to provide additional comprehensive, yet concise, information on diabetes. Immediately following the table of contents is a list of tables and figures with the title and page number for each table and figure by chapter. There are five appendixes, including tables of diabetes prevalence in the United States (diagnosed and undiagnosed), U.S. maps of diabetes prevalence for two time periods (1996–1998 and 1998–2000), and the American Diabetes Association's guide to standards

of care. A list of abbreviations of common diabetes terms or related organizations and a glossary of terms used in the monograph are located after the appendixes. Glossary listings for the major diabetes organizations and frequently cited diabetes studies include a Web site address.

Following chapter 7 is an epilogue in which the editors present personal comments on the insights they gained from their experience with the project.

Terminology

The racial and ethnic categories used in this document are in keeping with those set forth in the Office of Management and Budget's Statistical Policy Directive No. 15, Race and Ethnic Standards for Federal Statistics and Administrative Reporting. Hence, these names are used: American Indian or Alaska Native, Asian/Pacific Islander, black not of Hispanic origin, Hispanic, and white not of Hispanic origin. However, because some authors used different terminology for race and ethnicity, data are presented here as reported in the publications cited.

Many diabetes terms or abbreviations used in this publication may be found in the list of abbreviations or in the glossary in the back of the monograph.

References

1. Vinicor F. Is diabetes a public health disorder? *Diabetes Care* 1994;17(Suppl 1):22–7.

2. Harris MI. Summary. In: National Diabetes Data Group, editors. Diabetes in America. 2nd ed. Bethesda, MD: National Institutes of Health, 1995:1–13. (NIH Publication No. 95-1468)

3. Centers for Disease Control and Prevention. *National Diabetes Fact Sheet: National Estimates and General Information on Diabetes in the United States.* Atlanta: U.S. Department of Health and Human Services, Centers for Disease Control and Prevention, 1997.

4. American Diabetes Association. Economic consequences of diabetes mellitus in the U.S. in 1997. *Diabetes Care* 1998;21(2):296–309.

5. Slovic P. Perception of risk. *Science* 1987;236(4799): 280–5.

6. Litzelman DK, Slemenda CW, Langefeld CD, et al. Reduction of lower-extremity clinical abnormalities in patients with non–insulin-dependent diabetes mellitus. A randomized, controlled trial. *Ann Intern Med* 1993;119(1):36–41.

7. Ferris FL 3rd. How effective are treatments for diabetic retinopathy? *JAMA* 1993;269(10):1290–1.

8. The Diabetes Control and Complications Trial Research Group. The effect of intensive treatment of diabetes on the development and progression of long-term complications in insulin-dependent diabetes mellitus. *N Engl J Med* 1993;329(14):977–86.

9. Rost KM, Flavin KS, Schmidt LE, McGill JB. Self-care predictors of metabolic control in type 1 patients. *Diabetes Care* 1990;13(11):1111–13.

10. Brown SA. Studies of educational interventions and outcomes in diabetic adults: a meta-analysis revisited. *Patient Educ Couns* 1990;16(3):189–215.

11. The Diabetes Control and Complications Trial Research Group. Lifetime benefits and cost of intensive therapy as practiced in the Diabetes Control and Complications Trial. *JAMA* 1996;276(17):1409–15.

12. U.S. Public Health Service. *Women's Health: Report of the Public Health Service Task Force on Women's Health Issues.* Vol. 1. U.S. Department of Health and Human Services, 1985.

13. Coustan DR. Gestational diabetes. In: National Diabetes Data Group, editors. *Diabetes in America.* 2nd ed. Bethesda, MD: National Institutes of Health, 1995:703–17. (NIH Publication No. 95-1468)

14. Buchanan TA. Pregnancy in preexisting diabetes. In: National Diabetes Data Group, editors. Diabetes in America. 2nd ed. Bethesda, MD: National Institutes of Health, 1995:719–33. (NIH Publication No. 95-1468)

15. Kenny SJ, Aubert RE, Geiss LS. Prevalence and incidence of non–insulin-dependent diabetes. In: National Diabetes Data Group, editors. Diabetes in America. 2nd ed. Bethesda, MD: National Institutes of Health, 1995:47–67. (NIH Publication No. 95-1468)

16. Tull ES, Roseman JM. Diabetes in African Americans. In: National Diabetes Data Group, editors. Diabetes in America. 2nd ed. Bethesda, MD: National Institutes of Health, 1995:613–30. (NIH Publication No. 95-1468)

17. Stern MP, Mitchell BD. Diabetes in Hispanic Americans. In: National Diabetes Data Group, editors. *Diabetes in America.* 2nd ed. Bethesda, MD: National Institutes of Health, 1995:631–59. (NIH Publication No. 95-1468)

18. Fujimoto WY. Diabetes in Asian and Pacific Islander Americans. In: National Diabetes Data Group, editors. Diabetes in America. 2nd ed. Bethesda, MD: National Institutes of Health, 1995:661–81. (NIH Publication No. 95-1468)

19. Gohdes D. Diabetes in North American Indians and Alaska Natives. In: National Diabetes Data Group, editors. *Diabetes in America.* 2nd ed. Bethesda, MD: National Institutes of Health, 1995:683–701. (NIH Publication No. 95-1468)

20. Gu K, Cowie CC, Harris MI. Mortality in adults with and without diabetes in a national cohort of the U.S. population, 1971–1993. *Diabetes Care* 1998;21(7): 1138–45.

21. Garcia MJ, McNamara PM, Gordon T, Kannel WB. Morbidity and mortality in diabetics in the Framingham population. Sixteen-year follow-up study. *Diabetes* 1974;23(2):105–11.

22. Barrett-Connor EL, Cohn BA, Wingard DL, Edelstein SL. Why is diabetes mellitus a stronger risk factor for fatal ischemic heart disease in women than in men? The Ranch Bernardo Study. *JAMA* 1991;265(5):627–31.

23. Manson JE, Colditz GA, Stampfer MJ, et al. A prospective study of maturity-onset diabetes mellitus and risk for coronary heart disease and stroke in women. *Arch Intern Med* 1991;151(6):1141–7.

24. Heyden S, Heiss G, Bartel AG, Hames CG. Sex differences in coronary mortality among diabetics in Evans County, Georgia. *J Chronic Dis* 1980;33(5):265–73.

25. Abbott RD, Donahue RP, Kannel WB, Wilson PW. The impact of diabetes on survival following myocardial infarction in men vs women. The Framingham Study. *JAMA* 1988;260(23):3456–60.

26. Eaker ED, Chesbro JH, Sacks FM, Wenger NK, Whisnant JP, Winston M. Cardiovascular disease in women. *Circulation* 1993;88:1999–2009.

27. Lee WL, Cheung AM, Cape D, Zinman B. Impact of diabetes on coronary artery disease in women and men: a meta-analysis of prospective studies. *Diabetes Care* 2000;23(7):962–8.

28. Harris MI, Klein R, Cowie CC, Rowland M, Byrd-Holt DD. Is the risk of diabetic retinopathy greater in non-Hispanic blacks and Mexican Americans than in non-Hispanic whites with type 2 diabetes? A U.S. population study. *Diabetes Care* 1998;21(8):1230–5.

29. Rewers MR, Hamman RF. Risk factors for non–insulin-dependent diabetes. In: National Diabetes Data Group, editors. Diabetes in America. 2nd ed. Bethesda, MD: National Institutes of Health, 1995:179–220. (NIH Publication No. 95-1468)

30. Keppel KG, Taffel SM. Pregnancy-related weight gain and retention: implications of the 1990 Institute of Medicine guidelines. *Am J Public Health* 1993;83(8):1100–3.

31. Parker JD, Abrams B. Differences in postpartum weight retention between black and white mothers. *Obstet Gynecol* 1993;81:768–74.

32. Kahn HS, Williamson DF, Stevens JA. Race and weight in U.S. women: the roles of socioeconomic and marital status. *Am J Public Health* 1991;81(3):319–23.

33. Ford ES, Williamson DF, Liu S. Weight change and diabetes incidence: findings from a national cohort of U.S. adults. *Am J Epidemiol* 1997;146(3):214–22.

34. Knowler WC, Pettitt DJ, Savage PJ, Bennett PH. Diabetes incidence in Pima Indians: contributions of obesity and parental diabetes. *Am J Epidemiol* 1981;113(2):144–56.

35. Will JC. Self-reported weight loss among adults with diabetes: results from a national health survey. *Diabet Med* 1995;12(11):974–8.

36. Hazuda HP, Haffner SM, Stern MP, Eifler CW. The effects of acculturation and socioeconomic status on obesity and diabetes in Mexican Americans. The San Antonio Heart Study. *Am J Epidemiol* 1988;128:1289–1301.

37. UK Prospective Diabetes Study Group. Tight blood pressure control and risk of macrovascular and microvascular complications in type 2 diabetes UKPDS 38. *BMJ* 1998;317(7160):703–13.

38. Lawrence SC, Bendixen K. His and hers: male and female anatomy in anatomy texts for U.S. medical students, 1890–1989. *Soc Sci Med* 1992;35(7):925–34.

39. Stanton AL. The psychology of women's health: barriers and pathways to knowledge. In: Stanton AL, Gallant SJ, editors. *The Psychology of Women's Health*. Washington, DC: American Psychological Association, 1995.

40. Travis CB. *Women and Health Psychology: Biomedical Issues*. Hillsdale, NJ: Erlbaum, 1988.

41. Bennett JC. Inclusion of women in clinical trials—policies for population subgroups. *N Engl J Med* 1993;329:288–92.

42. *Report of the Office of Research on Women's Health, Fiscal Years 1993–1995.* Bethesda, MD: National Institutes of Health, 1997. (Publication No. 97-3702)

43. Tinker LF. Diabetes mellitus—a priority health care issue for women. *J Am Diet Assoc* 1994;94(9):976–85.

44. American Diabetes Association. Clinical Practice Recommendations, 1998. Gestational diabetes mellitus. *Diabetes Care* 1998;21(Suppl 1):S60–S61.

45. Reisinger AL. *Health Insurance and Access to Care: Issues for Women.* New York: The Commonwealth Fund Commission of Women's Health, 1995.

46. Frank JW. The determinants of health: a new synthesis. *Current Issues in Public Health* 1995;1(6):233–40.

47. Lynch JW. Social position and health. *Ann Epidemiol* 1996;6(1):21–3.

48. Krieger N. Embodying inequality: a review of concepts, measures, and methods for studying health consequences of discrimination. *Int J Health Serv* 1999;29(2): 295–352.

2

A PROFILE OF WOMEN IN THE UNITED STATES

G.L.A. Beckles, MBBS, MSc, K-A. Ffrench, MPH, D. Hill, MPH, L.D. McNair, PhD

Currently, the issue of individual lifestyles is receiving great attention from both the public health community and the popular press. Women and men are urged not to smoke, to eat less fat, to engage in regular exercise, and to follow healthy practices to prevent various diseases and use fewer health services. Unfortunately, emphasizing individual behavior may mean that important social and economic factors that affect people's health are neglected.[1-4] Factors such as income, employment status, living arrangements, recency of immigration, and degree of acculturation may all impair the ability of people to keep themselves healthy or to take care of themselves when they are ill. Approaches to risk reduction that fail to take account of the limits of personal choice may therefore do little to change the health status of the group.[5-8] This profile of women in the United States presents a review of recent data on important features of the social and environmental context in which women develop and live with chronic diseases such as diabetes. The public health implications of the findings are summarized within the framework of the core public health functions for thought and action. Thus, the text should be helpful to public health officials as they seek to elaborate interventions and policies appropriate for women at different stages of life. It also suggests areas for research to reduce the impact of diabetes on women, to assist in the formulation of policies, and to identify where more effort is needed to assure the availability and adequacy of health care and preventive services.

2.1. Population Size and Growth

Of the 262.8 million residents of the United States in 1995, 134.4 million, or 51.2%, were female.[9]

Among all females, 16.8% were children under 12 years of age, 8.1% were adolescents aged 12–17 years, 40.2% were reproductive-aged women 18–44 years, 20.1% were in the middle years (45–64), and 14.8% were elderly women 65 years of age or older. Thirteen percent of elderly women were 85 years of age or older.

Between 1995 and 2010, the female population is projected to grow by 17.7 million;[10] more than three-quarters of that growth will comprise women aged 45–64 years. After 2010, the total female population is projected to grow more slowly than in earlier years.[10] However, as younger women age out of their reproductive years, the number of middle-aged and older women will continue to increase, thereby enlarging the population at risk for diabetes and other chronic diseases.

2.2. Population Composition

Age and Sex

The greater number of females than males in the total population is the result of a long-term pattern of greater life expectancy for females in all age groups that continued in the United States through the late 1980s.[11,12] Around 1990, however, death rates among U.S. females began to stabilize while rates for males started to decline rapidly. As a result, the survival "advantage" of females decreased at all ages under 85 years (Table 2-1). For example, between 1979–1981 and 1995, the additional life expectancy of females compared with males fell from 7.5 to 6.4 years among infant girls and from 4.2 to 3.4 years among 65-year-old women.

Table 2-1. Expectation of life, by age and sex—United States, 1979–81, 1990, 1995

| Age (years) | Year | Expectation of life (years) | | |
		Females	Males	Difference
0	1979–81	77.6	70.1	7.5
	1990	78.8	71.8	7.0
	1995	78.8	72.4	6.4
15	1979–81	63.8	56.5	7.3
	1990	64.7	57.9	6.8
	1995	64.7	58.4	6.3
25	1979–81	54.2	47.4	6.8
	1990	55.0	48.7	6.3
	1995	55.0	49.2	5.8
35	1979–81	44.5	38.2	6.3
	1990	45.3	39.6	5.7
	1995	45.4	40.1	5.3
45	1979–81	35.2	29.2	6.0
	1990	35.9	30.7	5.2
	1995	36.0	31.3	4.7
55	1979–81	26.4	21.1	5.3
	1990	27.0	22.3	4.7
	1995	27.0	22.9	4.1
65	1979–81	18.4	14.2	4.2
	1990	18.9	15.1	3.8
	1995	18.9	15.5	3.4
75	1979–81	11.6	8.9	2.7
	1990	12.0	9.4	2.6
	1995	11.9	9.7	2.2
85	1979–81	6.4	5.1	1.3
	1990	6.4	5.2	1.2
	1995	6.4	5.3	1.1

Source: Reference 12.

Despite this recent change in projected survival among women, which is consistent with a trend that emerged in many industrialized countries during the 1980s,[13] the greater longevity among women is projected to persist well into the middle of the 21st century.

A major consequence of the greater longevity of females is that women outnumber men, especially in the older age groups.[9] This excess of females increases steeply with age, and is most marked among the elderly; in 1995, for example, there were 176 women aged 75 years or older for every 100 men of comparable age (Table 2-2). This sex differential accounts, in part, for the increasing numbers of elderly American women who live alone (Figure 2-1).

Table 2-2. Age-specific female-male ratios, by race/Hispanic origin—United States, 1995

Age group (years)	All	White	Black	American Indian	Asian/Pacific Islander	Hispanic*
<18	0.95	0.95	0.97	0.97	0.96	0.91
18–24	0.96	0.95	1.02	0.96	1.01	0.91
25–44	1.01	0.99	1.13	1.01	1.09	0.92
45–54	1.05	1.03	1.21	1.07	1.15	1.06
55–64	1.10	1.08	1.30	1.13	1.18	1.14
65–74	1.25	1.23	1.40	1.21	1.35	1.26
≥75	1.76	1.76	1.90	1.75	1.38	1.60
All ages	1.05	1.04	1.11	1.02	1.07	0.97

*Hispanic may be of any race.

Source: Reference 9.

Racial and Ethnic Diversity

The U.S. female population is racially and ethnically heterogeneous.[14] In 1995, almost three-quarters (73.6%) were classified as non-Hispanic white; the remaining 26.4% belonged to other racial or ethnic groups (Figure 2-2). A total of 13.3 million females (of any race) were of Hispanic origin; of the more than 22 million non-Hispanic nonwhite women, 16.7 million were black, 4.5 million were Asian/Pacific Islander, and 982,000 were American Indian or Alaska Native.[9] By 2010, minority females are projected to account for one-third of U.S. females: Hispanics, 20.6 million; non-Hispanic blacks, 19.8 million; Asians/Pacific Islanders, 7.6 million; American Indians, 1.2 mil-

Figure 2-1. Percentage of women who lived alone, by age—United States, 1970, 1980, 1995

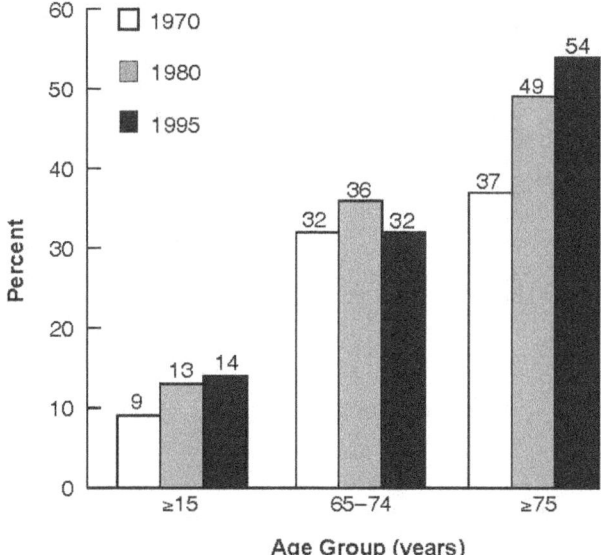

Source: Reference 24.

Figure 2-2. Percentage distribution of female population, by race/Hispanic* origin—United States, 1995 and 2010 (projected)

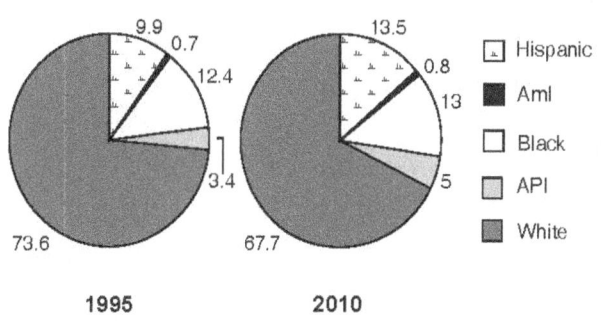

*Hispanic may be of any race.
AmI = American Indian; API = Asian/Pacific Islander.

Sources: References 9, 10.

lion (Figure 2-2).[10] These classifications do not adequately describe the considerable heterogeneity among American women; each racial or ethnic group is itself diverse. For example, the Asian American group may include descendants of Chinese, Japanese, and Filipinos who migrated to the United States between the mid-1800s and 1910 as well as recent immigrants from countries as varied as India, Vietnam, Korea, Laos, Cambodia, and Thailand.[15-17] Hispanics are also a diverse population that includes descendants of Spanish colonists who settled in the southwestern United States in the 1500s as well as persons who originated more recently from Mexico, Central and South America, and the Spanish-speaking Caribbean.[16,18,19] Finally, black Americans are becoming increasingly heterogeneous; most are descendants of slaves transported to the United States during the 17th to 19th centuries. But since the mid-1960s, there has been a

marked increase in immigration from English- and French-speaking Caribbean and African countries.[16,20,21] The percentage of foreign-born blacks is projected to increase nationwide to 10% of the total black population by the year 2010;[20] however, foreign-born persons already account for more than 20% of the black population in New York and 10% in Florida.[20]

Minority populations are expected to grow at a faster rate than the U.S. population as a whole.[10] From 1995 to 2010, the number of Hispanic and Asian American women in their middle years or older is expected to double, and the number of black women is expected to increase by two-thirds and American Indian women by almost half (Figure 2-3).

Figure 2-3. Projected percentage change in the number of females, by age and race/Hispanic origin—United States, 1995–2010

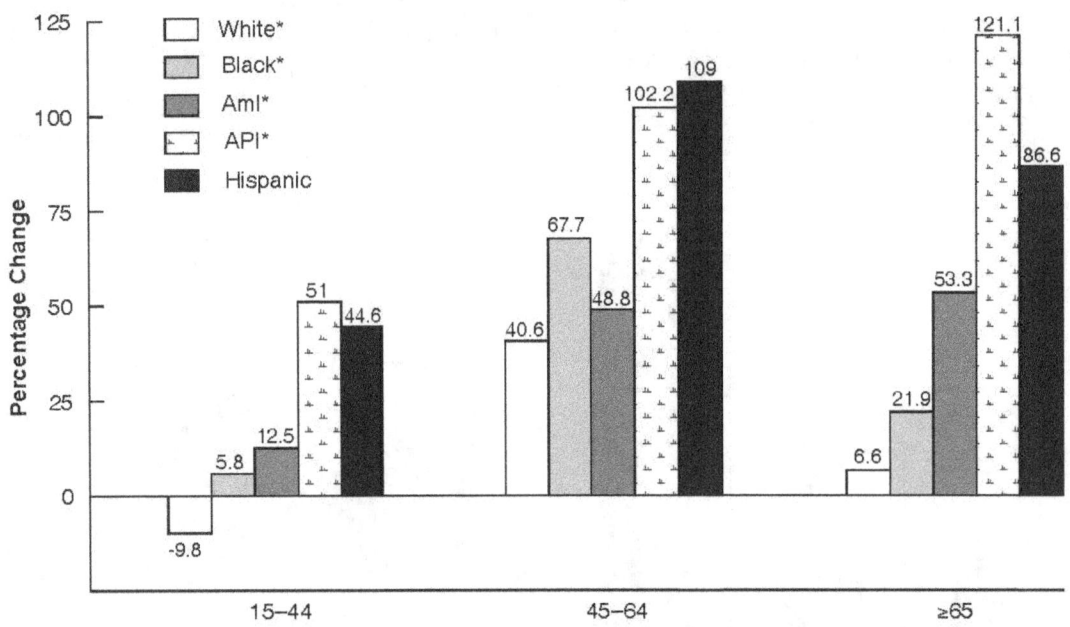

* Non-Hispanic.
AmI = American Indian; API = Asian/Pacific Islander.

Source: Reference 10.

Immigration will make a greater contribution to the increase among Hispanics and Asians/Pacific Islanders than other groups.[21] However, compared with the white population, the minority population is composed of a substantially higher proportion of children and adolescents (33% versus 24%) and lower proportion of adults aged 65 years (5%–10% versus 16%) (Figure 2-4). As a result, on average, minority females are 6 to 10 years younger than their non-Hispanic white counterparts.[9] Thus, even if the birth rate fell immediately to the level of the death rate and immigration were stopped, the current youth of the minority groups provide considerable population momentum for future increases in the numbers of middle-aged and elderly black, American Indian, Asian/Pacific Islander, and Hispanic women, the age groups most susceptible to diabetes and other chronic diseases. Already, the burden of diabetes falls disproportionately on persons in these racial and ethnic groups.[22] The rapid

Figure 2-4. Population age structures: minority and non-Hispanic white females—United States, 1995

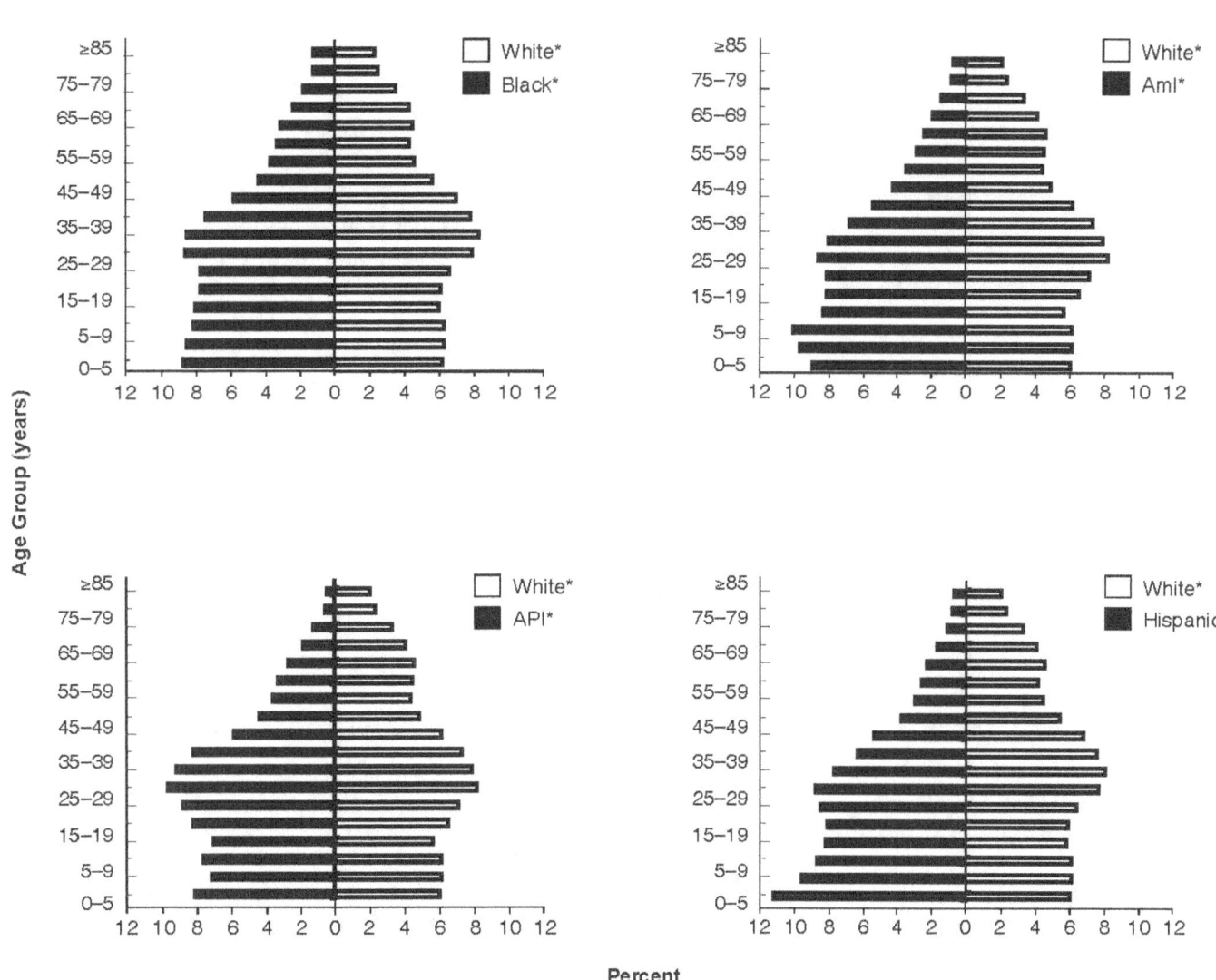

* Non-Hispanic.
AmI = American Indian; API = Asian/Pacific Islander.

Source: Reference 9.

growth of these susceptible subpopulations presages a sharp rise in the burden of diabetes. Increasingly, greater numbers of women with diabetes will be women with special cultural needs.

As in the general population, minority women outnumber minority men. Compared with whites, however, the sex imbalance among blacks and Hispanics begins at much younger ages and increases more steeply with age (Table 2-2). In addition, it has been widening since the 1970s,[23] whereas among whites the differential has narrowed recently.[9] The greater number of females in the black population is particularly striking; in 1995, women outnumbered men by 13% in the relatively young 25–44 age group and by 40% in the 65–74 age group (Table 2-2). As in the white population, sex differentials for each minority population were highest in the 75 or older age group, where there were 190 black, 175 American Indian, 138 Asian/Pacific Islander, and 160 Hispanic women per 100 men.

The population dynamics described herein point to several important implications for health policy, for the planning of diabetes services for women, and for the planning of research. First, the expected rapid growth in the numbers of high-risk women (middle-aged, elderly, minority) suggests that even under a simple assumption of constant prevalence, a substantial increase in the number of women with diabetes can be anticipated. Therefore, health officials need to reexamine the ability of the health care system to meet the future needs of these women for both primary and specialty diabetes services. Second, the importance of culturally appropriate prevention education for the population and the medical profession needs to be emphasized. Third, research efforts must expand to achieve an understanding of the mechanisms and pathways by which factors such as duration of residence in the United States and degree of acculturation alter risks for diabetes among minority groups. Finally, as the feminization of old age continues into this century, government at all levels as well as universities, foundations, and other organizations must expand their

efforts to understand the living arrangements, economic sufficiency, access to health care services, and health and well-being of elderly women.

Geographic Characteristics

Regional distribution. The percentage of the population that is white is distributed in fairly uniform fashion across the country but minority populations are geographically concentrated, a legacy of the historical circumstances and migration patterns of the various groups.[15,16] In 1995, for example, more than half all black females lived in the South, and in five southern states (Louisiana, Mississippi, Alabama, Georgia, South Carolina) and the District of Columbia, they made up more than one-quarter of the population.[16] Black females also have a substantial presence (19% of the total) in the Northeast and Midwest, where they account for at least 15% of the populations in three states (Illinois, Michigan, and New York). Two-fifths of Asian/ Pacific Islander females live in a single state: California; one-tenth live in Hawaii, and one-tenth live in New York.[16,17] American Indian females have a sizable presence only in Alaska, New Mexico, and Oklahoma.[16] Nearly two-thirds of Hispanic females live in just five states: California, Texas, New Mexico, Arizona, and Colorado; most of the remainder live in New York or New Jersey (a total of 12%), Florida (8%), or Illinois (about 5%).[16,19] These patterns of geographic concentration are expected to continue well into the 21st century.[19,21] Thus, the societal impact of the increased burden of diabetes anticipated among these susceptible groups is likely to have a major regional component.

Area of residence. In 1995, half of all American females lived in distinct areas—30.2% as urban populations in central cities (strictly metropolitan areas), and 20% as rural populations (strictly nonmetropolitan areas).[24,25] The remaining 49.8% lived in areas contiguous with the central (largest) city.[26] Black (54.9%) and Hispanic (48.8%) females were about twice as likely as white females (25.6%) to live inside central cities. This is true at all ages, but the difference is greatest at the extremes of the life span (Figure 2-5). Among females younger than 18 years, almost half of the black and Hispanic girls live in central cities, compared with about one-fourth of whites. At age 75 years or older, one-third of black and two-fifths of Hispanic women live in central cities compared with about one-seventh of whites.

Figure 2-5. Percentage of females who lived in central cities, by age and race/Hispanic* origin—United States, 1995

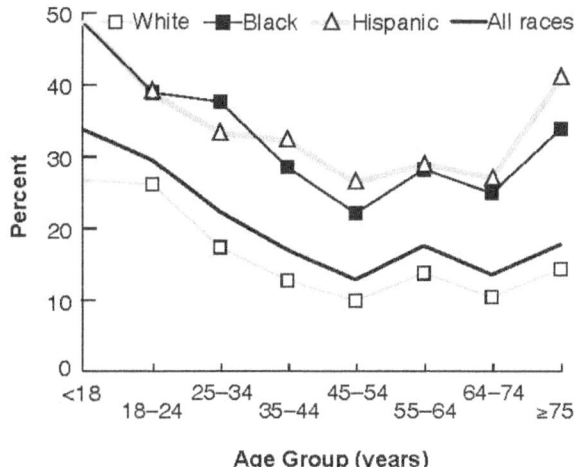

* Hispanic may be of any race.

Source: Reference 24.

Although many fewer (approximately 26 million in 1995) U.S. females live in nonmetropolitan or primarily rural areas, they represent about 1 in 5 white, 1 in 7 black, and 1 in 11 Hispanic females. Among women aged 18 years or older who live in these areas, half of white and 60% of black and Hispanic women are of childbearing age while nearly one-fifth of white, one-fifth of black, and one-tenth of Hispanic women are elderly.

Data on geographic characteristics often provide clues about the health status of populations and can help to identify vulnerable, underserved populations. In the United States, region of birth[26-30] and

area of residence[31-35] are strongly associated with the principal causes of death (e.g., cardiovascular disease, diabetes, cancer). Wherever they may live, black American women born in the South have relatively higher mortality rates for diabetes than black women born in other regions of the country.[30] Similarly, women who live in the South are more likely than women who live in other regions to report that they have diabetes.[36] Women who live in rural areas are at high risk for diabetes because they are more likely than urban residents to be obese and to be inactive;[26] in addition, they are more likely to have severely limited access to high-quality health care and social services because of poverty or transportation barriers.[37]

Social and Economic Characteristics

Social position, or socioeconomic status (SES), is a powerful determinant of health status.[1,6-8,38-39] Compared with persons of higher SES, persons of low SES have reduced life expectancy[40] and are more likely to have chronic diseases;[41-43] they also have higher levels of risk factors for and behaviors related to chronic disease.[44-46] The effect of SES on health status is not simply a threshold effect, but is graded and continuous in all populations studied.[4,32,38,39] In addition, these effects are cumulative[47] and may persist throughout the life course.[4,5,30,48] In the United States, as in other industrialized countries, the disparity in health between persons of low and high SES is increasing steadily.[49]

The three indicators most often used to measure SES are educational attainment, occupation, and income.[50,51] Educational attainment is considered to influence lifestyle behaviors and values and to provide access to prestigious occupational ranking, income, and power. It has high validity and, after early adulthood, is less likely to vary over a lifetime. Also, educational attainment has stronger association with cardiovascular health-related behaviors than either occupation or income.[50,51] Its strong and consistent correlation with health practices or "lifestyle" behaviors may explain its relation to morbidity and mortality. Occupation is considered to be related to differential exposure to noxious environments and to reflect access to medical care and housing. Income and wealth are thought to influence opportunities for access to more and better education and health care resources, material living standards, and other social amenities. We will use these three indicators to describe the social status of the female population.

Education. The percentage of American women who have completed high school increased steeply between 1970 and 1995.[52,53] White women are still more likely than women in the minority groups to have had this much education, but the racial/ethnic gap closed substantially between 1970 and 1995 (Figure 2-6). During this period, percentages of high school completion increased from 55.0% to 80.0% among white women, from 34.2% to 53.8% among Hispanic women, and from 32.5% to 74.1% among black women. For all three groups, even more dramatic increases occurred in the percentages of women who completed 4 or more years of college: this percentage more than doubled among whites (8.4% to 21.0%), doubled

among Hispanics (4.3% to 8.4%), and almost tripled among blacks (4.6% to 12.9%). The improvement in college completion for Hispanic women notwithstanding, there have been discouraging trends in this population.[52] First, the level of high school completion decreased sharply from 1980 to 1990 (65.8% to 50.1%), then increased to only 53.8% in 1995. Second, the percentage of Hispanic women who completed college did not change from 1985 to 1995.

Overall in the United States in the 1980s, women began to outnumber men as recipients of all earned degrees conferred, except for first professional (e.g., medical doctors, lawyers) and doctoral degrees.[52,53] In these areas as well, however, there have been dramatic improvements: in 1970, women earned only 1 of every 20 first professional degrees and about 1 of every 8 doctoral degrees; by 1995, 2 of 5 degrees in each of these categories were earned by women.[52,53] This reduction in the gender gap in higher education occurred in all racial or ethnic minority groups but was greatest among Hispanics and American Indians, somewhat less so among

Figure 2-6. Percentage of women completing high school and college, by race/Hispanic* origin—United States, 1970, 1985, 1995

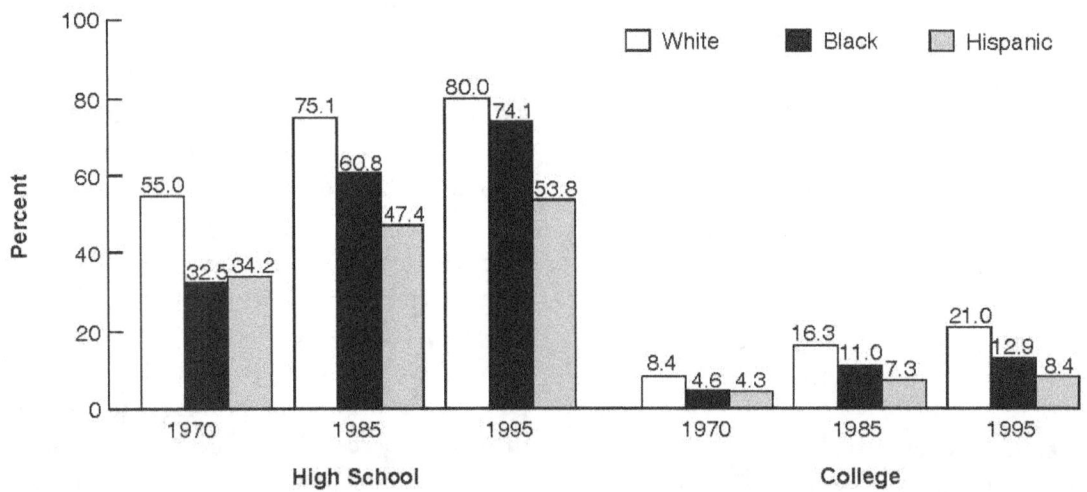

* Hispanic may be of any race.

Source: Reference 52.

Asian Americans, and even less among blacks. Black women, however, had already closed the gender gap as early as 1975; by 1995, black women earned 70% more bachelor's degrees, 20% more doctoral degrees, and 34% more first professional degrees than black men.

Despite the great improvements made by women in recent years, the sexes still have many differences in educational attainment. In 1994, for example, more than two-thirds of the bachelor's degrees earned in the fields of the humanities, education, library and archival sciences, health sciences, and public affairs were awarded to women, but they received fewer than one-third of the higher degrees awarded in business management and administrative services, computer/information sciences, engineering and engineering technologies, and physical sciences and science technologies.[52,53] Many of the fields in which women predominate are characterized by a relatively modest remuneration.[53-55]

Employment. A striking phenomenon of the last third of the 20th century is the movement of women into the paid labor force; between 1970 and 1995, the proportion of females over 15 years of age who participated in the labor force grew from 43% to 59%.[55] An upward trend was seen in all age groups under 65 years of age, but the steepest rise was seen among women aged 25–54 years, three-quarters of whom were in the labor force by 1995.[53,55] Among women 55 years or older, participation rates either remained steady or declined until the mid-1980s, when they began to increase. By 1995, about half of all women aged 55–64 years and about 10% of elderly women were participating. Overall participation was somewhat lower for Hispanic (53%) than for black or white women (59%), but among teenagers (16–19 years) whites had higher rates (55%) than blacks and Hispanics (40%).

Reflecting the increased participation, the percentage of the total paid labor force made up of women rose from 38.1% to 46% from 1970 to 1995.[53] The total number employed full-time and the number who either worked part-time or who were unemployed but looking for work rose by 90% to 100%. Women living with a spouse were about as likely as separated women to be in the workforce (61% versus 62%); however, divorced women had higher rates of participation (74%). In 1995, about 25 million women with children under 18 years of age were in the civilian labor force; of those with children under 6 years of age, two-thirds worked full-time.[55]

Income. In 1995, women had lower incomes than men at all ages (Table 2-3) and at all levels of educational attainment (Figure 2-7). This pattern held in all racial or ethnic groups. Between 1970 and 1995, however, women's earnings increased from 59.2% to 73.8% of men's earnings among year-round, full-time workers; similar trends were also seen for hourly earnings. Although the gender gap in earnings closed among all racial and ethnic groups, the smaller current gaps among blacks and Hispanics reflect the lower earnings of men in these groups more than gains made by women.[54]

Hispanic and black women have lower earnings than their white or Asian American counterparts.

Table 2-3. Median annual income of persons aged 15 years or older, by age and sex—United States, 1995

Age group (years)	Males ($)	Females ($)
15–24	6,913	5,310
25–34	23,609	15,557
35–44	31,420	17,397
45–54	35,586	17,723
55–64	29,980	12,381
≥65	16,484	9,355
Total	22,562	12,130

Source: Reference 57.

Figure 2-7. Median annual income of adults aged 25 years or older, by sex and educational attainment—United States, 1995

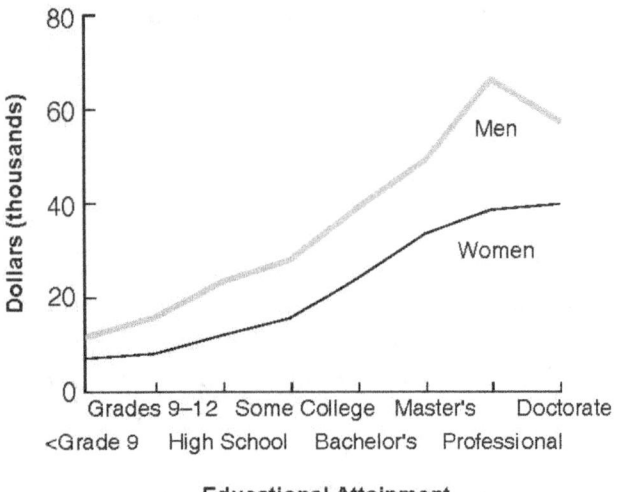

Source: Reference 57.

Figure 2-8. Median annual earnings of women who worked full-time year round, by race/Hispanic* origin—United States, 1970–95

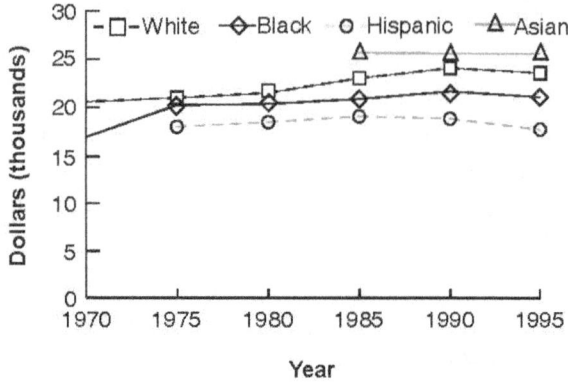

* Hispanic may be of any race.

Source: Reference 57.

In 1995, median annual earnings among year-round, full-time female workers ranged from $17,200 for Hispanic women to $24,900 for Asian American women (Figure 2-8). From 1975 to 1990, the gap between the earnings (in constant dollars) of black and white women widened steadily but did not change from 1990 to 1995. In this period, the gap between Hispanic and white women increased steadily.

Poverty among women is a particular concern. In 1995, 13.5 million American women were living below the official poverty level. Thus women account for about 3 of every 5 poor adults aged 18 years or older.[55-57] Most poor women (61.3%) are in their reproductive years, but nearly 20% are elderly. At all ages past adolescence, women are more likely than men to be poor (Table 2-4). The sex differential narrows during the middle years, but by the time a woman reaches 65 years of age, she is twice as likely as an elderly man to live in poverty (Table 2-4). In general, women are also more likely to be poor if they have not completed high school, work part-time, are single heads of households, live alone, or live in central cities or nonmetropolitan areas.[53,55,56]

Although most poor women (69%) are white, because of their relatively larger population, they account for about 12% of the white population. However, despite the increasing improvement in educational attainment and income, the poverty statistics for minority women continue to be especially grave. In 1995, almost one-third of black and Hispanic women lived below the federal poverty level compared with about one-eighth of white women (Table 2-4).[57] At all ages, black and Hispanic women are 2–3 times as likely as white women to live in poverty (Figure 2-9). The percentage in poverty is lower for Asian/Pacific Islander women (15% in 1995), but there are wide disparities among Asian subgroups.[15,17] Asian women who have immigrated to the United States since 1965 are much more likely to be poor than earlier immigrants: in 1990, poverty levels ranged from 6% among Japanese American women to 66% among Laotians.[15,17]

Table 2-4. Percentage of persons who lived below the poverty level, by age, sex, and race/ Hispanic* origin—United States, 1995

Age group (years)	All Female	Male	White Female	Male	Black Female	Male	Hispanic* Female	Male
<18	21.2	20.4	16.7	15.8	41.8	41.9	41.3	38.7
18–24	21.7	15.0	18.7	13.2	36.4	23.9	34.8	26.6
25–34	15.4	10.0	12.6	8.9	31.8	15.3	28.4	21.7
35–44	10.9	8.0	8.6	7.1	23.5	13.2	26.7	19.6
45–54	8.5	7.0	6.8	5.7	19.8	16.4	21.0	18.3
55–59	12.4	8.1	9.9	7.4	28.0	13.3	25.4	20.2
60–64	11.4	8.8	10.1	8.2	22.6	15.6	29.2	20.8
65–74	11.1	5.6	9.3	5.0	26.1	11.4	26.6	15.4
≥75	16.5	7.2	14.6	6.1	37.6	22.8	33.2	17.2
Total ≥18	**13.4**	**9.0**	**11.1**	**7.8**	**28.1**	**16.3**	**28.2**	**21.4**
Total ≥65	**13.6**	**6.2**	**11.7**	**5.4**	**31.1**	**15.4**	**28.9**	**16.0**
All ages	**15.4**	**12.2**	**12.4**	**9.9**	**32.4**	**25.7**	**32.9**	**27.7**

*Hispanic may be of any race.

Source: Reference 57.

Figure 2-9. Percentage of females who lived below the federal poverty level, by age and race/Hispanic* origin—United States, 1995

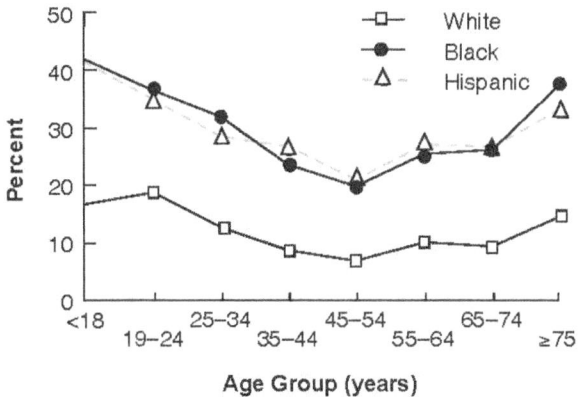

* Hispanic may be of any race.

Source: Reference 57.

This summary suggests very clearly that the health of millions of American women is being threatened by economic insecurity. From the perspective of diabetes, it is particularly disturbing that poverty is so common during childhood, when type 1 diabetes usually emerges; during the reproductive years, when gestational diabetes poses a threat; and among the very elderly, who frequently become blind, undergo amputations, or develop heart disease and stroke because of diabetes. The very high levels of poverty at all ages for black and Hispanic women, who have an elevated risk for diabetes in general, are especially compelling because they suggest that many of these women have limited access to medical and preventive services. Finally, there is an urgent need to focus research and careful thinking on the impact of poverty on the development of diabetes and its complications. The emphasis should be to identify modifiable community-level and individual-level determinants of risk for use in prevention efforts, especially among all women in the childbearing and older age groups.

Health-Related Behaviors

Several potentially modifiable health behaviors influence the occurrence of diabetes and are associated with its complications rates. In particular, the risk of developing diabetes increases progressively with increasing weight,[58-60] weight gain,[61,62] body fat distribution,[63] and decreased physical activity.[64-67]

Overweight. In the United States, overweight is a major (and worsening) public health problem for all age and racial or ethnic groups (Table 2-5). In the Third National Health and Examination Survey (NHANES III, 1988–1994), 10.5% of adolescent girls aged 12–17 years were overweight as defined by a body mass index (weight in kilograms divided by height in meters squared, kg/m^2) at or above the sex- and age-specific 95th percentile; an additional 10.7% were at or above the sex- and age-specific 85th percentile cutoff.[68,69] Approximately half of women aged 20 years or older were overweight as defined by a body mass index of 25.0 kg/m^2 or higher (Table 2-5). Based on these estimates, about 52 million adolescent and adult women are overweight.

Table 2-5. Percentage of adolescent females and women who were overweight in various national surveys, by age and race/Hispanic origin—United States, 1988–96

Population	Percentage*		Sample description (survey)
Adolescent females	≥85th Percentile	≥95th Percentile	
Total[†]	21.4	10.5	Ages 12–17 years (NHANES III, 1988–94)
Non-Hispanic white	20.3	9.3	
Non-Hispanic black	29.9	16.0	
Mexican American	23.4	14.1	
Total	25.9	11.6	Ages 13–18 years (National Longitudinal Study of Adolescent Health, 1996)[‡]
Total	25.9	–	Ages 12–22 years (National Longitudinal Study of Adolescent Health, 1996)
Non-Hispanic white	22.6	–	
Non-Hispanic black	34.0	–	
Non-Hispanic American Indian	40.0	–	
Non-Hispanic Asian American	15.0	–	
Hispanic American	29.1	–	
Women	Overweight		
Total[†]	48.0		Ages ≥20 years (NHANES III, 1988–94)[‡]
Non-Hispanic white	45.7		
Non-Hispanic black	66.8		
Mexican American	67.8		
Total[†]	20.2		Ages ≥18 years (National College Health Risk Behavior Survey, 1995)[§]
Non-Hispanic white	18.5		
Non-Hispanic black	35.8		
Hispanic	16.8		
18–24 years	13.9		
≥25 years	29.0		

* Percentages for adolescents are for ≥ 85th and ≥ 95th percentiles of body mass index. Percentages for women are for body mass index ≥ 25.0 kg/m^2.

[†] Includes racial and ethnic groups not shown.

[‡] Body mass index calculated from measured values of weight and height.

[§] Body mass index calculated from self-reported values of weight and height.

Sources: References 68–71.

Overweight is particularly common among adolescents and women in several minority groups (Table 2-5). In NHANES III, non-Hispanic black (16.0%) and Mexican American (14.1%) adolescent girls were more likely to be overweight (95th percentile of body mass index) than non-Hispanic whites (9.3%).[68,69] The National Longitudinal Study of Adolescent Health later confirmed these differences; in this survey the prevalence of overweight (85th percentile of body mass index) was highest for American Indian (40.0%), non-Hispanic black (34.0%), and Hispanic (29.1%) adolescent girls; intermediate for non-Hispanic white girls (22.6%); and lowest for Asian American girls (15.0%).[70] However, the prevalence of overweight varied widely among Hispanic and Asian American subgroups. Among Hispanic girls, overweight was highest among Mexican Americans (32.0%), lowest among Cuban Americans (21.4%), and intermediate for Puerto Ricans (28.0%) and girls of Central or South American origin (26.9%); among Asian American girls, Chinese American (10.9%) and Filipino American (12.8%) girls were about half as likely to be overweight as girls of all other Asian origins combined (20.6%).[70]

Differences in prevalence of overweight by race or ethnicity among adolescent girls are similar to those observed among women in several surveys.[68,71-76] In NHANES III, for example, more than two-thirds of non-Hispanic black (66.8%) and Mexican American (67.8%) women aged 20 years or older were overweight compared with about two-fifths (45.7%) of non-Hispanic white women (Table 2-5). Other surveys have reported similar or higher levels of overweight among American Indian[72-74] and Pacific Islander women (60%).[75] In contrast, estimates for Asian women ranged from 12.0% among Chinese Americans to 26.0% among Filipino Americans.[75]

Today, overweight among girls and women must be seen as a serious public health concern that is already well entrenched. Both the average weight of adolescent girls and women and the prevalence of overweight have shifted upward progressively since the early 1960s, with the steepest rise occurring after the late 1970s.[69,76-78] Over the ensuing two decades, the prevalence of overweight doubled among adolescent girls and rose by more than 40% among women in all racial or ethnic groups measured. Also of concern is that long-term increases in both weight and adiposity have also been seen among preadolescent girls.[77,79]

Overweight in childhood and adolescence persists into adulthood;[80-82] overweight adolescent girls, for example, are 40% to 60% more likely than their peers of normal weight to become overweight women.[81] In addition, many overweight adolescents can expect to become even more overweight after childbearing begins because prepregnancy weight and parity predict future weight gain.[83,84] The magnitude of recent trends suggests a populationwide impact of changes in social and environmental factors. One study, for example, found that a trend toward increased body mass and weight gain among young women aged 18–30 years was concurrent with increased average daily energy intake and decreased physical activity and physical fitness.[78]

Physical activity. Although lack of exercise is a risk factor for diabetes and other major illnesses among women, most American women do not get regular exercise.[85,86] NHANES III found that 59% of women aged 20 years or older engaged in little (less than 3 times per week) or no leisure-time physical activity.[85] In this study, Mexican American (46%) and non-Hispanic black (40%) women were about twice as likely as non-Hispanic white women (23%) to report no leisure-time physical activity. Overall, very few women (3%) participated in vigorous activity (3 or more times per week). Results from the Behavioral Risk Factor Surveillance System surveys for the years 1992–1994, which included more racial and ethnic groups than NHANES III, confirmed that study's findings: 43.6% of black, 33.8% of Asian/Pacific Islander, 34.6% of American Indian, and 41.4% of Hispanic women aged 18 or older reported engaging in no regular leisure-time physical activity, compared with 29.3% of whites.[72] Older women are less likely than younger women to undertake regular leisure-time physical activity. In NHANES III, the percentages of women reporting no leisure-time physical activity at all increased from 17% at ages 20–29, to 30% at age 50, to 44% at age 70. Even among adolescents and college students, age seems to be related to exercise habits.[71,87] For example, among a nationally representative sample of high school students, the percentages of girls participating in vigorous activity fell from 61.6% in grade 9 to 42.4% in grade 12; for moderate physical activity, the percentages declined from 27.0% to 13.7% (Table 2-6).

Socioeconomic status (SES), degree of acculturation, and generation of residence are also strongly related to whether women are overweight or do not engage in regular exercise.[46,86,88,89] Women who either have not completed high school or who live below the poverty level are twice as likely to be overweight as better educated or more affluent (300% or more

of the poverty level) women. Similarly, about half of women living in poverty or near poverty and more than half of those who have not completed high school do not exercise at all; by comparison, fewer than one-third of women who are either more affluent or have at least some college do not exercise. Furthermore, adolescent girls of all racial and ethnic origins are less likely to be sedentary as the educational attainment of the responsible adult with whom they live rises or as the family income increases.[46]

A fuller explanation of the differences between white and minority women is needed. At all levels of socioeconomic status, overweight and physical inactivity are more prevalent among minority than among white women;[86,89] cultural differences may well play an important role. For example,

Table 2-6. Percentage of female high school and college students who participated in vigorous* or moderate[†] physical activity, were enrolled in a physical education class, and played on an intramural sports team, by age, race/Hispanic origin, and grade—United States, 1995

Population	Vigorous physical activity	Moderate physical activity	Physical education class	Intramural sports team
High school				
Total	52.1	20.5	56.8	42.4
Non-Hispanic white	56.7	16.8	61.7	47.1
Non-Hispanic black	41.3	26.4	44.4	34.9
Hispanic	45.2	27.6	44.6	27.3
Grade 9	61.6	27.0	80.8	43.7
Grade 10	59.3	22.9	71.4	47.9
Grade 11	47.2	19.6	41.2	39.4
Grade 12	42.4	13.7	39.1	38.8
College				
Total	33.0	19.3	20.1	10.3
Non-Hispanic white	34.7	18.2	19.8	10.7
Non-Hispanic black	27.6	24.6	18.1	7.8
Hispanic	30.6	20.4	19.4	6.3
18–24 years	35.3	20.8	25.5	16.4
≥25 years	29.7	17.0	11.8	1.4

* Activities that caused sweating and hard breathing for at least 20 minutes on ≥ 1 of 7 days preceding the survey.

[†] Walked or bicycled for at least 30 minutes on ≥ 5 of 7 days preceding the survey.

Sources: References 71, 87.

differences in prevalence of obesity between black and white women are virtually constant across levels of SES, whereas differences between Hispanic and white women decrease sharply with increasing affluence.[86,90] Black women may perceive overweight to be more acceptable than do white women and may be encouraged by their social environment to maintain their weight.[91] Among Mexican American women, however, increasing affluence is strongly associated with assimilation into the mainstream non-Hispanic white U.S. society, which may account for the reduction in body mass.[90]

The effects of acculturation on risk behaviors have also been found in national surveys of adolescents and women.[70,86] For example, second-generation (at least one foreign-born parent) adolescents are more likely than their first-generation (born in a foreign country to foreign-born parents) counterparts to be overweight (30.6% versus 23.1% for Hispanics and 22.0% versus 8.3% for Asian Americans) (Table 2-7).[70] Furthermore, second-generation adolescents have levels of obesity equivalent to those of U.S.-born adolescents with U.S.-born parents. In addition, foreign-born women who have resided in the United States for at least 15 years are likely to report levels of overweight similar to those of U.S.-born women, whereas those resident for less than 15 years report lower levels (Table 2-7).

This summary provides evidence of disturbing trends in obesity and physical inactivity, especially among younger females. Results of the few studies reported here do not establish cause and effect between socioeconomic status, duration or generation of residence, and behavioral risk factors among adolescent girls and women. Still, they offer some evidence of major increases in the average weight and level of physical inactivity among women at all stages across the lifespan, from preadolescence to later adulthood. The magnitude of the increases in these major determinants of diabetes risk suggests a populationwide impact of changes in social and environmental factors. With the current emphasis on health promotion, health officials and researchers need to pay more attention to under-

Table 2-7. Percentage of adolescent females and women who were overweight* or did not exercise, by race/Hispanic origin, generation,† and duration of residence—United States, 1995

Population	Overweight	No physical activity
Adolescent females (grades 7–12)		
Non-Hispanic white	22.6	–
Non-Hispanic back	34.0	–
Hispanic	29.1	–
First generation	23.1	–
Second generation	30.6	–
Third generation	31.0	–
Asian American	15.0	–
First generation	8.3	–
Second generation	22.0	–
Third generation	20.3	–
Women (aged ≥18 years)		
Born in U.S.	37	37
Not born in U.S.		
Resident ≥15 years	35	55
Resident <15 years	25	69

* Body mass index (kg/m²) ≥ 85th percentile for age and sex.

† First generation = child and both parents not born in U.S.; Second generation = child born in U.S., at least one parent not born in U.S.; Third generation = child and both parents born in U.S.

Sources: References 70, 86.

standing the processes that precipitate (and protect against) changes in these health behaviors and environmental exposures.

2.3. Psychosocial Determinants of Health Behaviors and Health Outcomes
The general status of the health of U.S. women presents an apparent paradox. While living 7 years longer than men on average, their more frequent reports of illness and utilization of health services suggest that they experience poorer health than men.[92-95] Sex-related differences in socialization, social environment, and health attitudes and

behaviors may account for much of the observed discrepancy between men and women.

There are three general categories of psychosocial influences on women's overall health in the United States. The first category includes factors related to the social environment (e.g., influence of marital and family status, role strain and conflict, and social support; community norms regarding health-related attitudes and behaviors). The second group of psychosocial determinants involves those factors influencing women's interactions with the health care system, such as access to services and relationships with health care providers. The final category includes psychological variables related to the development of health beliefs, such as locus of control and confidence in health interventions. Taken together, these factors provide a context for understanding the influence of social and psychological factors on women's health behaviors and outcomes.

The Social Environment
The social environment, broadly conceptualized as social networks encompassed by family, marital, and social relationships, exerts a strong influence on women's health-related behaviors and outcomes. It is primarily within this environment that individuals learn attitudes about health and help-seeking, as well as observe the practice of health-related behaviors.[95-97] According to a recent report of the Public Health Service Task Force on Women's Health Issues,[98] the family can provide an important source of social support as well as an arena within which women exert significant effects on family health. For this reason, women's experiences in the family are of particular interest when examining the social context of health behaviors.

The Task Force identified two aspects of women's roles within the family that merit attention for their contribution to women's health experiences:
1) women's increased employment outside of the home, combined with primary responsibility for child rearing and home-related responsibilities, and 2) increases in divorce, which result in higher numbers of woman-headed households. The effects of

these changes in women's roles within the family include direct as well as indirect effects on health. For many, with divorce comes a decline in household income, which may restrict access to health services and bring additional financial stress. Similarly, significant changes in women's employment and family roles are often accompanied by greater demands placed on those women who are already experiencing role overload and conflict.[97] Such stresses can lead to greater vulnerability to physical as well as psychological problems. Thus, women's social position, as represented by the roles played within their households, can have a significant impact on their health status.

Social support. Social support is a mechanism for promoting and restoring health related to the psychological consequences of one's roles within the household. Social support can be conceptualized as the extent and quality of one's social relationships and networks that provide the following functions: esteem (or emotional support), informational support, companionship, and instrumental support.[99] Thus, social support can serve a number of functions that are related to enhanced psychological well-being.

The effects of social support on the relationship between stress and illness have been widely studied.[99,100] Lower levels of social support have consistently predicted higher rates of morbidity and mortality.[93,100,101] Although these findings are robust, the process accounting for the positive effects of social support remains unclear. The influence of social support on health may operate through several possible pathways.[93] For example, the relationship may be due to indirect or direct influences of social support and social networks on actual health behaviors,[102,103] either by providing resources that increase access to health services (e.g., transportation, financial support), or by increasing the likelihood of health-promoting or health-damaging behaviors.[104] Alternatively, the relationship between social support and health may be explained by the psychological consequences of increased social support.[93] That is, increased social support may be related to a greater sense of control and self-esteem,[102,105] which in turn can increase the probability of health-promoting behaviors. For example, it has been shown that women receive and use social support more than men do.[106,107] This is consistent with women's higher rates of health-promoting behaviors and lower rates of mortality but not with their higher rates of morbidity.

Women's roles in providing increased levels of social support can also contribute to their higher morbidity rates.[99] For example, women tend to be involved with a wider range of people, are more responsive to others, and are more likely to provide caregiving services.[108] Women are also more likely to provide social support to others and more likely to initiate and sustain support networks.[101,109] This pattern of increased social support, both in terms of initiating support for oneself and providing it to others, can have contradictory effects on women's health. By increasing opportunities for women to experience the negative consequences of the caregiving role, increased social support can place greater demands on their emotional and physical resources.[93] In sum, social support may influence the health of women and men differently. These apparently discrepant effects on health highlight the significance of women's roles in social networks.

Women's multiple social roles are viewed as potent contributors to overall levels of health. It appears that it is not the mere presence or absence of multiple roles that influences women's health outcomes, but other aspects of such roles that may mediate this relationship. For example, marriage is associated with better health for women and men, and people who are both married and employed have the best health. On the other hand, women who are employed but not married and also have children have poorer levels of health than nonmarried working women without children.[110] For women who are married and employed, having children does not negatively influence health outcome. Therefore, the stresses associated with motherhood pose a greater health risk to women who are not married than to those who are married.[110]

These findings are consistent with research indicating that married women having multiple roles (e.g., wife, worker, mother) experience positive health benefits.[110,111] However, other research has found that women working outside the home have worse health than do men who work.[112,113] The discrepancy between these findings underscores the necessity to consider the overall context of women's social roles when attempting to isolate the contribution of specific factors on overall health.

Socioeconomic factors. An inverse relationship exits between SES and health; lower SES is associated with higher rates of morbidity and mortality.[114,115] Women, in particular, experience disproportionately more health problems that result from poverty than do men. This relationship may be a function of two different, yet potentially related, mechanisms. On the one hand, lower SES is associated with decreased access to health services, which can negatively affect health outcome. Alternatively, those in lower SES groups are more likely to perceive some life events as more negative and uncontrollable than those in higher SES groups.[116] This cognitive style is also associated with lower health ratings.[116] Hanner suggests a similar relationship among education, health status, self-esteem, and the likelihood of engaging in health-promoting behaviors.[117] SES may have a direct influence on health outcomes through its impact on health resource and services options. For example, inadequate insurance coverage and access to services have been cited as major barriers to health care for Asian American,[118] Hispanic,[119] and Native American women.[120] Conversely, SES may affect health outcomes indirectly by influencing psychosocial variables such as health locus of control and self-esteem.

For black women, the relationship between SES and health is moderated by the influences of ethnicity and gender, which have also been associated with variations in SES.[115] Because the SES of blacks tends to be lower than that of whites,[121] and the SES of women is generally lower than that of men,[122] African American women are particularly vulnerable to the negative effects of SES on health. The weathering hypothesis put forth by Geronimus is consistent with this perspective.[123] According to Geronimus, deteriorating reproductive health outcomes for African American women in their early adult years are a function of their "cumulative socioeconomic disadvantage."

This relationship between SES and health is also illustrated by racial variation in the mortality rates for specific diseases. The diseases that cause death for African American women at higher rates than for white women are also the diseases often linked to SES (e.g., diabetes, lung disease, cerebrovascular disease, cirrhosis of the liver).[124] Even HIV/AIDS, which was once primarily associated with homosexuality, has a strong economic determination. Groups that currently have a high risk of contracting HIV (either through sex or injection drug use) include groups that tend to be economically vulnerable: poor women and men, prostitutes, and young people living in high-risk social environments.[125] Thus, SES represents a number of significant social and environmental factors that have powerful effects on the health status of women of color.

Risk behaviors such as tobacco and alcohol use are also related to social and economic influences, and thus can lead to negative health outcomes for women. In fact, examining risk behaviors may illuminate our understanding of how social and economic influences are exerted upon health. Women who are younger, divorced, have higher levels of education, and are employed report higher rates of alcohol consumption.[126] Relatedly, white women tend to consume more alcohol at all ages than do African American women.[126]

There are also racial and SES-related differences in rates of women's tobacco use.[127] In general, the prevalence of cigarette smoking is highest among American Indian or Alaska Native women, intermediate among non-Hispanic white and non-Hispanic black women, and lowest among Asian and Hispanic women; women who have a high school education or less are more likely than their counter-

parts to report current cigarette smoking. Although sex differences in health risk behaviors have long been noted,[93] such variation among women points to the influences of social and economic factors on health-promoting versus health-damaging behaviors. Social norms regarding alcohol and tobacco use may vary as a function of SES-related variables and thus increase the likelihood that some groups of women will be at greater risk of engaging in these behaviors. For example, Baines cites the ceremonial use of tobacco as a cultural norm influencing tobacco use and therefore risk for cardiovascular disease, cancer, and related medical conditions in Native American women.[120]

In summary, a number of behaviors related to sociodemographic characteristics and social roles are associated with women's health outcomes. Although the relationships among these factors are not consistently linear, they do demonstrate the need for considering these aspects of women's social environments as they affect health-related behaviors,[128] particularly as they influence the development of community norms regarding health behaviors. The pattern of variation in women's risk behaviors in relation to socioeconomic status demonstrates that health status is a function of one's social context in addition to individual characteristics. Thus, the social environment exerts a powerful influence on health status, through both 1) the effects of community norms and the influences of social roles and 2) SES-related factors.

Interactions with the Health Care System

Access. A person with adequate access to health care services can make timely use of personal health services to achieve the best possible outcomes.[129-131] Health insurance coverage, having a usual source of care, and satisfaction with care are among the indicators of access that have been studied extensively.[131-138] These studies have shown that health insurance coverage is necessary but not sufficient for adequate access to health care services. Nevertheless, a major barrier to health care is cost, and health insurance provides people with the means to overcome financial barriers to care.[129,130,139]

Most full-time workers have access to health care through private insurance, primarily employment-based; unemployed people and those who work for low wages often have no coverage. In the mid-1960s, the jointly sponsored federal-state Medicaid and federally sponsored Medicare programs were implemented to provide health insurance protection to low-income persons, the disabled, and persons 65 years of age or older.[140]

Data from several national surveys confirm that the majority of females are covered by some form of health care insurance.[131,132,141] These surveys have also shown that minority women, poor women (family income-to-poverty ratio less than 1.00), and those near poverty (family income-to-poverty ratio between 1.00 and 1.24) are less likely than other women to be covered.[131,132,141,142] For example, the 1996 Current Population Survey (CPS) found that only about 7 of 10 Hispanic women and 8 of 10 black women were covered compared with 9 of 10 white women (Figure 2-10).[142] The CPS also found that, regardless of racial or ethnic group, poor women were less likely to be insured.

Most women (about 70%) have private coverage, primarily employment-based; however, minority women are considerably less likely than white women to have private coverage (Figure 2-11). Women also rely more heavily than men on government health insurance programs. In 1996, approximately one-quarter of females were covered through Medicaid and Medicare compared with just one-fifth of males.[142] Black and Hispanic women are more than twice as likely as white women to rely on Medicaid coverage (28.0% and 24.5% versus 10.9%). More women than men are covered through Medicare simply because women live longer. The percentages of women covered by Medicare are consistent with the proportions of elderly women in each racial or ethnic group (Figure 2-11).

One reason why women rely more heavily than men on government programs, especially Medicaid, is because they are more likely to be poor.[53,141] Figure 2-11 demonstrates clearly that poverty is strongly

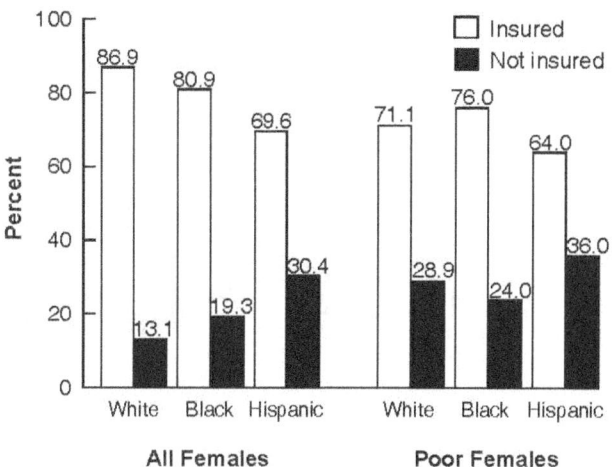

Figure 2-10. Health insurance coverage among all females and poor* females, by race/Hispanic[†] origin—United States, 1996

* Poor = family income-to-poverty ratio less than 1.00.
[†] Hispanic may be of any race.

Source: Reference 142.

related to reduced levels of private coverage and to increased levels of coverage through a government program. Thus, irrespective of racial or ethnic origin, poor women are more likely than other women to be covered through the Medicaid program: whites, 42.6% versus 10.6%; blacks, 59.7% versus 51.2%; Hispanics, 51.4% versus 24.5% (Figure 2-11). Because Medicaid is primarily a program for poor mothers and their children, it is used most prominently during the childbearing years when women are most at risk of being poor.[55,56] The high levels of poverty among minority women, their youth, and high fertility may combine to make them more vulnerable to dependence on health care coverage through Medicaid.

Women are more prone than men to discontinuous employment and part-time and low-paying jobs, which frequently makes them less likely to receive employment benefits that would include health insurance coverage. In addition, because they are more than twice as likely as men to be covered as a

Figure 2-11. Type of health care insurance coverage among all females and poor* females, by race/Hispanic† origin—United States, 1996

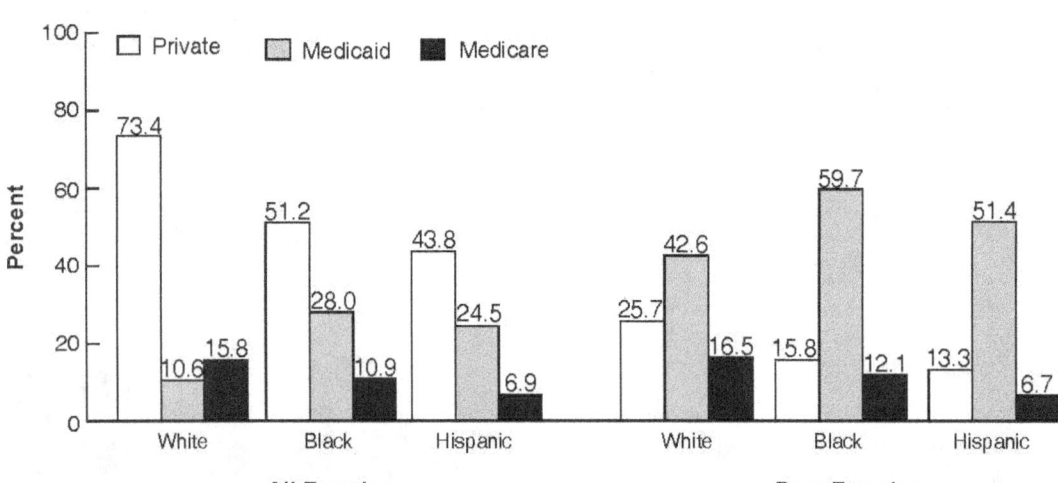

* Poor = family income-to-poverty ratio less than 1.00.
† Hispanic may be of any race.

Source: Reference 142.

dependent, they are more vulnerable to loss of coverage through separation, divorce, and widowhood.[53,55,141] As of 1996, 19.4 million females (14% of the female population) were uninsured; of these, 14.6 million were white, 3.5 million were black, 4.4 million were Hispanic of any race, and 7.6 million were considered poor or near poor.[142] Women of minority racial and ethnic origin and women of low SES were overrepresented among the uninsured. Black and Hispanic women, who constituted 24% of all women in 1996, accounted for 41% of the uninsured; poor and near-poor women, who comprised 21% of all women in that year, accounted for 40% of the uninsured. Sex-specific data on health insurance coverage are very limited. However, the 1995 National Health Interview Survey found that 14.3% of adolescent girls aged 10–18 years were without health care coverage.[143] Among adolescents aged 12–17 years, 3.8 million (16.1%) were uninsured, representing nearly 13.9% of whites, 20% of blacks, 30% of Hispanics, and 30% of those in poverty.

Thus, socioeconomic and demographic factors such as income, ethnicity, marital status, age, and educa-

tional attainment affect a woman's ability to obtain health care coverage. States have broad discretion in determining eligibility criteria for Medicaid, but these criteria vary between states and can change from year to year within states.[140] Consequently, Medicaid does not provide comprehensive health care coverage for many poor and minority reproductive-aged women who are at increased risk for gestational diabetes and early-onset type 2 diabetes. In contrast, Medicare provides coverage for 95% of the nation's aged, but beneficiaries are responsible for charges for services not covered by the program, including most prescription drugs and long-term nursing care. States can use Medicaid funds to "buy in" Medicare coverage to provide coverage for prescription drugs, nursing home care, premiums, and cost sharing for low-income Medicare beneficiaries.[138] Recent data indicate that Medicare beneficiaries covered by Medicaid are more likely than those not covered to be women, nonwhite, nursing home residents, and poor (annual incomes less than $10,000). But older beneficiaries covered by Medicaid are less likely to receive recommended preventive care and to be satisfied with the quality of care they receive. Thus, both Medicaid and Medicare fall short of providing important coverage that women need, especially poor women and working women who support children. Furthermore, even when women are employed and supporting children, they may earn too much to qualify for programs such as Medicaid but too little to afford private insurance.

In addition to concerns about lack of coverage, policy makers, health care professionals responsible for assuring access, and researchers need to consider that underinsurance is also an important issue for women.[130,144,145] This review suggests strongly that regardless of the type of coverage, large numbers of women do not have adequate protection against the cost of health care. Absence of appropriate insurance coverage forces women to forego needed services, especially preventive services that provide early detection, successful treatment, and continuity of care essential for effective management of serious diseases such as diabetes.[146]

Utilization. Women seek health services more frequently and use a greater variety of these services than do men.[92] One explanation may be that women are socialized to provide the bulk of home health services and social support,[93,98,106] which makes them more aware of health-related problems and thus more ready to seek medical services for such problems. At the same time, their socialization as caretakers and providers of social support may protect women from negative health outcomes in the long run. Thus, it should not be surprising that unmarried women have fewer negative health consequences than unmarried men, because men are not socialized to seek health services.[92]

Three differences in the socialization of women and men have been advanced that relate to health behavior:[92]

- Females are socialized to be aware of their physical discomforts; males are taught to ignore them. The likely result is that women are more aware of their physical conditions.

- Women are more willing than men to discuss physical complaints with health care providers and others;[92] men are more likely to keep such complaints to themselves. This difference appears consistent with sex-typed behavior: discussing personal information, particularly about illness, is more consistent with the female role. Such behavior on the part of boys can easily be viewed as evidence of weakness.

- Women appear more likely to curtail their activity level when ill, reflecting their greater attention to signs of illness and disease. Women are also more likely than men to believe that health service providers and their interventions will be effective, and they are more likely to believe that preventive behaviors will have positive results. Not surprisingly, women are more likely than men to engage in preventive behaviors, such as using vitamins, obtaining a physical exam when they are well, not smoking cigarettes, and refraining from heavy alcohol use.

The more frequent use of health services by women can be seen as a function not merely of their having greater illness rates, but also a different socialization toward health and illness. Although women can be broadly characterized as disposed to taking action on their health complaints, here also ethnic differences are apparent. Social factors such as language, lack of insurance coverage, cultural values, and opinions on the role of health professionals are all important. Asian American women, for example, are frequently reluctant to discuss their sexuality.[118] Not surprisingly, Asian American women use preventive health services such as Pap smears and breast exams less often than other groups of women and have low survival rates for breast and cervical cancer.[118]

Patient/provider relationship. Women have access to greater amounts of health communications than men, and they ask more health-related questions of their providers.[92,147-149] They also receive more empathy from their providers.[149,150] One might conclude that women are generally more satisfied than men with the relationship they have with their providers, and one might expect that women have a greater belief that health services are effective. In trying to characterize attitudes of women about their providers and about the effectiveness of health care, however, one must again consider ethnicity. For example, Asian American, Hispanic, and Native American women all experience barriers to obtaining health care services that often translate into lower utilization, thereby blunting the effects of a positive orientation about health care.[118] For example, a culturally sanctioned belief among Hispanic women is that individuals are responsible for their own health outcomes, and this factor tends to discourage care-seeking.[119] Among Native American women, cultural norms related to interpersonal communications and attitudes about health and wellness affect the provider/patient relationship; if physicians do not pay attention to these norms, they may harm their relationship with the patient and thus create a barrier to care.[120]

Personality Characteristics

Self-esteem. Higher self-esteem is associated with increased likelihood that a person will engage in health-promoting behaviors.[96,105,151] Not surprisingly, higher self-esteem is related to decreased levels of smoking and alcohol and drug use[152] and to increased exercise;[151] lower self-esteem is associated with greater frequency of risk behaviors related to HIV transmission.[153] In addition, women high in self-esteem have been found to perceive themselves at lower risk for HIV infection than women low in self-esteem.

One might surmise that women with high self-esteem are more interested in maintaining their health, but most research on the health effects of self-esteem has not considered the ethnicity of female participants. Thus, generalizing these findings to all groups of women is premature.

Health locus of control. Based on the concept of internal and external locus of control,[154] individual attitudes toward control over personal health can be attributed to belief in the role of internal forces that an individual can direct, the role of external forces directed by powerful others (such as health professionals), or the role of chance (i.e., fate or luck). High levels of internal control among women have been positively correlated with preventive health behaviors,[155] health-promoting behavior (such as exercise),[92,156] and help-seeking and reports of overall good health.[92] Conversely, low internal control has been associated with less preventive behavior, higher reports of illness, and less confidence in the outcomes of treatment interventions.[155] The concepts of internal control, the role of professional control, and the impact of fate may be especially relevant to diabetes. Persons with this disorder often curse their fate, yet they must be prepared to control their own health status through careful self-management and trust in professionals for oversight and guidance. At this point, however, it is not clear whether findings about internal control can be applied to minority women, as studies have generally not focused on them. Furthermore, there is evidence that this model may not fit Hispanic women, whose strong belief that health is under individual control has been cited as reducing their access to care.[119]

Connection with traditional health beliefs. Higher educational attainment is associated with higher levels of internal control for both women and men.[157] Correspondingly, women with lower education and SES have been found to believe more strongly in fate and chance than women of higher SES.[116] Thus, women of lower SES may be at greater risk of holding health beliefs that are not conducive to health-promoting behaviors.

It would be easy to conclude that inappropriate health beliefs lead to negative health outcomes, and that the solution is to educate women both formally and informally. The issue is not quite straightforward, however. For example, it is not clear whether such beliefs result from one's health status or actually give rise to health outcomes.[114] Second, health beliefs should not be considered purely individual characteristics, or traits, that might be susceptible to adjustment. Rather, it may be useful to conceptualize them as a component of overall health socialization that varies in relation to a woman's particular social context (e.g., SES, socialization within family and community of origin, current social roles and networks).[158] Specifically, the attitudes and expectations one holds about the import of health-promoting and health-damaging behavior reflect one's general notions about health.

The evidence presented above suggests that women's health orientation, as shaped by socialization experiences, influences their levels of knowledge about health issues, perceptions of symptoms, interest in seeking care or treatment, and confidence in the benefits of treatment. Together, such psychological variables ultimately affect morbidity and mortality rates as well as women's general experiences within the health care system. Clearly, psychosocial factors strongly affect women's health through attitudes, behaviors, and social influences, and these influences must be included in any accurate description and explanation of women's health status.

2.4. Public Health Implications

The findings from this literature review demonstrate that the social status of U.S. women improved markedly since the early 1970s. Over the ensuing decades, however, several social and environmental themes emerged or persisted—including some that pertain specifically to diabetes—that currently affect the health status of women. Many of these themes recur across the lifespan, combine to increase women's risk for diabetes, and can impede both individual and societal efforts to prevent this disease. Many of these issues are common to all women; others are peculiar to specific subgroups.

Issues common to all women include

- The large increase expected in the number of women at risk for diabetes.

- A trend toward increasing prevalence of major risk factors for diabetes (i.e., overweight and lack of physical activity).

- Economic insecurity and risk for poverty at all ages over 18 years of age.

- The growth in the number of older women, or the "feminization of old age."

- The increasing number of elderly women who live alone.

Other issues common to specific groups of women include those that are related to demographic changes among women of minority racial and ethnic origin. Between 1995 and 2010, the number of minority women—American Indian, Asian/Pacific Islander, black, and Hispanic—will increase by approximately 15 million. Also affecting this increase is the impact of immigration and acculturation. Among adolescents and women, duration of residence and acculturation are associated with the development of a diabetogenic risk profile.

The public health implications of these issues identified are organized according to the three core functions of public health practice as recommended by the Institute of Medicine: assessment, policy development, and assurance.[159] These core functions provide a framework for thought and action on the impact of diabetes on women's health.

Assessment

Surveillance. The magnitude of the increasing trends in major risk factors for diabetes (overweight, weight gain, and low levels of physical activity), especially among adolescent and young adult women, suggests a populationwide impact of changes in social and environmental factors and calls for more systematic monitoring of these major risk factors for diabetes using a life-stage approach.

Women at highest risk of developing diabetes and its complications may be the least likely to have access to preventive health care services. Therefore, there is a need for systematic monitoring and reporting of health insurance coverage, changes in Medicaid (including buy-ins to Medicare), and other state-based insurance programs to provide information on their impact on access to care among women, notably during adolescence and the reproductive and elderly years.

The greatest growth in the size of the female population is expected in the age and ethnic groups at highest risk for diabetes; much of this change will be concentrated regionally. The reporting of the expected increase in the prevalence and incidence of diabetes in women by regional concentration, nativity, duration and generation of residence, and degree of acculturation would provide useful information for allocating resources and for planning and programming appropriate services for this population.

Socioeconomic status, region or area of residence, and place of birth are often as strongly associated with health status as currently used risk markers (e.g., race, ethnicity). Appropriate and valid indicators of social status and social context are needed for routine use in assessing the burden of diabetes and its complications among women of all racial and ethnic groups.

Research. More intensive study is needed to determine the contribution of cumulative gestational weight gain to overweight among middle-aged women, to identify modifiable determinants of the sharp decline in physical activity among school-aged girls, and to identify types of physical activity that appeal to women in various age, cultural, and socioeconomic groups.

In addition, among immigrant adolescent girls and older women, factors such as acculturation and duration of residence are positively associated with having a diabetogenic profile. Additional research is needed to identify protective health behaviors among immigrant groups, to develop intervention strategies aimed to preserve these behaviors, and to develop effective strategies for translating this knowledge to other groups of women.

An increasing number of elderly women are at risk for poverty and are living alone. This population will require additional community-based services and support to carry out daily activities and to access appropriate health services. The assessment of community barriers to self-management of diabetes and other chronic diseases could provide data for programmatic activity and identify potentially modifiable determinants of such barriers.

Policy Development

The planning and programming of appropriate services and interventions for women will require input from many agencies at the federal, state, and local levels. For instance, collaboration between the appropriate health and education agencies will be required to develop and implement programs aimed at 1) ensuring that schools comply with federal recommendations for healthy diets and the availability of healthy foods, and 2) integrating education on the importance of healthy eating habits and physical education into school curricula for all grades, especially in junior and senior high schools.

Women who are at risk for poverty are also least likely to have adequate health care insurance coverage. Ensuring financial access to adequate preventive care for women with diabetes and other chronic diseases is an important strategy for reducing the burden of disease in high-risk populations. This would benefit individuals and society at large.

Assurance

In general, women are the initial providers of primary care to family members or to their extended family. Women are socialized to be more aware of health-related problems and thus are more likely to seek medical services for their problems.[93] This is in addition to the fact that many women work and provide support to family and community members. At the same time, self-care or preventive care may not be a priority for many women who work outside of or in the home, women who are heads of households, women who are poor or nearly poor, and women responsible for providing for their parents and members of their extended family. To facilitate healthy behaviors in this population, innovative models of health care delivery that include features such as extended hours, culturally competent providers, and access to preventive care services and education in traditional and nontraditional settings would make the use of services—especially preventive care services—more accessible.

Efforts at the state and local levels to increase access through the provision of quality care services for persons with diabetes and other chronic diseases are important for women at all ages in the life cycle. Extending this approach to elderly women would further necessitate intersectoral collaboration (e.g., among health, social services, organizations in the voluntary sector) to promote increased awareness and availability of community services that specifically target the needs of elderly women who live alone.

References

1. Lynch JW. Social position and health. *Ann Epidemiol* 1996;6(1):21–3.

2. Becker MH. A medical sociologist looks at health promotion. *J Health Soc Behav* 1993;34(1):1–6.

3. Davison C, Frankel S, Smith GD. The limits of lifestyle: re-assessing "fatalism" in the popular culture of illness prevention. *Soc Sci Med* 1992;34(6):675–85.

4. Adler NE, Boyce T, Chesney MA, et al. Socioeconomic status and health. The challenge of the gradient. *Am Psychol* 1994;49:15–24.

5. Lynch JW, Kaplan GA, Salonen JT. Why do poor people behave poorly? Variation in adult health behaviors and psychological characteristics by stages of the socioeconomic life course. *Soc Sci Med* 1997;44(6):809–19.

6. Kaplan GA. People and places: contrasting perspectives on the association between social class and health. *Int J Health Serv* 1996;26(3):507–19.

7. Link BG, Phelan J. Social conditions as fundamental causes of disease. *J Health Soc Behav* 1995;Spec No: 80–94.

8. Williams DR. Socioeconomic differentials in health: a review and redirection. *Soc Psychol Q* 1990;53:81–99.

9. Deardorff KE, Hollmann FW, Montgomery PM. *U.S. Population Estimates by Age, Sex, Race, and Hispanic Origin: 1990–1995.* Population Paper Listings, No. 41. Washington, DC: Population Division, U.S. Bureau of the Census, 1996.

10. U.S. Bureau of the Census. *Population Projections of the United States, by Age, Sex, Race, and Hispanic Origin: 1995 to 2050.* Current Population Reports, Series P25, No. 1130. Washington, DC: U.S. Government Printing Office, 1996.

11. McFalls, JA Jr. Population: a lively introduction. Updated 3rd ed. *Popul Bull* 1998;53(3):1–47.

12. Kranczer S. Mixed life expectancy changes. *Stat Bull* 1996;77(4):29–36. Data used with permission from publisher.

13. Waldron I. Recent trends in sex mortality ratios for adults in developed countries. *Soc Sci Med* 1993;36(4): 451–62.

14. Wallman KK, Hodgdon J. Race and ethnic standards for federal statistics and administrative reporting. Directive No. 15. *Stat Reporter,* 1977(July):450–4.

15. Leigh WA, Lindquist MA. *Women of Color Health Data Book.* Washington, DC: Office of Research on Women's Health, 1998. (NIH Publication No. NIH 98-4247)

16. Centers for Disease Control and Prevention. *Chronic Disease in Minority Populations.* Atlanta: Centers for Disease Control and Prevention, 1994.

17. Takeuchi DT, Young KNJ. Overview of Asian Pacific Islander Americans. In: Zane NWS, Takeuchi D, Young KNJ, editors. *Confronting Critical Health Issues of Asian and Pacific Islander Americans.* Thousand Oaks, CA: Sage, 1994:3–21.

18. De Vita CJ, Pollard KM. Increasing diversity of the U.S. population. *Stat Bull Metrop Insur Co* 1996;77(3): 12–17.

19. del Pinal JH. Hispanic Americans in the United States: young, dynamic, and diverse. *Stat Bull Metrop Insur Co* 1996; 77(4):2–13.

20. Reid J. Immigration and the future of the U.S. black population. *Popul Today* 1986;14(2):6–8.

21. Smith JP, Edmonston B, editors. *The New Americans: Economic, Demographic, and Fiscal Effects of Immigration.* Washington, DC: National Academy Press, 1997.

22. Carter JS, Pugh JA, Monterrosa A. Non–insulin-dependent diabetes mellitus in minorities in the United States. *Ann Int Med* 1996;125(3):221–32.

23. Markides KS. Consequences of gender differentials in life expectancy for black and Hispanic Americans. *Int J Aging Hum Dev* 1989;29(2):95–102.

24. U.S. Census Bureau. <http://www.census.gov/population/censusdata/urdef.txt>. Released October 1995.

25. Office of Technology Assessment. *Health Care in Rural America,* OTA-H-434. Washington, DC: U.S. Government Printing Office, 1990.

26. U.S. Census Bureau. <http://www.census.gov/population/www/estimates/metrodef.html>. Last revised: May 9, 1997.

27. Greenberg MR, Schneider D. Region of birth and mortality of blacks in the United States. *Int J Epidemiol* 1992;21(2):324–8.

28. Fang J, Madhavan S, Alderman MH. Nativity, race, and mortality: influence of region of birth on mortality of U.S.-born residents of New York City. *Hum Biol* 1997; 69(4):533–44.

29. Schneider D, Greenberg MR, Lu LL. Region of birth and mortality from circulatory diseases among black Americans. *Am J Public Health* 1997;87(5):800–4.

30. Schneider D, Greenberg MR, Lu LL. Early life experiences linked to diabetes mellitus: a study of African-American migration. *J Natl Med Assoc* 1997;89(1): 29–34.

31. Sorlie PD, Backlund E, Johnson NJ, Rogot E. Mortality by Hispanic status in the United States. *JAMA* 1993; 270(20):2464–8.

32. Haan MN, Kaplan GA, Camacho T. Poverty and health. Prospective evidence from the Alameda County study. *Am J Epidemiol* 1987;125(6):989–98.

33. Anderson RT, Sorlie PD, Backlund E, Johnson N, Kaplan GA. Mortality effects of community socioeconomic status. *Epidemiology* 1997;8(1):42–7.

34. Waitzman NJ, Smith KR. Phantom of the area: poverty-area residence and mortality in the United States. *Am J Public Health* 1998;88(6):973–6.

35. Sternberg S. Study shows yawning gaps in U.S. health care. Longevity affected by environment. *USA TODAY,* December 4, 1997, pp. 1A and 11A.

36. Centers for Disease Control and Prevention. *Diabetes Surveillance 1997.* Atlanta, GA: Centers for Disease Control and Prevention, 1997.

37. Bushy, A. Health issues of women in rural environments: an overview. *J Am Womens Assoc* 1998;53(2): 53–6.

38. Susser MW, Watson W. *Sociology in Medicine.* 3rd ed. New York: Oxford University Press, 1985.

39. Marmot MG, Kogevinas M, Elston MA. Social/economic status and disease. *Annu Rev Public Health* 1987;8:111–35.

40. Rogot E, Sorlie PD, Johnson NJ. Life expectancy by employment status, income, and education in the National Longitudinal Mortality Study. *Public Health Rep* 1992;107(4):457–61.

41. Pincus T, Callahan LF, Burkhauser RV. Most chronic diseases are reported more frequently by individuals with fewer than 12 years of formal education in the age 18–64 U.S. population. *J Chronic Dis* 1987;40(9): 865–74.

42. Baquet CR, Horm JW, Gibbs T, Greenwald P. Socioeconomic factors and cancer incidence among blacks and whites. *J Natl Cancer Inst* 1991;83(8):551–7.

43. Kaplan GA, Keil JE. Socioeconomic factors and cardiovascular disease: a review of the literature. *Circulation* 1993;88:1973–98.

44. Winkleby MA, Fortmann SP, Barrett DC. Social class disparities in risk factors for disease: eight-year prevalence patterns by level of education. *Prev Med* 1990; 19(1):1–12.

45. Brunner EJ, Marmot MG, Nanchahal K, et al. Social inequality in coronary risk: central obesity and the metabolic syndrome. Evidence from the Whitehall II study. *Diabetologia* 1997;40(11):1341–9.

46. Lowry R, Kann L, Collins JL, Kolbe LJ. The effect of socioeconomic status on chronic disease risk behaviors among U.S. adolescents. *JAMA* 1996;276(10):792–7.

47. Lynch JW, Kaplan GA, Shema SJ. Cumulative impact of sustained economic hardship on physical, cognitive, psychological, and social functioning. *N Engl J Med* 1997; 337(26):1889–95.

48. Marmot MG, Shipley MJ. Do socioeconomic differences in mortality persist after retirement? 25 year follow-up of civil servants from the first Whitehall study. *BMJ* 1996;313(7066):1177–80.

49. Pappas G, Queen S, Hadden W, Fisher G. The increasing disparity in mortality between socioeconomic groups in the United States, 1960 and 1986. *N Engl J Med* 1993;329(2):103–9.

50. Liberatos P, Link BG, Kelsey JL. The measurement of social class in epidemiology. *Epidemiol Rev* 1988;10: 87–121.

51. Winkleby MA, Jatulis DE, Frank E, Fortmann SP. Socioeconomic status and health: how education, income, and occupation contribute to risk factors for cardiovascular disease. *Am J Public Health* 1992;82(6): 816–20.

52. U.S. Bureau of the Census. *Statstical Abstract of the United States, 1997.* Washington, DC, 1997.

53. Costello C, Stone AJ, editors. *The American Woman 1994–95: Where We Stand.* New York: W.W. Norton & Company, Inc., 1994.

54. Jacobs EE, editor. *Handbook of U.S. Labor Statistics.* First Edition. Maryland: Berman Press, 1997.

55. Bianchi SM, Spain D. Women, work, and family in America. *Popul Bull* 1996;51(3):24–7.

56. O'Hare WP. A new look at poverty in America. *Popul Bull* 1996;51(2):1–44.

57. U.S. Bureau of the Census. "Current Population Survey: March Supplement, 1995;" <http://ferret.bls.census.gov/macro/031996/pov/4_001.htm>.

58. National Institutes of Health Consensus Development Panel. Health implications of obesity. *Ann Intern Med* 1985;103(1):147–51.

59. Pi-Sunyer FX. Medical hazards of obesity. *Ann Intern Med* 1993;119:655–60.

60. Colditz GA, Willet WC, Stampfer MJ, et al. Weight as a risk factor for clinical diabetes in women. *Am J Epidemiol* 1990;132(3):501–13.

61. Hanson RL, Narayan KMV, McCance DR, et al. Rate of weight gain, weight fluctuation, and incidence of NIDDM. *Diabetes* 1995;44(3):261–6.

62. Ford ES, Williamson DF, Liu S. Weight change and diabetes incidence: findings from a national cohort of U.S. adults. *Am J Epidemiol* 1997;146(3):214–22.

63. Haffner SM, Stern MP, Mitchell BD, Hazuda HP, Patterson JK. Incidence of type II diabetes in Mexican-Americans predicted by fasting insulin, and glucose levels, obesity, and body-fat distribution. *Diabetes* 1990; 39(3):283–8.

64. Manson JE, Rimm EB, Stampfer MJ, et al. Physical activity and incidence of non–insulin-dependent diabetes mellitus in women. *Lancet* 1991;338(8770):774–8.

65. Haapanen N, Miilunpalo S, Vuori I, Oja P, Pasanen M. Association of leisure-time physical activity with the risk of coronary heart disease, hypertension, and diabetes in middle-aged men and women. *Int J Epidemiol* 1997; 26(4):739–47.

66. Colditz GA, Coakely E. Weight, weight gain, activity, and major illnesses: the Nurses' Health Study. *Int J Sports Med* 1997;18(Suppl 3):S162–70.

67. Lee IM, Paffenbarger RS Jr, Hennekens CH. Physical activity, physical fitness, and longevity. *Aging (Milano)* 1997;9:2–11.

68. CDC. Update: National Center for Health Statistics. <http://www.cdc.gov/nchs/fastats/overwt.htm>. Last accessed December 2000.

69. Troiano RP, Flegal KM, Kuczmarski RJ, Campbell SM, Johnson CL. Overweight prevalence and trends for children and adolescents. *Arch Pediatr Adolesc Med* 1995; 149(10):1085–91.

70. Popkin BM, Udry JR. Adolescent obesity increases significantly in second and third generation U.S. immigrants: the National Longitudinal Study of Adolescent Health. *J Nutr* 1998;128(4):701–6.

71. CDC. CDC surveillance summaries. *MMWR* 1997 ;46(SS-6):1–56.

72. Hahn RA, Teutsch SM, Franks AL, Chang M-H, Lloyd EE. The prevalence of risk factors among women in the United States by race and age, 1992–1994: opportunities for primary and secondary prevention. *J Am Med Womens Assoc* 1998;53(2):96–104, 107.

73. Ellis JL, Campos-Outcalt D. Cardiovascular disease risk factors in Native Americans: a literature review. *Am J Prev Med* 1994;10(5):295–307.

74. Strauss KF, Mokdad A, Ballew C, et al. The health of Navajo women: findings from the Navajo Health and Nutrition Survey, 1991–1992. *J Nutr* 1997;127(10 Suppl):2128S–33S.

75. Crews DE. Obesity and diabetes. In: Zane NWS, Takeuchi DT, Young KNJ, editors. *Confronting Critical Health Issues of Asian and Pacific Islander Americans.* Thousand Oaks, CA: Sage, 1994:174–208.

76. Kuczmarski RJ, Flegal KM, Campbell SM, Johnson CL. Increasing prevalence of overweight among U.S. adults: the National Health and Nutrition Examination Surveys, 1960 to 1991. *JAMA* 1994;272(3):205–11.

77. Freedman DS, Srinivasan SR, Valdez RA, Williamson DF, Berenson GS. Secular increases in relative weight and adiposity among children over two decades: the Bogalusa Heart Study. *Pediatrics* 1997;99(3):420–6.

78. Lewis CE, Smith DE, Wallace DD, Williams OD, Bild DE, Jacobs DR Jr. Seven-year trends in body weight and associations with lifestyle and behavioral characteristics in black and white young adults: the CARDIA Study. *Am J Public Health* 1997;87(4):635–42.

79. Campaigne BN, Morrison JA, Schumann BC, et al. Indexes of obesity and comparisons with previous national survey data in 9- and 10-year-old black and white girls: the National Heart, Lung, and Blood Institute Growth and Health Study. *J Pediatr* 1994;124:675–80.

80. Srinivasan SR, Bao W, Wattigney WA, Berenson GS. Adolescent overweight is associated with adult overweight and related multiple cardiovascular risk factors: the Bogalusa Heart Study. *Metabolism* 1996;45(2):235–40.

81. Serdula MK, Ivery D, Coates RJ, Freedman DS, Williamson DF, Byers T. Do obese children become obese adults? A review of the literature. *Prev Med* 1993;22(2):167–77.

82. Guo SS, Roche AF, Chumlea WC, Gardner JD, Siervogel RM. The predictive value of childhood body mass index values for overweight at age 35 y. *Am J Clin Nutr* 1994;59(4):810–19.

83. Wolfe WS, Sobal J, Olson CM, Frongillo EA Jr, Williamson DF. Parity-associated weight gain and its modification by sociodemographic and behavioral factors: a prospective analysis in U.S. women. *Int J Obes Relat Metab Disord* 1997;21(9):802–10.

84. Smith DE, Lewis CE, Caveny JL, Perkins LL, Burke GL, Bild DE. Longitudinal changes in adiposity associated with pregnancy. The CARDIA Study. Coronary Artery Risk Development in Young Adults Study. *JAMA* 1994;271(22):1747–51.

85. Crespo CJ, Keteyian SJ, Heath GW, Sempos CT. Leisure-time physical activity among U.S. adults. Results from the Third National Health and Nutrition Examination Survey. *Arch Intern Med* 1996;156(1):93–8.

86. Brown ER, Wyn R, Cumberland WG, et al. *Women's Health-Related Behaviors and Use of Clinical Preventive Services.* New York: The Commonwealth Fund, 1995.

87. Kann L, Warren CW, Harris WA, et al. Youth risk behavior surveillance—United States, 1995. *MMWR* 1996;45(SS-4):1–84.

88. CDC. Prevalence of selected risk factors for chronic disease by education level in racial/ethnic populations—United States, 1991–1992. *MMWR* 1994;43(48):894–9.

89. Winkleby MA, Kraemer HC, Ahn DK, Varady AN. Ethnic and socioeconomic differences in cardiovascular disease risk factors: findings from the Third National Health and Nutrition Examination Survey, 1988–1994. *JAMA* 1998;280(4):356–62.

90. Hazuda HP, Mitchell BD, Haffner SM, Stern MP. Obesity in Mexican American subgroups: findings from the San Antonio Heart Study. *Am J Clin Nutr* 1991;53(6 Suppl):1529S–34S.

91. Stevens J, Kumanyika SK, Keil JE. Attitudes toward body size and dieting: differences between elderly black and white women. *Am J Public Health* 1994;84(8):1322–5.

92. Corney RH. Sex differences in general practice attendance and help-seeking for minor illness. *J Psychosom Res* 1990;34(5):525–34.

93. Shumaker SA, Hill DR. Gender differences in social support and physical health. *Health Psychol* 1991;10(2):102–111.

94. Verbrugge LM. The twain meet: empirical explanations of sex differences in health and mortality. *J Health Soc Behav* 1989;30(3):282–304.

95. Verbrugge LM, Wingard DL. Sex differentials in health and mortality. *Women Health* 1987;12(2):103–45.

96. Duffy ME. Determinants of health promotion in midlife women. *Nurs Res* 1988;37(6):358–62.

97. Doyal L. *What Makes Women Sick: Gender and the Political Economy of Health.* Basingstoke, England: Macmillan, 1995.

98. U.S. Department of Health and Human Services. *Women's Health. Report of the Public Health Service Task Force on Women's Health Issues. Vol. II.* Washington, DC: U.S. Government Printing Office, 1996.

99. Reifman A, Biernat M, Lang E. Stress, social support, and health in married professional women with small children. *Psych Women Quart* 1991;15:431–5.

100. Antonucci TC. Social support: theoretical advances, recent findings, and pressing issues. In: Sarason IG, Sarason BR, editors. *Social Support: Theory, Research, and Applications.* Boston: Martinus Nijhoff, 1985:21–7.

101. Antonucci TC, Akiyama H. An examination of sex differences in social support in mid and late life. *Sex Roles* 1987;17:737–49.

102. Cohen S. Psychosocial models of the role of social support in the etiology of physical disease. *Health Psychol* 1988;7(3):269–97.

103. Dean K. Self-care components of lifestyles: the importance of gender, attitudes, and the social situation. *Soc Sci Med* 1989;29(2):137–52.

104. Kaplan RM, Hartwell SL. Differential effects of social support and social network on physiological and social outcomes in men and women with type II diabetes mellitus. *Health Psychol* 1987;6(5):387–98.

105. Muhlenkamp AF, Sayles JA. Self-esteem, social support, and positive health practices. *Nurs Res* 1986;35(6):334–8.

106. Flaherty J, Richman J. Gender differences in the perception and utilization of social support: theoretical perspectives and an empirical test. *Soc Sci Med* 1989;28(12):1221–8.

107. Vaux, A. *Social Support: Theory, Research, and Intervention.* New York: Praeger, 1988.

108. Kessler RC, McLeod JD, Wethington E. The costs of caring: a perspective on the relationship between sex and psychological distress. In: Sarason IG, Sarason BR, editors. *Social Support: Theory, Research, and Applications.* Boston: Martinus Nijhoff, 1985:491–506.

109. Belle D. *Lives in Stress: Women and Depression.* Beverly Hills, CA: Sage, 1987.

110. Verbrugge LM. Gender and health: an update on hypotheses and evidence. *J Health Soc Behav* 1985;26(3):156–82.

111. Haavio-Mannila E. Inequalities in health and gender. *Soc Sci Med* 1986;22(2):141–9.

112. Haynes SG, Feinleib M, Kannel WB. The relationship of psychosocial factors to coronary heart disease in the Framingham Study. III. Eight-year incidence of coronary heart disease. *Am J Epidemiol* 1980;111(1):37–58.

113. Zappert LT, Weinstein HM. Sex differences in the impact of work on physical and psychological health. *Am J Psychiatry* 1985;142(10):1174–8.

114. Anderson NB, Armstead CA. Toward understanding the association of socioeconomic status and health: a new challenge for the biopsychosocial approach. *Psychosom Med* 1995;57(3):213–25.

115. McNair LD, Roberts GW. Social and behavioral influences on African American women's health. In: Blechman E, Brownell K, editors. *Behavioral Medicine and Women: A Comprehensive Handbook.* New York: Guilford, 1998:821–25.

116. Raja SN, Williams S, McGee R. Multidimensional health locus of control beliefs and psychological health for a sample of mothers. *Soc Sci Med* 1994;39(2):213–20.

117. Hanner ME. Factors related to promotion of health-seeking behaviors in the aged. Unpublished doctoral dissertation, The University of Texas at Austin, 1986.

118. Helstrom AW, Coffey C, Jorgannathan P. Asian American women's health. In: Blechman EA, Brownell KD, editors. *Behavioral Medicine and Women: A Comprehensive Handbook.* New York: Guilford, 1998:826–32.

119. Woodward AM. Hispanic women and health care. In: Blechman EA, Brownell KD, editors. *Behavioral Medicine and Women: A Comprehensive Handbook.* New York: Guilford, 1998:833–7.

120. Baines DR. Native American women and health care. In: Blechman EA, Brownell KD, editors. *Behavioral Medicine and Women: A Comprehensive Handbook.* New York: Guilford, 1998:839–42.

121. Jaynes G, Williams R. *A Common Destiny: Blacks and American Society.* Washington, DC: National Academy Press, 1989.

122. Amott T, Matthaei J. The promise of comparable worth: a socialist-feminist perspective. In: Kesselman A, McNair LD, Schniedewind N, editors. *Women: Images and Realities. A Multicultural Anthology.* Mountain View, CA: Mayfield Press, 1995:177–82.

123. Geronimus AT. The weathering hypothesis and the health of African American women and infants: evidence and speculations. *Ethn Dis* 1992;2(3):207–21.

124. Beckles GLA, Blount SB, Jiles RB. African Americans. In: *Chronic Disease in Minority Populations.* Atlanta: Centers for Disease Control and Prevention, 1994.

125. McNair LD, Roberts GW. Pervasive and persistent risks: factors influencing African American women's HIV/ AIDS vulnerability. *J Black Psychol* 1997;23:180–91.

126. National Institute on Alcohol Abuse and Alcoholism. *Sixth Special Report to the U.S. Congress on Alcohol and Health.* Washington, DC: Government Printing Office, 1990. (DHHS Publication No. [ADM] 87-1519)

127. U.S. Department of Health and Human Services. *Women and Smoking. A Report of the Surgeon General.* Rockville, MD: U.S. Department of Health and Human Services, Public Health Service, Office of the Surgeon General, 2001.

128. Woods NF, Lentz M, Mitchell E. The new woman: health-promoting and health-damaging behaviors. *Health Care Women Int* 1993;14(5):389–405.

129. Institute of Medicine, Committee on Monitoring Access to Personal Health Care Services. Millman ML, editor. *Access to Health Care in America.* Washington, DC: National Academy Press, 1993.

130. Bashshur R, Smith DG, Stiles RA. Defining underinsurance: a conceptual framework for policy and empirical analysis. *Med Care Rev* 1993;50(2):199–218.

131. Ammons L. Demographic profile of health-care coverage in America in 1993. *J Natl Med Assoc* 1997;89(11): 737–44.

132. Vistnes JP, Monheit AC. *Health Insurance Status of the U.S. Civilian Noninstitutionalized Population.* Rockville, MD: Agency for Health Care Policy Research, 1997. (AHCPR Publication No. 97-0030. MEPS Research Findings No. 1)

133. Weinick RM, Zuvekas SH, Drilea S. *Access to Health Care—Sources and Barriers, 1996.* Rockville, MD: Agency for Health Care Policy and Research, 1997. (AHCPR Pub. No. 98-001. MEPS Research Findings No. 3)

134. Moy E, Bartman BA, Weir MR. Access to hypertensive care. Effects of income, insurance, and source of care. *Arch Intern Med* 1995;155(14):1497–1502.

135. Sox CM, Swartz K, Burstin HR, Brennan TA. Insurance or a regular physician: which is the most powerful predictor of health care? *Am J Public Health* 1998;88(3): 364–70.

136. Ettner SL. The timing of preventive services for women and children: the effect of having a usual source of care. *Am J Public Health* 1996;86(12):1748–54.

137. Lambrew JM, DeFriese GH, Carey TS, Ricketts TC, Biddle AK. The effects of having a regular doctor on access to primary care. *Med Care* 1996;34(2):138–51.

138. Merrell K, Colby DC, Hogan C. Medicare beneficiaries covered by Medicaid buy-in agreements. *Health Aff* 1997;16(1):175–84.

139. Weissman JS, Stern R, Fielding SL, Epstein AM. Delayed access to health care: risk factors, reasons, and consequences. *Ann Intern Med* 1991;114(4):325–31.

140. Waid MO. *Brief Summaries of Medicare & Medicaid.* Baltimore, MD: U.S. Department of Health and Human Services, Health Care Financing Administration, AHCAG, 1997.

141. Reisinger AL. *Health Insurance and Access to Care: Issues for Women.* New York: The Commonwealth Fund Commission on Women's Health, 1995.

142. U.S. Bureau of the Census. <http://ferret.bls.census.gov/ macro/031997/noncash/6_000.htm>. Current Population Survey, March 1997. Last accessed March 2001.

143. Newacheck PW, Brindis CD, Cart CU, Marchi K, Irwin CE. Adolescent health insurance coverage: recent changes and access to care. *Pediatrics* 1999;104:195–202.

144. Monheit AC. Underinsured Americans: a review. *Annu Rev Public Health* 1994;15:461–85.

145. Short PF, Banthin JS. New estimates of the underinsured younger than 65 years. *JAMA* 1995;274(16): 1302–6.

146. Brown ER, Wyn R, Cumberland WG, et al. *Women's Health-Related Behaviors and Use of Clinical Preventive Services.* New York: The Commonwealth Fund Commission on Women's Health, 1995.

147. Weisman CS, Teitelbaum MA. Women and health care communication. *Patient Educ Couns* 1989;13(2):183–99.

148. Pendleton DA, Bochner S. The communication of medical information in general practice consultations as a function of patients' social class. *Soc Sci Med* 1980; 14A(6):669–73.

149. Hooper EM, Comstock LM, Goodwin JM, Goodwin JS. Patient characteristics that influence physician behavior. *Med Care* 1982;20(6):630–8.

150. Hall JA, Irish JT, Roter DL, Ehrlich CM, Miller LH. Gender in medical encounters: an analysis of physician and patient communication in a primary care setting. *Health Psychol* 1994;13(5):384–92.

151. McAuley E, Jacobson L. Self-efficacy and exercise participation in sedentary adult females. *Am J Health Promot* 1991;5(3):185–91.

152. Corbin WR, McNair LD, Carter J. Self-esteem differences among problem drinking males and females. *J Alcohol and Drug Education* 1996;42:1–14.

153. McNair LD, Carter JA, Williams MK. Self-esteem, gender, and alcohol use: relationships with HIV risk perception and behaviors in college students. *J Sex Marital Ther* 1998;24:29–36.

154. Pender NJ. *Health Promotion in Nursing Practice.* 2nd ed. Norwalk, CT: Appleton-Century-Crofts, 1987.

155. Seeman M, Seeman TE. Health behavior and personal autonomy: a longitudinal study of the sense of control in illness. *J Health Soc Behav* 1983;24(2):144–60.

156. Liao KLM, Hunter M, Weinman J. Health-related behaviors and their correlates in a general population sample of 45-year-old women. *Psychol and Health* 1995; 10:171–84.

157. Galanos AN, Strauss RP, Pieper CF. Sociodemographic correlates of health beliefs among black and white community-dwelling elderly individuals. *Int J Aging Hum Dev* 1994;38(4):339–50.

158. Rotter JB. Generalized expectancies for internal versus external control of reinforcement. *Psychol Monogr* 1966; 80(1):1–28.

159. Institute of Medicine. *The Future of Public Health.* Washington, DC: National Academy Press, 1988.

Case Studies

Type 1 Diabetes:

At 5:30 p.m. on a weeknight, Sarah gets off her fourth phone call since coming home from school after track practice. She squeezed in a snack between and during calls. She and three girlfriends have made plans to go cosmic bowling late on Friday night—a lot of people from school will be there. A friend will drive. Her parents just got home. Now Sarah will have a quick dinner with her family before leaving to babysit. After returning, she has to complete her homework and try to get to bed at a reasonable hour. She will start her day at 5:30 a.m., making sure she has enough time to "look good" before taking the school bus.

Sarah takes her insulin four to six times a day with meals and snacks, and at bedtime. She tries very hard to be inconspicuous with her diabetes management, even though she knows that she must consider her diabetes constantly with every decision and plan that she makes. This routine is fairly automatic now, since she was diagnosed with type 1 diabetes 12 years ago, when she was 4. Sarah carries her insulin and glucometer in her backpack. She checks her blood sugar levels before meals, and periodically, four to seven times a day. She gets tired of pricking her fingers.

Sarah knows how important it is to control her blood sugar levels to prevent complications such as kidney failure and blindness. Still, Sarah has mixed feelings sometimes because the better her blood sugar control is, the more weight she gains. Sarah is heavier than most of her friends, and her clothes don't fit. Summertime at the beach is the worst.

Sometimes Sarah is hassled at school for having her syringes. She recalls the policy statement on the JDRF Web site and the discussion at the ADA-sponsored camp she attended this summer regarding testing and the use of medications in schools. She hopes the policies in her school will change; in the meantime, Sarah has asked her doctor at her appointment today about the possibility of getting an insulin pump. It would be so much more convenient, and it would probably improve her blood sugar control. Sarah received her shot for birth control today, so she knows that her blood sugar levels will be more difficult to control for 1 to 2 weeks. She tries not to worry too much about having blood sugar levels that may be too low or too high. Sarah learns continually how to take care of her diabetes and her health.

Type 2 Diabetes:

LaTonya comes into the house out of breath. She's wearing sweatpants and a loose shirt. She has been walking along the road for 45 minutes, alone, avoiding dogs and cars. It was boring; none of her friends would come along. Hungrily, she looks through the kitchen cabinets, trying to find a snack that will be low in calories, sugar, and fat; taste great; and also satisfy her appetite.

It seems that her favorite foods for as long as she can remember have included lots of fat and sugar. It has been a challenge for LaTonya to introduce new foods and beverages into her daily diet and to ask her family and friends to support her by buying new foods and learning healthier ways to prepare favorite foods. The dietitian at the clinic has helped her figure out foods to choose that will help control her diabetes and work well with her medication and activity schedule.

Since her doctor told her that she had type 2 diabetes last year, near her 13th birthday, she has been trying hard to lose some weight and to exercise. It has been difficult because she has been heavy as long as she can remember. Her four younger brothers and sisters are having chips and soft drinks, watching cartoons in the other room. She's going to try her hardest to eat only healthy foods tonight even though her old favorites seemed so flavorful, and her new snack foods taste so plain.

3

THE ADOLESCENT YEARS

J.M. Norris, MPH, PhD, G.J. Klingensmith, MD

This chapter presents a summary of data and information in the current literature on diabetes in female adolescents and women aged 10–19 years. Adolescence characterizes a time of marked physical and psychological transition for young women. The majority of adolescents who are diagnosed with diabetes in these early years have type 1 diabetes; recently, however, an increasing number of adolescents are being diagnosed with type 2 diabetes. The latter condition is likely to increase the burden of type 2 diabetes now and for years to come. This chapter describes the economic, sociocultural, and environmental context in which adolescents with diabetes live and the impact of this disease on the health of adolescents and young women, including increased mortality, psychosocial and behavioral issues (e.g., eating disorders, insulin manipulation), and frequent hospitalization. The public health implications of these findings are framed by the three core functions of public health: assessment, which includes surveillance and research; policy development; and assurance. Highlights include discussions on institutional behaviors and other environmental factors that predispose adolescents to the development of diabetes and its complications. Interagency collaboration is presented as an important strategy for public health action.

The primary form of diabetes among children and adolescents aged 10–19 years is type 1 diabetes, formerly known as insulin-dependent diabetes mellitus. Therefore, most data presented in this chapter refer to type 1 diabetes unless otherwise noted. Recently, however, research suggests that type 2 diabetes, formerly called non–insulin-dependent diabetes mellitus, is emerging as a public health problem among adolescents, particularly in certain ethnic subgroups.[1]

For women, adolescence is a time of transition, both psychological and physical, which may have a negative impact on the health of those with diabetes. Psychological changes during adolescence may affect how one copes with diabetes and its care regimen, and the physical changes during adolescence may make it more difficult to control diabetes regardless of the level of adherence to the diabetes care regimen.

3.1. Prevalence, Incidence, and Trends

Prevalence

In 1990, the estimated prevalence of type 1 diabetes in the United States among persons younger than 20 years was 1.7 per 1,000.[2] Thus, approximately 123,000 persons in this age group have diabetes. Because the risk of diabetes is similar among boys and girls in this age range, an estimated 61,500 girls younger than 20 years have type 1 diabetes. The prevalence of type 1 diabetes is slightly higher among white girls than among those of other races.[2] The prevalence of type 2 diabetes among young persons has not been measured in most populations. One exception is the Pima Indians of Arizona, a population at very high risk for type 2 diabetes; the prevalence of type 2 diabetes among girls increased from 7.2 per 1,000 during 1967–1976 to 28.8 per 1,000 during 1987–1996 among those aged 10–14 years, and from 27.3 per 1,000 to 53.1 per 1,000 among those aged 15–19 years during the same time periods.[3] The most recent prevalence estimates for the Pima Indians aged 15–19 years is 50.9 per 1,000, a rate that stands in sharp contrast to that of 1.7 per 1,000 for type 1 diabetes among those aged 0–19 years. Recent data indicate that type 2 diabetes is being diagnosed more frequently among adolescents in other minority groups, and as such, is a major cause for public health concern.[1]

Incidence

The incidence of type 1 diabetes among girls aged 10–19 years varies by race and ethnicity.[4-7] In the early to mid-1980s, among white girls aged 10–14 years, the incidence was 22.4 per 100,000 per year.[4] This incidence was slightly higher than that among Hispanic (18.3/100,000/year)[4] and black (8.3/100,000/year)[5] girls in the same age group. However, among girls aged 15–19 years, the incidence of type 1 diabetes was slightly higher among blacks (10.9/100,000/year)[5] than among whites (8.1/100,000/year) and Hispanics (7.0/100,000/year).[4] In all racial/ethnic groups, the risk of type 1 diabetes was lower among girls aged 15–19 years than among those aged 10–14 years.[4,5] In Chicago, during 1985–1990, the annual incidence of type 1 diabetes in black girls was 22.4 per 100,000 among those aged 10–14 years and 13 per 100,000 among those aged 15–17 years.[6] This same study showed a type 1 diabetes incidence in Hispanic girls of 15.5 per 100,000 among those aged 10–14 years and 11.6 per 100,000 among those aged 15–17 years. In Allegheny County, Pennsylvania, between 1990 and 1994, the annual incidence of type 1 diabetes among those aged 10–14 years was 23.6 per 100,000 among nonwhites (includes blacks and other groups) compared with 24.9 per 100,000 among whites.[7] Interestingly, the type 1 diabetes incidence among those aged 15–19 years was higher in nonwhites compared with whites (30.4/100,000 versus 11.2/100,000, respectively). This was seen in both male and female patients.[7]

A review of the medical records of children and adolescents with diabetes at a hospital in Cincinnati found that the incidence of type 2 diabetes among girls aged 10–19 years was 9 per 100,000 in 1994.[8] In this population, black girls accounted for 69% of girls with type 2 diabetes but only 9.7% of those with type 1 diabetes. Incidence of type 2 diabetes among those aged 10–19 years rose from 1.2 per 100,000 in 1992 to 7.2 per 100,000 in 1994.

Overall, type 2 diabetes accounted for 3%–10% of new cases from 1982 to 1992, but for 33% in 1994.[8]

Trends

The incidence of type 1 diabetes varies both seasonally and yearly. In the United States, the incidence of type 1 diabetes declines during the warm summer months.[4-7] Because this seasonal pattern occurs only among school-aged children, it suggests that factors related to attending school (e.g., infections, stress) may be related to the etiology or clinical diagnosis of type 1 diabetes.

A subsequent report from Allegheny County, Pennsylvania, suggests that there is an epidemic of diabetes in nonwhite adolescents.[7] The incidence among nonwhites aged 15–19 years during 1990–1994 (30.4/100,000) was more than 2 times higher than during 1985–1989 (13.8/100,000) and more than 3 times higher than during 1980–1984 (7.6/100,000). The dramatic increase was not seen in whites. The authors did not give sex-specific data so it is unclear whether boys and girls had similar increases. This epidemic of diabetes may be either the result of an increasing incidence of type 1 diabetes among nonwhites or of another type of diabetes, such as type 2 diabetes, that has been misclassified as type 1 diabetes.[7] Data from Chicago did not show an increasing incidence of type 1 diabetes in either black or Hispanic girls aged 0–17 years between 1985 and 1990.[6]

The incidence of adolescent type 2 diabetes appears to be increasing over time among both boys and girls. In the Cincinnati study, the rate of type 2 diabetes among adolescents increased 10-fold between 1982 and 1994, from 0.7 per 100,000 to 7.2 per 100,000.[8]

3.2. Sociodemographic Characteristics

Of adolescent girls with type 1 diabetes in the United States, 92% are white, about 4% are black, and the remaining 4% are Hispanic or Asian American.[9] This racial distribution is very different from that of adolescent girls with type 2 diabetes;

in the Cincinnati study, 69% were black, and the remainder were white.[8]

Type 1 diabetes is thought to result from the interaction between genetic susceptibility and exposures that can cause diabetes. (See Section 3.4.) Some, if not all, of the genetic predisposition for type 1 diabetes lies in the possession of the human leukocyte antigen markers DR3 and DR4. Differences in the frequency of these high-risk genetic markers in ethnic and racial groups in the United States may explain, in part, the racial/ethnic disparities in the distribution of type 1 diabetes.[10]

The majority of girls with diabetes live in (24%) or just outside (52%) a metropolitan area.[9,11] The education of adolescent girls with diabetes resembles that of the general population of adolescent girls without diabetes[9] but specific data are not available.[11] Data on the marital status, employment, and personal income of adolescent girls with diabetes are also not available. The education and income distribution of the families of adolescent girls with diabetes resembles that of the general population.[9,11] Data on the socioeconomic status of American Indian adolescent girls with diabetes are not available. However, given that American Indian families are more likely to live below the poverty level than are families in the general U.S. population (27% versus 10%),[12] American Indian adolescent girls with diabetes are more likely to be living in poverty than are girls with diabetes in the general population.

3.3. Impact of Diabetes on Health Status

Complications of Diabetes: Type 1

Adolescent girls with type 1 diabetes are at risk for both acute and chronic complications; acute complications are more common and have greater impact. Diabetic ketoacidosis is the most prevalent acute complication and commonly occurs at the onset of type 1 diabetes. Its underlying cause is insulin deficiency. In a cohort of children and adolescents aged 9–16 years with diabetes who were monitored for 8 years, 30% of the girls had at least one episode of ketoacidosis.[13] Episodes are characterized by excessive thirst and urination followed by nausea and vomiting. If untreated, diabetic ketoacidosis can lead to coma and death.

Hypoglycemia, another acute complication of diabetes, may range from very mild lowering of blood glucose levels with minimal or no symptoms to severe hypoglycemia resulting in very low glucose levels, nerve damage, coma, and death if not treated. Estimates of the incidence of hypoglycemia vary because different glucose levels have been used to define cases. In the same cohort of children and adolescents aged 9–16 years cited above, 21% had at least one episode of hypoglycemia, and adolescent boys (26%) were more likely to have hypoglycemia than adolescent girls (7%).[13]

The chronic complications of diabetes include eye disease, kidney disease, nerve damage, heart disease, and circulatory problems. Diabetic eye disease, or retinopathy, is characterized by alterations in the small blood vessels of the retina. The most severe form of diabetic retinopathy, proliferative diabetic retinopathy, can lead to blindness if untreated.[14] By age 20, 40%–60% of persons with diabetes have some retinopathy, and 2% have the more severe proliferative diabetic retinopathy.[14-16] At least one study has found that adolescent girls have a higher risk of progressing to proliferative retinopathy than adolescent boys.[17] Although the presence of retinopathy among adolescents is usually asymptomatic, it is a predictor of proliferative retinopathy and future vision loss if untreated.

Diabetic kidney disease, or nephropathy, is diagnosed by measuring albumin levels in the urine. Microalbuminuria, or low levels of albumin in the urine, is a precursor to proteinuria (macroalbuminuria), or high levels of urinary protein. Persistent proteinuria signals a decline in renal function that leads to end-stage renal disease, a relatively common cause of death among persons with type 1 diabetes. Almost 22% of adolescents with diabetes have some form of albuminuria: 18% have microalbuminuria, and 4% have persistent proteinuria.[18]

Among 164 adolescents with diabetes, adolescent girls were nearly 60% more likely than boys to develop microalbuminuria after 8 years of follow-up (24% and 15%, respectively).[19] However, a separate study of the progression of microalbuminuria among adolescents (mean age 17 years) with type 1 diabetes found no difference between girls and boys in the risk of progression of microalbuminuria.[20]

The presence and progression of both nephropathy and retinopathy are associated with sustained hyperglycemia.[14,16,20-23] The higher prevalence of both diabetic retinopathy and nephropathy among adolescent girls than among boys may be related to the difficulties that adolescent girls have in maintaining diabetes control during puberty or to the earlier onset of puberty in girls.[24]

A significant comorbidity of diabetes in adolescence is periodontal disease, a condition rarely otherwise seen during adolescence.[25,26] Periodontal disease typically coincides with the onset of puberty among children with type 1 diabetes. Hormonal changes, particularly in young women with diabetes, appear to trigger this onset.[25]

The prevalence of periodontal disease among adolescents with diabetes is 11%–16% compared with 1% in the adolescent population at large.[25] It is easier to attribute dental disease to diabetes in this life stage because in the general population, the occurrence of such illness is typically more common at older ages.[26]

The adolescent years are characterized by the rapid physical growth and hormonal changes of puberty, which can affect diabetes management. During this time, increasing insulin resistance and associated physiological changes make diabetes control more difficult.[27] The difference between adolescents and adults with diabetes was clearly shown in the Diabetes Control and Complications Trial (DCCT), in which the average hemoglobin A_{1c} (a measure of long-term blood glucose control) of adolescents was significantly higher than that of adults who were receiving the same care.[28] In addi-

tion to the hormonal changes complicating diabetes management, the adolescent years are marked by psychological changes. Adolescents are establishing independence from their family, and peer relationships become more important. Adolescent pressures to conform to peer standards may interfere with routine diabetes management and the planning constraints that diabetes care requires. Moreover, although adolescents may intellectually understand the relationship between current diabetes management and long-term health, translating this knowledge into consistent day-to-day behavior is difficult for teens and young adults.[29]

The DCCT has suggested that intensive therapy to control glucose levels in adolescents effectively delays the onset and slows the progression of both diabetic retinopathy and nephropathy.[28] Unfortunately, intensive therapy doubles a person's risk of becoming overweight. The increased risk of weight gain could hinder adherence to this regimen, particularly among adolescent girls.

Although research regarding the full array of complications of type 1 diabetes is necessary for adolescent populations, it will be equally important to know the type of diabetes that causes them. This distinction is important because misclassification of type 2 as type 1 appears to be common.[1]

Complications of Diabetes: Type 2
Among black and Hispanic adolescents, the onset of type 2 diabetes often resembles that of type 1.[1] Complications among children with type 2 diabetes will closely resemble those complications associated with type 1: retinopathy and nephropathy as well as cardiovascular disease and neuropathy. However, it is instructive to note that type 2 diabetes is expected to mirror type 1 in outcomes, such as limitations on usual activities, school absences, days spent in bed, use of medications, hospitalization, and increased physician contacts.[1]

Risk of Death
Between 1960 and 1980, the mortality rate among girls aged 10–19 years with type 1 diabetes was

1.92 per 1,000 person-years, which is almost 5 times greater than the mortality rate of the general population of girls in this age group.[30] More recently, a Swedish study reported the mortality rate among adolescent girls with diabetes to be 0.49 per 1,000 person-years, which still represents a 2.5-fold increased risk of death.[31] Another study has estimated that the life expectancy of a person aged 10–19 years with diabetes will be reduced by 17 years.[32]

Fifty percent of the deaths among adolescents with diabetes are due to acute complications, some of which occur at the onset of the disease. Other causes of death in this age group are causes unrelated to diabetes (31%), other diabetes complications (9%), kidney disease (5%), and cardiovascular disease (5%).[30]

Adolescent girls have been found to have a significantly greater risk than adolescent boys of dying of ketoacidosis at the onset of type 1 diabetes.[33] An early study of persons with type 1 diabetes diagnosed between 1965 and 1980 reported that 8 persons died at the onset of diabetes. All of these persons were adolescents (aged 8–17 years), and 7 of the 8 were girls.[33] These results parallel those of another study from the same research center that suggested that the onset of diabetes was more severe among girls than boys.[34] However, reasons for this more severe onset in girls were not clear. Moreover, this difference may no longer exist. A more recent study found no difference between adolescent boys and girls in deaths at onset.[31]

Hospitalizations

Persons with diabetes are more likely to be hospitalized than persons without diabetes. Reasons for hospitalization are primarily related to treatment and metabolic control and to complications of diabetes, most commonly kidney disease, eye disease, stroke, and ischemic heart disease. A review of national survey data found that among U.S. girls and women younger than age 20, diabetes was listed on the hospital discharge record for approximately 25,000 hospitalizations per year and was the primary reason for almost 20,000 of these

hospitalizations. The average hospital stay was 5 days.[35] In a separate study, girls aged 10–14 years with diabetes were 8 times as likely to be admitted to the hospital and had 6 times as many days in the hospital as girls without diabetes. Girls aged 15–19 years with diabetes were 3 times as likely to be hospitalized and had 3 times as many days in the hospital as girls the same age without diabetes.[36]

Until recently, children and adolescents were routinely hospitalized when type 1 diabetes was diagnosed, primarily to stabilize their glucose levels and provide diabetes education. In the past 20 years, however, many health care providers have been using outpatient management at the time of diagnosis.[37] This trend has reduced hospitalization costs and lessened disruption to the child and family. Hospitalizations after onset of diabetes were also frequent among children and adolescents until recently. A 1982 study found that 39% of girls aged 10–19 years with preexisting diabetes had one or more hospital admissions within a year. Poor metabolic control and infection accounted for over 50% of these hospital admissions.[38] With the advent of home blood glucose monitoring and outpatient educational programs, the need for hospitalization to improve metabolic control has decreased.[38-40]

From 2% to 10% of all hospitalizations for diabetes are attributed to diabetic ketoacidosis.[41] Rates of hospitalization for diabetic ketoacidosis are higher among children and adolescents than among adults. The annual incidence of hospital admissions for diabetic ketoacidosis among children younger than 15 years is 53.6 per 1,000.[42] In a study of adolescents aged 15–18 years, girls of all races had more diabetes hospitalizations than did boys, primarily due to diabetic ketoacidosis.[43] The researchers speculated that compared with young men, young women may have more frequent high-risk behaviors (e.g., low levels of physical activity, insulin omission, or disordered eating), and be less likely to comply with medical treatment, be more likely to have biologic factors that negatively affect glucose control. These issues are discussed later in this chapter.

Several studies have suggested that diabetic adolescents of lower socioeconomic status may be at increased risk for hospitalizations.[38,43-45] A Rhode Island study found that diabetic adolescents living in poverty had a higher frequency (71%) of readmission to the hospital than adolescents in all other socioeconomic groups.[38] The authors speculated that children in poverty may have difficulty practicing effective self-care or interacting with health care providers.

Risk of hospitalization is also associated with emotional and behavioral problems in adolescent girls with diabetes, suggesting that they may be demonstrating high-risk behaviors resulting in poor metabolic control.[40,46]

Based on available data,[30,31,36] estimates of population attributable risk fractions suggest that eliminating diabetes from the U.S. adolescent population would eliminate 2.5%–6.3% of the deaths and 3.2%–10.5% of the hospitalizations in this age group.

Disabilities

Because adolescents with diabetes have generally had the disease for a relatively short time, physical disabilities associated with type 1 diabetes are rare among adolescents. However, diabetes can have a psychological impact on adolescents—particularly adolescent girls—that may result in mental health disabilities. However, of the three studies to examine this issue, only one addresses girls specifically. One study of school performance found that adolescents with diabetes performed more slowly on a series of visual-motor tasks and had lower scores on tests of reading, spelling, and arithmetic than adolescents without diabetes.[47] This disparity could be due to more absences from school among adolescents with diabetes or to a diabetes-related impairment of psychosocial development, cognitive functioning, or even visual impairments. Another study found selective impairment in cognitive functioning among adolescents (aged 10–19 years) with diabetes, particularly among those who were

younger than age 5 when diabetes was diagnosed and those with poor metabolic control.[48] A third study suggested that girls may be more likely than boys to have impaired cognitive functioning: adolescent girls with diabetes performed more poorly on several neuropsychological measures and had poorer verbal intelligence scores than adolescent boys with diabetes.[49]

Depression is another risk factor for adolescents with diabetes, particularly girls. Twelve percent of a cohort of adolescents with diabetes described themselves as "possibly depressed."[50] In this study, and in a study of adolescent girls with diabetes, the prevalence of depression was associated with the level of self-esteem.[50,51] In another study of adolescents with diabetes, girls were found to have a higher rate of depression and anxiety than boys.[52] Because these studies did not include adolescents without diabetes for comparison, it is unclear whether this prevalence is higher than in the general population.

However, studies that have compared the mental health of adolescents with diabetes with that of adolescents in the general population show conflicting results. In one study, adolescents with diabetes experienced more depression, dependency, and withdrawal than those without diabetes.[53] However, their overall self-perceived competence in multiple areas and their peer relationships were not different from those of other adolescents. A second study found that psychiatric disorders, such as somatic symptoms, sleep disturbances, compulsions, and depressive moods, were more prevalent among adolescent girls with diabetes than among those without diabetes;[54] however, these findings did not hold true in another study.[55] Adolescent girls with diabetes have also been shown to have higher rates of suicidal ideation than girls without diabetes.[56] The higher depression rates among adolescent girls with type 1 diabetes may not be related to diabetes itself but rather to the increased strain of having a chronic disease.[57]

Two studies of the impact of diabetes on adolescents' quality of life found that both adolescent girls and boys with diabetes were generally satisfied and not worried, and that diabetes had only a modest impact on their lives.[58,59] However, other studies have found that adolescents view diabetes as a controlling or limiting factor in their lives and a threat to their health status and their future.[60] Adolescents have reported that dietary restrictions and the need to inject insulin and test blood make them feel alienated from their peers.[61] At least two studies have found that adolescent girls report a more negative impact of diabetes on their lives than do adolescent boys.[61,62] However, whether this finding reflects a sex difference in the severity of the disease or in the perception of its impact is not clear.

3.4. Health-Related Behaviors

Environmental Exposures

Several environmental exposures have been examined as potential causes of diabetes. At least one study has suggested that lack of breast-feeding and early introduction of cow's milk protein may increase a child's risk for type 1 diabetes,[63] but contradictory findings have been reported.[64,65] Childhood diets high in cow's milk protein, cereal protein, and total protein have been associated with increased risk for type 1 diabetes.[66,67] Although consumption of nitrates, nitrites, or nitrosamines during childhood has been associated with type 1 diabetes,[67-69] these findings have also been contradicted.[66] Coffee,[70] sugar,[71] and milk consumption[72] are positively correlated with type 1 diabetes rates: countries that consume the greatest amounts of these foods also have the highest rates of type 1 diabetes. Studies suggest that exposure to picornaviruses,[73] herpes viruses,[74,75] mumps,[76] rubella,[77] and retroviruses[78] may also trigger type 1 diabetes in children and adolescents. Finally, negative events in the first 2 years of life, events that result in difficult adaptation, deviant behavior during childhood, and a chaotic family life have been associated with an increased risk for type 1 diabetes in children and adolescents.[79-81]

Although lifestyle choices, such as smoking and physical inactivity, do not appear to play a role in the development of type 1 diabetes, they may affect a person's risk for the long-term complications of the disease. The three health risk factors that have the greatest negative impact on persons with diabetes are smoking, obesity, and insufficient physical activity. In addition to being risk factors for the complications of type 1 diabetes, obesity, a high-fat diet, and lack of physical activity have been identified as risk factors for type 2 diabetes among adults[82] and may increase an adolescent's risk for type 2 diabetes.

Smoking

Tobacco use continues to be a health risk in all segments of society. Among high school students, the prevalence of cigarette smoking is 30%–40%.[83] Among high school girls, the prevalence of tobacco use is significantly lower among blacks (12.2%) than among non-Hispanic whites (39.8%) and Hispanics (32.9%).[83]

Tobacco use, particularly cigarette smoking, has been shown to increase the risk for cardiovascular disease in the general population. Both persons with type 1 and those with type 2 diabetes have an increased incidence of cardiovascular events, including circulatory problems and heart disease.[84] Many studies have shown that, among persons with type 1 diabetes, smoking increases the risk of death attributable to cardiovascular disease and may also increase the incidence of microvascular disease, including nephropathy and retinopathy.[85-87]

Because of these increased risks, persons with diabetes have even more reason than the general population to refrain from using tobacco. However, most studies have not documented a lower prevalence of tobacco use among adolescents and young adults with diabetes than among those without diabetes.[88] The 1988 Behavioral Risk Factor Surveillance System found that the prevalence of smoking was actually greater among persons aged 18–34 years with diabetes (33.1%) than in the general population (28.7%).[89] Similarly, a study of young adults (average age 21 years) with diabetes at the University of Liverpool reported that patients whose diabetes developed before age 10 were as likely to smoke as those whose diabetes developed in adolescence or young adulthood.[88] The median age for initiating smoking was 16 years and also did not differ by age at onset of diabetes. In addition, this study found that only 31% of the patients admitted to smoking when questioned, whereas 48% had evidence of recent tobacco use from their urinalysis. This finding suggests that, regardless of smoking history, all young persons with diabetes should be counseled on the adverse health risks of tobacco use and should be given information about smoking cessation programs.

In addition to increased cardiovascular risks, increased acute illness has been documented among teens who are smokers. One study found that teens who smoked were 2 times more likely than teens who did not smoke to have been hospitalized and 3 times more likely to spend the day in bed. In addition, 24% of smokers but only 8% of nonsmokers reported themselves to be in poor health.[89] Data specifically for adolescents with diabetes were not available. However, multivariate analysis suggests that 50%–75% of the excess illness among young smokers with diabetes is related to the interaction between smoking and diabetes.[89] It is not clear whether this excess illness is a direct effect of smoking or whether smoking is an indicator of increased risk-taking behavior and poor compliance with diabetes-related management. In either case, tobacco use remains an identifiable risk factor for diabetes-related illness and death.

Obesity

The prevalence of obesity is increasing among the general population and among children and adolescents.[90,91] The National Health and Nutrition Examination Surveys of the U.S. population (NHANES I, II, and III) have documented increases in the prevalence of overweight and obesity in all segments of the population, including adolescent girls.[91-94] The percentage of female adolescents at or above the 85th percentile for age increased from 15.8% in NHANES II (1976–1980) to 22.7% in NHANES III (1988–1994).[91] Black girls are

disproportionately affected: 8.8% of all girls aged 12–18 years but 14.4% of black girls this age are in the very obese group. Thus not only are a greater percentage of adolescents overweight, but the degree of obesity has also increased, especially among girls of racial/ethnic minorities.

Obesity and type 1 diabetes. Adolescents with type 1 diabetes are at risk for excessive weight gain. Use of intensified insulin therapy carries with it an increased risk for weight gain,[28] which may contribute to an increase in the prevalence of obesity and increased body mass index (BMI) among adolescents with type 1 diabetes.[95] The DCCT suggested that a weight gain of 8–10 pounds per year was associated with intensified management.[96] Providing adolescents with dietary counseling before they begin and during therapy may be essential to the success of intensive diabetes management.

Persons with type 1 diabetes who attempt weight loss through standardized weight-loss programs have approximately the same success rate as the general population.[95] Weight management programs that improve body image and increase self-confidence and self-esteem may allow teens to practice better overall diabetes management.[95]

Obesity and type 2 diabetes. Type 2 diabetes is caused by insulin resistance in combination with decreased beta cell ability to respond to increasing hyperglycemia. Because obesity is associated with increased insulin resistance,[97] the increased prevalence of obesity among adolescent girls may play an important role in the dramatic increase in the incidence of type 2 diabetes among adolescents that began in the early 1990s.[8,98-102] In a Cincinnati study,[8] as many as 30% of adolescents whose diabetes was diagnosed in 1994 lacked evidence of islet cell autoimmunity and had a high BMI suggestive of type 2 diabetes rather than type 1 diabetes. In contrast, only 4% of teens whose diabetes was diagnosed in 1982 were considered to have type 2. This increase is consistent with the higher incidence of type 2 diabetes among adults and is thought to be related to the increasing levels of obesity in the U.S.

population.[90,97,103] Black, Hispanic, and American Indian youth are overrepresented among adolescents with type 2 diabetes, just as they are among obese adolescents.[8,100,101] However, factors other than obesity may determine risk for type 2 diabetes.[97]

Insufficient Physical Activity

Dietary evaluation of obese persons with type 2 diabetes suggests that their caloric intake is not markedly different from that of persons who are not obese.[104] However, persons who are not obese expend significantly more calories than obese persons. A study of the Pima Indians that explored the association between physical activity and risk for diabetes found that persons who had diabetes by age 35 reported having had significantly less leisure-time physical activity during their teenage years than those without diabetes.[105] Women with diabetes reported only 1 hour of leisure-time activity per week between the ages of 12 and 18 years, but those without diabetes reported 2–3 times as much activity. This study suggests that relatively minor increases in leisure-time activity, particularly among teenaged girls, may markedly decrease the risk for type 2 diabetes in adulthood. The importance of insufficient physical activity as a risk factor for type 2 diabetes appears to be related to the increased insulin resistance found in persons with low levels of physical activity.[27]

Adolescent girls with type 1 diabetes can also benefit from increased physical activity. Increased physical fitness improves insulin sensitivity and increases cardiovascular fitness.[29] Although much of the educational information given to patients with type 1 diabetes stresses the importance of exercise,[106] some studies suggest that young people with type 1 diabetes may not exercise as much as their age-matched peers without diabetes.[29] The reasons given by patients for the lower level of exercise were weather constraints, inadequate time, and difficulty of exercise.

Among adults of all racial and ethnic origins, women are much less likely than men to participate in regular or vigorous physical activity.[107] This sex difference is apparent by the start of high school[83] and increases markedly through the 12th grade. Among 12th-grade girls, only 9.1% of blacks but 18.8% of non-Hispanic whites and 20.9% of Hispanics report participating in vigorous physical activity 3 or more times a week. Participation rates for 12th-grade boys were 42.3% for blacks, 46.1% for whites, and 46.4% for Hispanics. These cultural differences in participation in vigorous physical activity need to be considered in planning strategies to engage girls with diabetes in physical fitness programs.

Pregnancy

The birth rate for teens has been dropping steadily throughout the 1990s.[108] Nevertheless, many teens choose to become sexually active, and their risk for pregnancy should be addressed by their health care providers.[109] The appropriate time to begin discussions about responsible family planning and the impact of diabetes on pregnancy and childbearing is during the middle school years as adolescent girls mature and experience menarche. This discussion can be quite positive, emphasizing the likelihood of a future normal pregnancy and of the birth of a healthy baby, if careful attention is paid to diabetes control prior to and throughout the pregnancy and delivery.[110] It is helpful to the adolescent and her parents to hear this discussion because popular culture often presents childbearing in a woman with diabetes as being difficult or impossible.

For the teen who chooses to be sexually active, confidential counseling on appropriate birth control or referral for these services should be part of the diabetes health care team's routine practice.[109] The importance of preconception counseling cannot be overemphasized to the teen, as well as the need for early notification of the diabetes health care team when an unplanned pregnancy is suspected. The risk of congenital anomalies in the offspring is reduced 10-fold by careful diabetes management in the 3 months prior to and during pregnancy.[110] The care of the pregnant patient with diabetes is one of the major recent advances in diabetes care, and the adolescent patient should be made aware of the importance of intensified diabetes management during this time of her life so she and her unborn child can benefit from this new information.

Adherence to Diabetes Management Tasks

As mentioned earlier in the chapter, the adolescent years are characterized by the rapid physical growth and hormonal changes of puberty, which can affect diabetes management. During this time, increasing insulin resistance and associated physiological changes make diabetes control more difficult.[111]

Care for both type 1 and type 2 diabetes has become more complex as practitioners have addressed issues raised by the DCCT. Patients with type 1 and type 2 are increasingly asked to monitor their blood glucose 3 or 4 times a day and to administer insulin 2 to 4 times a day. Recent surveys have shown that patients are responding to this advice by increasing the frequency of blood testing and insulin injections; however, most patients with type 1 diabetes still monitor their blood glucose fewer than 4 times per day and take only 2 doses of insulin per day.[112] Patients are also given a meal plan designed to provide a constant carbohydrate intake and consistency in meal timing. Those patients who are striving for more intensified diabetes management are encouraged to learn the associations between food intake, exercise, and insulin dose and their effects on blood glucose levels and to adjust their diabetes management accordingly throughout the day to achieve near-normal blood sugar levels.[28] Although mastery of these complex algorithms can improve diabetes control, complying with such a complicated regimen is difficult for even the most sophisticated and mature adult. The spontaneity and impulsiveness of adolescence compound the difficulties of compliance.

Studies have shown that knowledge correlates poorly with adherence to medical recommendations,[113] and this finding holds true for adolescents with diabetes.[114] Concrete objectives, such as insulin administration and self-monitoring of blood glucose, are considerably easier to comply with than the more complex behavioral lifestyle changes required for appropriate dietary and exercise programs.[115-117] However, studies show that adolescents with diabetes have difficulty consistently complying with insulin administration.[118,119] In one such study, a questionnaire completed anonymously by adolescents and their parents attending a diabetes clinic for a routine diabetes evaluation demonstrated that 25% of adolescents had missed at least one insulin injection in the 10 days preceding their clinic visit.[118] Almost 80% of the adolescents reported some mismanagement of their blood glucose monitoring, including altering the test strip to produce a lower blood glucose number, making up a test result rather than doing the test, or replacing a test result that was considered too high. Additionally, over 80% had eaten inappropriate foods at least once, and more than half had missed a meal or a snack at least once during the 10 days before the visit. Researchers did not obtain information about exercise and appropriate management of exercise. However, as teenagers are increasingly asked to adjust their caloric intake for activity, mismanagement of exercise is likely to be as common as mismanagement of dietary intake and blood glucose monitoring. The risks of diabetes mismanagement increase as adolescents become older and generally have more responsibility for their own diabetes management.[40,119] These findings underscore the importance of a gradual transition of diabetes management from parents to adolescents and of continued comanagement until independent management can be successfully established.[52,119]

There is a dearth of data on adherence to diabetes management plans. However, limited data indicate that glycemic control after diagnosis is typically poor, as evidenced by mean glycated hemoglobin values of 10% to 13%.[1] Among Pima Indian children and adolescents, microvascular disease (microalbuminuria) and cardiovascular risk factors (e.g., hypercholesterolemia, elevated blood pressure) were already common at diagnosis and the prevalences were higher at the 10-year follow-up.[120]

Teens who adhere to diabetes regimens have been shown to have higher self-esteem and greater confidence in their ability to accomplish diabetes management tasks.[119] This issue is particularly relevant to adolescent girls, since adolescence is a time when girls are more susceptible to feelings of low self-esteem and incompetence. Some research findings suggest that participation in activities such as team sports and diabetes camps may increase feelings of self-worth and competence among young women and may improve adherence to diabetes routines, including diet plans and exercise recommendations.

Recurrent Episodes of Ketoacidosis

A small subset of persons with diabetes have recurrent episodes of diabetic ketoacidosis. The risk for this syndrome is greatest among adolescents, is more common among women than men, and is associated with living in a single-parent home, with a stepparent, or outside the immediate family home.[40,44,121,122] Other risk factors are abusing drugs or alcohol or having a parent who does so, receiving public assistance, and being older than 14 years. No physiological factors are known to contribute to this syndrome.[40,44,121,122] Because these episodes of ketoacidosis generally resolve when an adult assumes responsibility for monitoring the adolescent's blood glucose levels and administering insulin doses, they are most likely caused by diabetes mismanagement.[118,121,122] The risk for recurrent episodes of ketoacidosis has also been shown to decrease when the adolescent is cared for by a multispecialty team that comprises a nurse educator, a dietitian, a counselor, and the diabetes physician.[44,121] In addition, frequent outpatient contact can decrease the hospital readmission rate for ketoacidosis among adolescents.[44,121]

Extreme inattention to the essentials of diabetes care during adolescence, as evidenced by recurrent ketoacidosis or recurrent severe hypoglycemia, is an indicator of excessive risk for the early development of diabetes complications and death. One study monitored 26 persons who had had recurrent diabetic ketoacidosis as adolescents (case patients) and compared them with a group matched for age and diabetes duration (control patients).[123] After 10.5 years of follow-up, 5 case patients had died of dia-

betes-related disorders (2 of diabetic ketoacidosis, 2 of hypoglycemia, and 1 of end-stage renal disease). No diabetes-related deaths were reported in the control group. Sixty-seven percent of the surviving case patients but only 25% of control patients had diabetes-associated complications.

Two of the case patients continued to have frequent diabetic ketoacidosis. Of the 28 pregnancies among the case patients, 13 (46%) involved complications, compared with 2 (7%) of the 27 pregnancies among the control group. Overall, case patients reported a lower quality of life than the control group. A separate 20-year follow-up study reported similar findings.[124] These studies point to the need to identify adolescents at risk for recurrent episodes of diabetic ketoacidosis or hypoglycemia and to develop effective intervention strategies to decrease the risks for acute illness, long-term complications, and death.

3.5. Psychosocial Determinants of Health Behaviors and Health Outcomes

Social Environment

Family and social support are important determinants of health behaviors and health outcomes of adolescents with diabetes. A child's diabetes has wide-ranging effects on the family. When a child's diabetes is diagnosed, parents have to come to terms with their child's loss of health and the medical concomitants of diabetes, such as episodes of hypoglycemia, hyperglycemia, ketoacidosis, and hospitalizations. Shock, bewilderment, anxiety, fear, insomnia, depression, and guilt are common immediate reactions of parents to the diagnosis of a child's diabetes. In general, most of these parental feelings resolve during the first year after diagnosis.[125] However, both maternal depression and overall emotional stress have been shown to increase over time.[45] One study found that families of adolescents with diabetes rated their general functioning to be worse than did families of healthy adolescents.[126] Another study suggested that an adolescent daughter's diabetes was perceived to draw the whole family closer but to have a negative effect on the spousal relationship.[127]

Few childhood diseases rival diabetes in the high degree of family involvement needed for day-to-day management: the regimen for daily diabetes care involves injections of insulin, monitoring of blood glucose levels, and changes in the composition and timing of the child's diet. For young children with diabetes, family members, primarily mothers, assume responsibility for diabetes care and continue to be involved in some aspects of care throughout adolescence. Adolescence is a particularly sensitive time because it marks the transition from family responsibility to adolescent independence. By age 13, most teenagers with diabetes can perform all regimen-specific tasks; however, they continue to need parental supervision and support to ensure that they adhere to the regimen and to assist them in solving diabetes management problems. Parents tend to give more responsibility for diabetes care to adolescent girls than to adolescent boys.[128] However, adolescents who have the most responsibility for their diabetes regimen have been shown to have the poorest diabetes control.[129] This finding may explain, in part, why adolescent girls have more problems with diabetes control than adolescent boys[24] and why better communication between adolescent daughters and their mothers is associated with better adherence to diabetes care.[130] Other family characteristics that influence adolescents' adherence to the diabetes regimen include family cohesion, parents' perception of family organization,[131] family communication,[128] and overall quality of family life.[132]

In addition to family support, social support is a critical factor in facilitating motivation and normal development and in helping adolescents with diabetes cope with an otherwise unpredictable and confusing situation.[133] Role models are a major form of social support. One study showed that adolescents improved their attitudes toward diabetes when they were able to interact with an adult with diabetes.[134] A relationship with an empathetic, respected adult who has successfully dealt with diabetes and built a life and career without allowing diabetes to interfere appears to alleviate the adolescent's sense of doom.

The support of friends and peers is also important to adolescents with diabetes. Although adolescents have reported that family members provide more support for their diabetes care than friends, they have also reported that family members and friends provide comparable levels of support for physical activity and that friends are more important than family members in helping them feel good about diabetes.[135]

Networks focusing on diabetes care seem to have a positive impact on adolescents with diabetes. The implementation of a comprehensive diabetes care network for adolescents reduced the frequency of diabetic ketoacidosis in one intervention study.[121] For adolescents, networks are largely made up of family and friends. Schools could also act as an important network for adolescents. Parents of children with diabetes have voiced their concern over the poor liaison they have with schools and teachers' lack of diabetes knowledge.[136]

Legal Environment

On occasion, the lack of knowledge on the part of school administrators and faculty has resulted in discriminatory practices affecting young people with diabetes, necessitating legal remedies to ensure educational access and accommodation of the needs of adolescents with diabetes.

Although adolescents with diabetes have a right to "free, appropriate public education,"[137] as established through the Rehabilitation Act of 1973, the Americans with Disabilities Act and the Individuals with Disabilities Education Act litigation has sometimes been required to ensure that children are safe, adequately trained faculty can address diabetes emergencies, and reasonable accommodation for diabetes management needs is provided.[137] Plans to ensure access and accommodation must be individualized to reflect the needs of the person with diabetes as well as the educational environment. That said, in school settings, minimum standard requirements specific to diabetes are generally lacking.

Interactions with the Health Care System

Access to care. Although families with and without a child with diabetes have similar health insurance coverage, the cost of health care is greater for families of a child with diabetes. In one study, out-of-pocket health care expenses for families of a child with diabetes were 49% higher than for families of nondiabetic children.[138] In addition, working parents of a child with diabetes were twice as likely to be absent from work for reasons related to child care and health.[138] Another study found that 10%–30% of families of a child with diabetes received no health insurance reimbursement for the cost of insulin, syringes, or blood testing strips.[139] Because the management of diabetes requires frequent blood glucose testing as well as regular contact with health care professionals, lack of coverage for blood glucose testing supplies and copayments represent barriers to health care, even for fully insured persons. Seventeen percent of families of a child with diabetes had out-of-pocket expenses that exceeded 10% of their income. Total family health care expenses as a share of household income were 50% higher for families of a child with diabetes than for families of a child without diabetes.[139] The higher out-of-pocket expenses are more detrimental to families of low socioeconomic status. And, of course, families without any health insurance face the greatest barriers to proper diabetes management and control.

Patient/provider relationship. Among teenagers with diabetes, the patient/provider relationship involves the parents as well as the physician and the patient. The patient/provider relationship strongly influences the amount of diabetes education the adolescent receives, the likelihood that the adolescent will keep diabetes care appointments, and the adolescent's general acceptance of the disease. A national survey suggested that over 90% of parents were satisfied with the treatment and information that they and their child had received at diagnosis.[136] A separate study found that after diagnosis, parents of adolescent girls had favorable attitudes toward the physician's personal qualities and professional competence and had neutral attitudes toward the cost

and convenience of health care.[140] The teenaged girls were even more satisfied than their parents with the physician's personal qualities. Girls in families who were satisfied with the physician's professional competence adhered better to the diabetes self-care regimen. In addition, the girls who were satisfied with their physician's professional competence had fewer diabetes-related hospitalizations.[140]

3.6. Concurrent Illness as a Determinant of Health Behaviors and Health Outcomes

Eating Disorders

During childhood and adolescence, the long-term sequelae of diabetes rarely cause major illnesses. The illnesses that affect children and adolescents with diabetes are predominantly related to psychosocial issues, especially those leading to extreme diabetes mismanagement. Eating disorders are one of the most critical associated disorders among teens with diabetes. The prevalence rate of eating disorders among the general population is reported to be between 1.3% and 11%,[141,142] and research suggests that the prevalence among young women with type 1 diabetes may be much higher.[143,144]

The two most common eating disorders among adolescent girls with diabetes are anorexia nervosa and bulimia nervosa. An examination of the characteristics of these disorders and the issues contributing to their development illustrates why young women with diabetes may be at increased risk for eating disorders. The definitions of these disorders have been established by the American Psychiatric Association and are in the *Diagnostic and Statistical Manual of Mental Disorders,* Fourth Edition (DSM-IV).[145]

Anorexia nervosa. Anorexia nervosa is characterized by all of the following factors:

- Weight that is at least 15% below that expected for age and height because of weight loss or failure to gain weight during the growth period.

- A fear of weight gain or fatness despite being underweight.
- Disturbed body image.
- Among postmenarcheal adolescents, interruption of menstrual cycles for at least 3 months.

Anorexia can involve restricting food intake alone or restricting accompanied by binge eating and purging.

The issues that persons with anorexia struggle with are an excessive need to meet perfectionist standards, a fear of emerging sexuality, and a fear of being unable to control life's demands. In teens and younger children, anorexia is frequently a symptom of the fear of growing up.[146]

Children or adolescents with diabetes are encouraged to have perfect diabetes control, even though this goal may be a physiological impossibility. Among adolescent girls with diabetes, parental expectations for them to perform all diabetes tasks perfectly and their own expectations of achieving perfect glucose control can lead to feelings of failure and the belief that they have lost control of the demands of daily life. The additional and inevitable emphasis on food and the sometimes rigid recommended eating schedules may increase the risk for anorexia. The frequent dissociation of normal hunger cues from eating and a deemphasis on the pleasure of food may cause adolescents with diabetes to view food as another entity to manage rather than a source of nourishment and comfort. The combination of food issues and the inability to achieve perfect blood glucose control appears to contribute to the development of anorexia in adolescents with diabetes.

Bulimia nervosa. Bulimia nervosa is characterized by all of the following:

- Repeated episodes of binge eating with frequent compensatory behaviors to prevent weight gain, which may include vomiting or misuse of laxatives and diuretics.

- Lack of control during binge episodes.
- Self-evaluation unduly influenced by weight.

Among adolescents with diabetes, compensatory behaviors to prevent weight gain may also include misusing insulin by eliminating or decreasing the insulin dose, thus eliminating the food through glycosuria. Unlike persons with anorexia nervosa, those with bulimia nervosa usually maintain a normal weight for age and height, though weight may fluctuate considerably.[146]

The central issue for persons with bulimia nervosa is a feeling of living behind a facade. An adolescent girl with bulimia tends to believe everyone thinks she is pretty or mature and capable, and she fears that others will find out that she is not really that perfect and will be angry and disappointed with her. Although perfect blood glucose control is not a realistic expectation for persons with diabetes, adolescent girls with bulimia and diabetes need to present a facade of perfection to hide their "failure" from parents and health care providers. Thus, bulimic girls with diabetes frequently report excellent blood glucose control and "no difficulties" with diabetes management but have very elevated hemoglobin A_{1c} levels. Because of the strong inverse correlation between bulimic symptoms (binging and purging) and metabolic control in teenage girls with diabetes,[147] persistent hyperglycemia should alert health care providers to suspect bulimia.

Predisposing factors for eating disorders. Families of children with eating disorders have been characterized as enmeshed and overprotective, unable to resolve conflict, and rigid in their interactions. These same characteristics have also been noted in families of persons with difficult-to-control diabetes.[148] Thus, the characteristics that make it difficult for a family to cope with a chronic illness may also predispose the affected member to an eating disorder.

In addition to diabetes management issues, diabetes treatment outcomes and outcome measures may be risk factors for disordered eating among adolescent girls with diabetes. The use of weight as a method of evaluating diabetes control is a major risk factor. Weight loss is an indicator of poor control and weight gain a possible indicator of lack of adherence to the prescribed food plan. This emphasis on weight is psychologically difficult for many adolescent girls and may be an additional trigger for eating disorders for the teen with diabetes.

Finally, the stress related to having a chronic illness can exacerbate other difficulties for both the patient and the family and make the eruption of a latent eating disorder more likely. Persons with diabetes who are struggling with issues of identity or adjustment brought about by the diagnosis of a chronic illness are at higher risk of developing eating disorders than are those who are coping fairly well with life.[149]

Frequency of eating disorders among adolescent girls with diabetes. Despite the apparent increased risk for factors predisposing teens with diabetes to eating disorders, the first case of anorexia nervosa in a person with diabetes was not reported until 1973.[150] Between 1973 and 1984, there were only 10 reports involving a total of 31 patients.[144] Those 10 studies, however, firmly established the coexistence of eating disorders among patients with type 1 diabetes. Since the mid-1980s, several prevalence studies[151-153] and treatment reports[151,154] have been published. Despite controversy over the precise rate of eating disorders among women with diabetes, current evidence suggests that this rate is at least equal to that among women in the general population and may be significantly higher.[143,155]

A series of studies that used paper-and-pencil questionnaires found a significantly higher incidence of anorexia and bulimia among patients with diabetes than among those without diabetes.[153,155,156] Although the results are quite compelling, these studies rely on paper-and-pencil measures and thus lack the diagnostic rigor of interview methods. Other studies that have included an interview in addition to paper-and-pencil measurements have found that the incidence of eating disorders among

young women with diabetes is equal to, but not higher than, that among the general population of young women.[157]

The use or misuse of insulin to manipulate weight must also be considered an eating disorder among girls and young women with diabetes. Many young women who do not meet DSM-IV criteria for eating disorders manipulate their insulin to alter their weight and experience significant eating problems, which are generally termed "subclinical eating disorders." For example, girls with excessive fear of hypoglycemia eat more to prevent hypoglycemia, but then they feel guilty for overeating. This reaction may precipitate a cycle of overeating but without increasing insulin because of fears of weight gain.[151] If insulin manipulation is included in the definition of an eating disorder, the incidence of eating disorders is much higher among women with diabetes than among the general population.[143,155,158]

The strict definitions for anorexia and bulimia nervosa include a time factor requiring the abnormal behavior to persist for 3 or more months before the diagnosis is established. However, because of the serious implications of eating disorders among adolescents with diabetes, any episodes of binging accompanied by compensatory purging behavior among young women with diabetes should warrant attention.

The major concern for diabetic young women with eating disorders is the high risk of secondary complications. One study reported finding 15 women with eating disorders among a cohort of 208 women with diabetes.[155] Of these 15, 11 had retinopathy (6 with proliferative changes), 6 had nephropathy, 6 had neuropathy, and 4 had painful neuropathy that remitted with weight gain.

A 4–5-year follow-up study of 91 young women with diabetes found highly or moderately disordered eating in 29% of these women.[143] Of those with highly disordered eating behavior, 86% had retinopathy at follow-up, compared with 24% of those without disordered eating behavior. These studies underscore the importance of identifying young diabetic women with eating disorders.

Treatment of eating disorders. Treatment of any eating disorder should use a coordinated team approach that includes a therapist, a nutritionist, and a physician or a nurse practitioner. Recovering from eating disorders is difficult for adolescent girls. Although in some ways these girls may make a real effort to recover, they frequently undermine their treatment by surreptitiously not adhering to the recommended treatment plan. Unfortunately, the prognosis remains guarded for diabetic adolescents with anorexia or bulimia.[159,160]

Among patients with diabetes, treatment of eating disorders must be closely coordinated with diabetes management. Allowing more flexibility in the target blood glucose range and adjusting food choices may be necessary until the eating disorder improves.[154] Otherwise, the treatment should not differ from that of patients without diabetes.

Other Psychiatric Disorders Affecting Diabetes Management

During adolescence, several psychiatric disorders may become apparent. The two that have the greatest implications for adolescents with diabetes are *bipolar disease* (manic-depression) and *panic attacks.* Adolescents with bipolar disease may be unable to organize themselves adequately to adhere to the schedule required for diabetes care. Because spontaneity and impulsiveness are hallmarks of adolescence, the diagnosis of mania may be delayed until the behavior is dangerous to the adolescent or to others. By this time, glucose control may have been poor for months or even years. Once appropriate treatment is instituted, diabetes control may not be adequate for many additional months because other issues in the life of the patient must also be brought into equilibrium.

Panic attacks classically appear in late adolescence and the early twenties.[146] Because the feelings of extreme anxiety that characterize panic attacks may mimic the epinephrine release of a hypoglycemic

episode, patients may react to them by decreasing their insulin doses. Only by carefully documenting blood glucose levels during an event can the correct diagnosis be reached and appropriate medication instituted. As long as the symptoms persist, good diabetes control is difficult because of the patient's fear of hypoglycemia. Excessive blood glucose testing, especially in the absence of documented hypoglycemia, should suggest the diagnosis of an anxiety disorder. One study of Pima Indians has reported that 8% of children with diabetes displayed symptoms of depression or eating disorders.[1]

Community Norms and Acculturation

Community norms and acculturation in the United States are structured around the majority white racial/ethnic group. Because most adolescent girls with type 1 diabetes are white, there are no studies on the effect of acculturation on health behaviors and outcomes in adolescents with diabetes. However, community norms have a large impact on the health behaviors of adolescent girls with and without diabetes. The desire of adolescents not to be different may affect adherence to diet and regular glucose monitoring. Society's emphasis on being thin may also negatively affect an adolescent girl's adherence to a diabetes regimen of tight metabolic control, which can result in weight gain.

3.7. Public Health Implications

Teenaged girls do not appear to fare as well with their diabetes as their male counterparts. They experience higher mortality and morbidity from this disease. With increasing trends in risk factors such as obesity, lack of physical activity, and smoking among adolescent women, the prevalence of diabetes and its complications will increase. The public health and medical communities must begin to work together to identify modifiable societal and individual-level factors that can be used to develop effective interventions for the prevention and control of diabetes in this age group.

Assessment

There is much that needs to be done to assess the special needs of adolescent girls with diabetes.

Further studies are needed to

- Elucidate the relationship between smoking and other risk-taking behaviors and acute illness and general health status.

- Identify the determinants of eating disorders.

- Assess the prevalence and determinants of the major complications of diabetes mellitus, including dental disorders.

- Assess the impact of community-level and individual-level socioeconomic status on the health status of adolescents with diabetes.

- Determine the prevalence and incidence of type 1 and type 2 diabetes in adolescents.

Policy Development

Professional organizations and advocacy groups can play an important role in the development and promotion of policy initiatives to reduce barriers to diabetes care and to improve adherence among adolescent girls with diabetes. Policies that empower adolescent girls to take control of their diabetes management, provide special diabetes education opportunities for teens, support smoking prevention and cessation programs, and ensure access to counseling and family planning services for sexually active teens with diabetes could prevent or delay the onset of major complications and reduce the burden of disease in this population. The development of guidelines for assessing eating disorders among adolescent girls with diabetes would enhance the recognition of disease processes and facilitate early identification and treatment. Body image and weight management are serious concerns for all adolescents; however, the manipulation of insulin for weight control is a behavior with serious consequences. Effective interventions for weight management need to be structured to focus on the improvement of self-confidence and body image. In addition, opportunities for physical activity that could become a lifelong practice would enhance the

attainment and maintenance of good glycemic control as well as weight management.

Furthermore, to facilitate self-management behaviors for adolescents with diabetes, it is important that a consensus is reached on policies regarding medicines and treatment of diabetes in school settings. The collaboration of advocates and policy makers from local communities, medicine, public health, and education sectors would enhance this process. Finally, policies are needed to provide reimbursement for insulin administration devices that are appropriate for adolescents.

Assurance

The transition into adulthood and independence from parents or other authority figures is marked with many challenges for adolescents, even more so for adolescents with diabetes. At the same time, support from family, peers, and other members of the community is essential to help control this disease. Maintaining a balance between these two opposing features of the needs of adolescents with diabetes is a challenge for the public health community. Opportunities for counseling and education should be provided in settings frequented by adolescents, including schools, churches, camps, community centers, and social and athletic clubs. Knowledge and awareness of the public health impact of diabetes and its complications need to be widespread in the community, especially among teachers in public schools, among leaders of the faith community, and among providers of social services. All schools should ensure healthy food choices. The health delivery system should assure the availability of providers who are sensitive to the needs of adolescent women and who are competent in the care of adolescents with type 1 and type 2 diabetes. This would improve adherence to diabetes self-care practices and improve clinical outcomes for women with diabetes in this age group.

References

1. Fagot-Campagna A, Pettitt DJ, Engelgau MM, et al. Type 2 diabetes among North American children and adolescents: an epidemiologic review and a public health perspective. *J Pediatr* 2000;136(3):664–72.

2. LaPorte RE, Matsushima M, Chang Y-F. Prevalence and incidence of insulin-dependent diabetes. In: National Diabetes Data Group, editors. *Diabetes in America.* 2nd ed. Bethesda, MD: National Institutes of Health, 1995:37–46. (NIH Publication No. 95-1468)

3. Dabelea D, Hanson RL, Bennett PH, Roumain J, Knowler WC, Pettitt DJ. Increasing prevalence of type II diabetes in American Indian children. *Diabetologia* 1998;41(8):904–10.

4. Kostraba JN, Gay EC, Cai Y, et al. Incidence of insulin-dependent diabetes mellitus in Colorado. *Epidemiology* 1992;3(3):232–8.

5. Wagenknecht LE, Roseman JM, Alexander WJ. Epidemiology of IDDM in black and white children in Jefferson County, Alabama, 1979–1985. Diabetes 1989;38(5):629–33.

6. Lipton RB, Fivecoate JA. High risk of IDDM in African American and Hispanic children in Chicago, 1985–1990. *Diabetes Care* 1995;18(4):476–82.

7. Libman IM, LaPorte RE, Becker D, Dorman JS, Drash AL, Kuller L. Was there an epidemic of diabetes in non-white adolescents in Allegheny County, Pennsylvania? *Diabetes Care* 1998;21(8):1278–81.

8. Pinhas-Hamiel O, Dolan LM, Daniels SR, Standiford D, Khoury PR, Zeitler P. Increased incidence of non–insulin-dependent diabetes mellitus among adoles-cents. *J Pediatr* 1996;128:608–15.

9. Cowie CC, Eberhardt MS. Sociodemographic character-istics of persons with diabetes. In: National Diabetes Data Group, editors. Diabetes in America. 2nd ed. Bethesda, MD: National Institutes of Health, 1995:85–116. (NIH Publication No. 95-1468)

10. Dorman JS, LaPorte RE, Stone RA. Worldwide differ-ences in the incidence of type 1 diabetes are associated with amino acid variation at position 57 of the HLA-DQ beta chain. *Proc Natl Acad Sci USA* 1990;87(19):7370–4.

11. Gay EC, Hamman RF, Carosone-Link PJ, et al. Colorado IDDM registry: lower incidence of IDDM in Hispanics. Comparison of disease characteristics and care patterns in biethnic population. *Diabetes Care* 1989;12(10):701–8.

12. Paisano EL. The American Indian, Eskimo, and Aleut population. In: *Current Population Reports. Special Studies Series.* Washington, DC: U.S. Department of Commerce, Economic and Statistics Administration, Bureau of the Census, 1995:23–189.

13. Dumont RH, Jacobson AM, Cole C, et al. Psychosocial predictors of acute complications of diabetes in youth. *Diabet Med* 1995;12(7):612–8.

14. Klein R, Klein B. Vision disorders in diabetes. In: National Diabetes Data Group, editors. *Diabetes in America.* 2nd ed. Bethesda, MD: National Institutes of Health, 1995:293–338. (NIH Publication No. 95-1468)

15. Fairchild JM, Hing SJ, Donaghue KC, et al. Prevalence and risk factors for retinopathy in adolescents with type 1 diabetes. *Med J Aust* 1994;160(12):757–62.

16. Bonney M, Hing SJ, Fung AT, et al. Development and progression of diabetic retinopathy: adolescents at risk. *Diabet Med* 1995;12(11):967–73.

17. Malone JI, Grizzard S, Espinoza LR, Achenbach KE, Van Cader TC. Risk factors for diabetic retinopathy in youth. *Pediatrics* 1984;73(6):756–61.

18. Quattrin T, Waz W, Duffy L, et al. Microalbuminuria in an adolescent cohort with insulin-dependent diabetes mellitus. *Clin Pediatr (Phila)* 1995;34:12–17.

19. Janner M, Knill SE, Diem P, Zuppinger KA, Mullis PE. Persistent microalbuminuria in adolescents with type 1 (insulin-dependent) diabetes mellitus is associated to early rather than late puberty. Results of a prospective longitudinal study. *Eur J Pediatr* 1994;153(6):403–8.

20. Rudberg S, Dahlquist GG. Determinants of progression of microalbuminuria in adolescents with IDDM. *Diabetes Care* 1996;19(4):369–71.

21. Jackson RL, Ide CH, Guthrie RA, James RD. Retinopathy in adolescents and young adults with onset of insulin-dependent diabetes in childhood. *Ophthalmology* 1982;89(1):7–13.

22. Cerutti F, Sacchetti C, Vigo A, et al. Course of retinopathy in children and adolescents with insulin-dependent diabetes mellitus: a 10-year study. *Ophthalmologica* 1989;198(3):116–23.

23. Weber B, Burger W, Hartmann R, Hovener G, Malchus R, Oberdisse U. Risk factors for the development of retinopathy in children and adolescents with type 1 (insulin-dependent) diabetes mellitus. *Diabetologia* 1986;29(1):23–9.

24. Hamburg BA, Inoff GE. Relationships between behavioral factors and diabetic control in children and adolescents: a camp study. *Psychosom Med* 1982;44(4):321–39.

25. Loe H, Genco RJ. Oral complications of diabetes. In: National Diabetes Data Group, editors. *Diabetes in America*. 2ⁿᵈ ed. Bethesda, MD: National Institutes of Health, 1995:501–6. (NIH Publication No. 95-1468)

26. Loe H. Periodontal disease. The sixth complication of diabetes mellitus. *Diabetes Care* 1993;16(1):329–34.

27. Mayer-Davis EJ, D'Agostino R Jr, Karter AJ, et al. Intensity and amount of physical activity in relation to insulin sensitivity: the Insulin Resistance Atherosclerosis Study. *JAMA* 1998;279(9):669–74.

28. DCCT Research Group. Effect of intensive diabetes treatment on the development and progression of long-term complications in adolescents with insulin-dependent diabetes mellitus: Diabetes Control and Complications Trial. *J Pediatr* 1994;125(2):177–88.

29. Loman DG, Galgani CA. Physical activity in adolescents with diabetes. *Diabetes Educ* 1996; 22:121–5.

30. Dorman JS, LaPorte RE, Kuller LH, et al. The Pittsburgh Insulin-Dependent Diabetes Mellitus (IDDM) Morbidity and Mortality Study. Mortality results. *Diabetes* 1984;33(3):271–6.

31. Sartor G, Nystrom L, Dahlquist GG. The Swedish Childhood Diabetes Study: a sevenfold decrease in short-term mortality? *Diabet Med* 1991;8(1):18–21.

32. Panzram G. Mortality and survival in type 2 (non–insulin-dependent) diabetes mellitus. *Diabetologia* 1987;30(3):123–31.

33. Dorman JS, LaPorte RE, Tajima N, Orchard TJ, Becker DJ, Drash AL. Differential risk factors for death in insulin-dependent diabetic patients by duration of disease. *Pediatr Adolesc Endocrinol* 1986;15:289–99.

34. Drash AL, LaPorte RE, Becker DJ, et al. Epidemiologic studies in children with diabetes mellitus and their families: the Allegheny County Registry experience. In: Chiumello G, Sperling M, editors. *Recent Progress in Pediatric Endocrinology*. New York: Raven Press, 1983:124–36.

35. Aubert RE, Geiss LS, Ballard DJ, Cocanougher B, Herman WH. Diabetes-related hospitalization and hospital utilization. In: National Diabetes Data Group, editors. *Diabetes in America*. 2ⁿᵈ ed. Bethesda, MD: National Institutes of Health, 1995:553–69. (NIH Publication No. 95-1468)

36. Sutton L, Plant AJ, Lyle DM. Services and cost of hospitalization for children and adolescents with insulin-dependent diabetes mellitus in New South Wales. *Med J Aust* 1990;152(3):130–6.

37. Kostraba JN, Gay EC, Rewers M, Chase HP, Klingensmith GJ, Hamman RF. Increasing trend in outpatient management of children with newly diagnosed IDDM. Colorado IDDM Registry, 1978–1988. *Diabetes Care* 1992;15(1):95–100.

38. Fishbein HA, Faich GA, Ellis SE. Incidence and hospitalization patterns of insulin-dependent diabetes mellitus. *Diabetes Care* 1982;5(6):630–3.

39. Davidson J, Alogna M. Assessment of program effectiveness at Grady Memorial Hospital. In: Steiner G, Laurence P, editors. *Educating Diabetic Patients*. New York: Springer Publishing Company, 1981:329–49.

40. Challen AH, Davies AG, Williams RJ, Baum JD. Hospital admissions of adolescent patients with diabetes. *Diabet Med* 1992;9(9):850–4.

41. Faich GA, Fishbein HA, Ellis SE. The epidemiology of diabetic acidosis: a population-based study. *Am J Epidemiol* 1983;117(5):551–8.

42. Rutstein DD, Berenberg W, Chalmers TC, Child CG 3rd, Fishman AP, Perrin EB. Measuring the quality of medical care. *N Engl J Med* 1976;294(11):582–8.

43. Cohn BA, Cirillo PM, Wingard DL, Austin DF, Roffers SD. Gender differences in hospitalizations for IDDM among adolescents in California, 1991. *Diabetes Care* 1997;20(11):1677–82.

44. Glasgow AM, Weissberg-Benchell J, Tynan WD, et al. Readmissions of children with diabetes mellitus to a children's hospital. *Pediatrics* 1991;88(1):98–104.

45. Kovacs M, Iyengar S, Goldston D, Obrosky DS, Stewart J, Marsh J. Psychological functioning among mothers of children with insulin-dependent diabetes mellitus: a longitudinal study. *J Consult Clin Psychol* 1990;58(2): 189–95.

46. Kovacs M, Charron-Prochownik D, Obrosky D. A longitudinal study of biomedical and psychosocial predictors of multiple hospitalizations among young people with insulin-dependent diabetes mellitus. *Diabet Med* 1995;12(2):142–8.

47. Ryan CM, Longstreet C, Morrow L. The effects of diabetes mellitus on the school attendance and school achievement of adolescents. *Child Care Health Dev* 1985;11(4):229–40.

48. Ryan CM. Neurobehavioural complications of type 1 diabetes. Examination of possible risk factors. *Diabetes Care* 1988;11(1):86–93.

49. Northam E, Bowden S, Anderson V, Court J. Neuropsychological functioning in adolescents with diabetes. *J Clin Exp Neuropsychol* 1992;14(6):884–900.

50. Close H, Davies AG, Price DA, Goodyer IM. Emotional difficulties in diabetes mellitus. *Arch Dis Child* 1986;61(4):337–40.

51. Sullivan BJ. Adjustment in diabetic adolescent girls: II. Adjustment, self-esteem, and depression in diabetic adolescent girls. *Psychosom Med* 1979;41(2):127–38.

52. La Greca AM, Swales T, Klemp S, Madigan S, Skyler JS. Adolescents with diabetes: gender differences in psychosocial functioning and glycemic control. *Childrens Health Care* 1995;24(1):61–78.

53. Grey M, Cameron ME, Lipman TH, Thurber FW. Psychosocial status of children with diabetes in the first 2 years after diagnosis. *Diabetes Care* 1995;18(10): 1330–6.

54. Blanze BJ, Rensch-Riemann BS, Fritz-Sigmund DI, Schmidt MH. IDDM is a risk factor for adolescent psychiatric disorders. *Diabetes Care* 1993;16(12):1579–87.

55. Lavigne JV, Traisman HS, Marr TJ, Chasnoff IJ. Parental perceptions of the psychological adjustment of children with diabetes and their siblings. *Diabetes Care* 1982;5(4):420–6.

56. Goldston DB, Kovacs M, Ho VY, Parrone PL, Stiffler L. Suicidal ideation and suicide attempts among youth with insulin-dependent diabetes mellitus. *J Am Acad Child Adolesc Psychiatry* 1994;33(2):240–6.

57. Jacobson AM. Depression and diabetes. *Diabetes Care* 1993;16(12):1621–3.

58. DCCT Research Group. Reliability and validity of a diabetes quality-of-life measure for the Diabetes Control and Complications Trial (DCCT). *Diabetes Care* 1988;11(9):725–32.

59. Striegel-Moore RH, Nicholson TJ, Tamborlane WV. Prevalence of eating disorder symptoms in preadolescent and adolescent girls with IDDM. *Diabetes Care* 1992;15(10):1361–8.

60. Kyngas H, Barlow J. Diabetes: an adolescent's perspective. *J Adv Nurs* 1995;22(5):941–7.

61. Eiser C, Flynn M, Green E, et al. Quality of life in young adults with type 1 diabetes in relation to demographic and disease variables. *Diabet Med* 1992;9(4): 375–8.

62. Challen AH, Davies AG, Williams RJ, Haslum MN, Baum JD. Measuring psychosocial adaptation to diabetes in adolescence. *Diabet Med* 1988;5(8):739–46.

63. Gerstein HC, VanderMeulen J. The relationship between cow's milk exposure and type 1 diabetes. *Diabet Med* 1996;13(1):23–9.

64. Norris JM, Beaty B, Klingensmith GJ, et al. Lack of association between early exposure to cow's milk protein and beta-cell autoimmunity. Diabetes Autoimmunity Study in the Young (DAISY). *JAMA* 1996;276(8): 609–14.

65. Norris JM, Scott F. A meta-analysis of infant diet and insulin-dependent diabetes mellitus: do biases play a role? *Epidemiology* 1996;7(1):87–92.

66. Verge CF, Howard NJ, Irwig L, Simpson JM, Mackerras D, Silink M. Environmental factors in childhood IDDM. A population-based, case-control study. *Diabetes Care* 1994;17(12):1381–9.

67. Dahlquist GG, Blom LG, Persson LA, Sandstrom AI, Walls SG. Dietary factors and the risk of developing insulin-dependent diabetes in childhood. *BMJ* 1990;300(6735):1302–6.

68. Virtanen SM, Jaakkola L, Ylonen K, et al. Nitrate and nitrite intake and the risk for type 1 diabetes in Finnish children. Childhood diabetes in a Finland study group. *Diabet Med* 1994;11(7):656–62.

69. Kostraba JN, Gay EC, Rewers M, Hamman RF. Nitrate levels in community drinking waters and risk of IDDM. An ecological analysis. *Diabetes Care* 1992;15(11): 1505–8.

70. Tuomilehto J, Tuomilehto-Wolf E, Virtala E, LaPorte RE. Coffee consumption as a trigger for insulin-dependent diabetes in childhood. *BMJ* 1990;300(6725):642–3.

71. Pozzilli P, Bottazzo GF. Coffee or sugar. Which is to blame in IDDM? *Diabetes Care* 1991;14(2):144–5.

72. Scott F. Cow milk and insulin-dependent diabetes mellitus: is there a relationship? *Am J Clin Nutr* 1990;51(3): 489–91.

73. Craighead JE, Huber SA, Sriram S. Animal models of picornavirus-induced autoimmune disease: their possible relevance to human disease. *Lab Invest* 1990;63(4): 432–46.

74. Pak CY, Eun HM, McArthur RG, Yoon JW. Association of cytomegalovirus infection with autoimmune type 1 diabetes. *Lancet* 1988;2(86a):1–4.

75. Sairenji T, Daibata M, Sorli CH, et al. Relating homology between the Epstein-Barr virus BOLF1 molecule and HLA-DQw8 beta chain to recent-onset type 1 (insulin-dependent) diabetes mellitus. *Diabetologia* 1991;34(1): 33–9.

76. Helmke K. Virus infections and diabetes mellitus. In: Becker Y, editor. *Virus Infections and Diabetes Mellitus*. Boston: Matinua Nijhoff Publishing, 1987:127–42.

77. Ginsberg-Fellner F, Witt ME, Yagihashi S, et al. Congenital rubella syndrome as a model for type 1 (insulin-dependent) diabetes mellitus: increased prevalence of islet cell surface antibodies. *Diabetologia* 1984; 27(Suppl):87–9.

78. Suenaga K, Yoon JW. Association of beta-cell-specific expression of endogenous retrovirus with development of insulitis and diabetes in NOD mouse. *Diabetes* 1988; 37(12):1722–6.

79. Thernlund GM, Dahlquist GG, Hansson K, et al. Psychological stress and the onset of IDDM in children. *Diabetes Care* 1995;18(10):1323–9.

80. Robinson N, Lloyd CE, Fuller JH, Yateman NA. Psychosocial factors and the onset of type 1 diabetes. *Diabet Med* 1989;6(1):53–8.

81. Robinson N, Fuller JH. Role of life events and difficulties in the onset of diabetes mellitus. *J Psychosom Res* 1985;29(6):583–91.

82. Hamman RF. Genetic and environmental determinants of non–insulin-dependent diabetes mellitus (NIDDM). *Diabetes Metab Rev* 1992;8(4):287–338.

83. Kann L, Warren CW, Harris WA, et al. Youth risk behavior surveillance—United States, 1995. *MMWR CDC Surveill Summ* 1996;45(SS-4):1–84.

84. Krolewski AS, Warram JH. *Epidemiology* of late complications of diabetes. In: Kahn CR, Weir GC, editors. *Joslin's Diabetes Mellitus.* 13th ed. Malver, PA: Lea & Febiger, 1994:605–19.

85. Chase HP, Jackson WE, Hoops SL, Cockerham RS, Archer PG, Obrien D. Glucose control and the renal and retinal complications of insulin-dependent diabetes. *JAMA* 1989;261(8):1155–60.

86. Chase HP, Garg SK, Marshall G, et al. Cigarette smoking increases the risk of albuminuria among subjects with type 1 diabetes. *JAMA* 1991;265(5):614–7.

87. Chaturvedi N, Stephenson J, Fuller J. The relationship between smoking and microvascular complications in the EURODIAB IDDM Complications Study. *Diabetes Care* 1995;18(6):785–92.

88. Masson EA, MacFarlane IA, Priestly CJ, Wallymahmed ME, Flavell HJ. Failure to prevent nicotine addiction in young people with diabetes. *Arch Dis Child* 1992; 67(1):100–2.

89. Gay EC, Cai Y, Gale SM, et al. Smokers with IDDM experience excess morbidity. The Colorado IDDM Registry. *Diabetes Care* 1992;15(8):947–52.

90. Kuczmarski RJ, Flegal KM, Campbell SM, Johnson CL. Increasing prevalence of overweight among U.S. adults. The National Health and Nutrition Examination Surveys, 1960 to 1991. *JAMA* 1994;272(3):205–11.

91. Troiano RP, Flegal KM. Overweight children and adolescents: description, epidemiology, and demographics. *Pediatrics* 1998;101(3Suppl):497–504.

92. National Center for Health Statistics. *Plan and Operation of the Health and Nutrition Examination Survey, United States,* 1971–1973. Vital Health Statistics, Series 1, No. 10, Washington, DC: U.S. Government Printing Office, 1973.

93. McDowell A, Engel A, Massey J, Maurer K. *Plan and Operation of the Second National Health and Nutrition Examination Survey, United States,* 1976–1980. Vital Health Statistics, Series 1, No. 15. Washington, DC: U.S. Government Printing Office, 1981.

94. National Center for Health Statistics. *Plan and Operation of the Third National Health and Nutrition Examination Survey,* 1988–1994. Department of Health and Human Services, Vital and Health Statistics, Series 1, No. 32. Hyattsville, MD: National Center for Health Statistics, 1994. (Publication No. PHS 94-1308)

95. Thomas-Dobersen DA, Butler-Simon N, Fleshner M. Evaluation of a weight management intervention program in adolescents with insulin-dependent diabetes mellitus. *J Am Diet Assoc* 1993;93(5):535–40.

96. The Diabetes Control and Complications Trial Research Group. The effect of intensive treatment of diabetes on the development and progression of long-term complications in insulin-dependent diabetes mellitus. *N Engl J Med* 1993;329(14):977–86.

97. Cowie CC, Harris MI, Silverman RE, Johnson EW, Rust KF. Effect of multiple risk factors on differences between blacks and whites in the prevalence of non–insulin-dependent diabetes mellitus in the United States. *Am J Epidemiol* 1993; 137(7):719–32.

98. Scott CR, Smith JM, Cradock MM, Pihoker C. Characteristics of youth-onset non–insulin-dependent diabetes mellitus and insulin-dependent diabetes mellitus at diagnosis. *Pediatrics* 1997;100(1):84–91.

99. Babu SR, Walravens P, Wang T, et al. Disease heterogeneity at the onset of diabetes in children evaluated with multiple "biochemical" autoantibody screening and DQ typing. *Diabetes* 1996;45(Suppl 2):201A.

100. Jones KL. Non–insulin-dependent diabetes in children and adolescents: the therapeutic challenge. *Clin Pediatr (Phila)* 1998;37(2):103–10.

101. Pettitt DJ, Bennett PH, Saad MF, Charles MA, Nelson RG, Knowler WC. Abnormal glucose tolerance during pregnancy in Pima Indian women. Long-term effects on offspring. *Diabetes* 1991;40(Suppl 2):126–30.

102. Dean HJ, Mundy RL, Moffatt M. Non–insulin-dependent diabetes mellitus in Indian children in Manitoba. *CMAJ* 1992;147(1):52–7.

103. Pinhas-Hamiel O, Zeitler P. Insulin resistance, obesity, and related disorders among black adolescents. *J Pediatr* 1996;129(3):319–20.

104. Ravussin E, Lillioja S, Knowler WC, et al. Reduced rate of energy expenditure as a risk factor for body-weight gain. *N Engl J Med* 1988;318(8):467–72.

105. Kriska AM, LaPorte RE, Pettitt DJ, et al. The association of physical activity with obesity, fat distribution, and glucose intolerance in Pima Indians. *Diabetologia* 1993;36(9):863–9.

106. Chase HP. *Understanding Insulin-Dependent Diabetes.* Denver: Department of Pediatrics, University of Colorado Health Sciences Center, 1995.

107. Crespo CJ, Keteyian SJ, Heath GW, Sempos CT. Leisure-time physical activity among U.S. adults. Results from the Third National Health and Nutrition Examination Survey. *Arch Intern Med* 1996;156(1): 93–8.

108. Guyer B, MacDorman MF, Martin JA, Peters KD, Strobino DM. Annual summary of vital statistics— 1997. *Pediatrics* 1998;102(6):1333–49.

109. Beschart J. Oral contraception and adolescent women with insulin-dependent diabetes mellitus: risks, benefits, and implications for practice. *Diabetes Educ* 1996;22(4): 374–8.

110. Freinkel N, Dooley SL, Metzger BE. Care of the pregnant woman with insulin-dependent diabetes mellitus. *N Engl J Med* 1985;313(2):96–101.

111. Amiel SA, Simonson DC, Sherwin RS, Lauritano AA, Tamborlane WV. Exaggerated epinephrine responses to hypoglycemia in normal and insulin-dependent diabetic children. *J Pediatr* 1987;110(6):832–7.

112. Mortensen HB, Hougaard P. Comparison of metabolic control in a cross-sectional study of 2,873 children and adolescents with IDDM from 18 countries. The Hvidore Study Group on Childhood Diabetes. *Diabetes Care* 1997;20(5):714–20.

113. La Greca AM. Behavioral aspects of diabetes management in children and adolescents. *Diabetes* 1982;31(Suppl 2):12A.

114. McCaul KD, Glasgow RE, Schafer LC. Diabetes regimen behaviors. Predicting adherence. *Med Care* 1987; 25(9):868–81.

115. Summerson JH, Konen JC, Dignan MB. Association between exercise and other preventative health behaviors among diabetics. *Public Health Rep* 1991;106(5):543–7.

116. Glasgow RE, McCaul KD, Schafer LC. Barriers to regimen adherence among persons with insulin-dependent diabetes. *J Behav Med* 1986;9(1):65–77.

117. Marrero DG, Fremion AS, Golden MP. Improving compliance with exercise in adolescents with insulin-dependent diabetes mellitus: results of a self-motivated home exercise program. *Pediatrics* 1988;81(4):519–25.

118. Weisberg-Benchell J, Glasgow AM, Tynan WD, Wirtz P, Turek J, Ward J. Adolescent diabetes management and mismanagement. *Diabetes Care* 1995;18(1):77–82.

119. Daviss WB, Coon H, Whitehead P, Ryan K, Burkley M, McMahon W. Predicting diabetic control from competence, adherence, adjustment, and psychopathology. *J Am Acad Child Adolesc Psychiatry* 1995;34(12): 1629–36.

120. Fagot-Campagna A, Burrows NR, Williamson DF. The public health epidemiology of type 2 diabetes in children and adolescents: a case study of American Indian adolescents in the Southwestern United States. *Clin Chim Acta* 1999;286(1-2):81–95.

121. Golden MP, Herrold AJ, Orr DP. An approach to prevention of recurrent diabetic ketoacidosis in the pediatric population. *J Pediatr* 1985;107(2):195–200.

122. Drozda DJ, Dawson VA, Long DJ, Freson LS, Sperling MA. Assessment of the effect of a comprehensive diabetes management program on hospital admission rates of children with diabetes mellitus. *Diabetes Educ* 1990; 16(5):389–93.

123. Kent LA, Gill GV, Williams G. Mortality and outcome of patients with brittle diabetes and recurrent ketoacidosis. *Lancet* 1994;344(8925):778–81.

124. Tattersall R, Gregory R, Selby C, Kerr D, Heller S. Course of brittle diabetes: 12-year follow-up. *BMJ* 1991; 302(6787):1240–3.

125. Jacobson AM, Hauser ST, Lavori P, et al. Adherence among children and adolescents with insulin-dependent diabetes mellitus over a 4-year longitudinal follow-up: I. The influence of patient coping and adjustment. *J Pediatr Psychol* 1990;15(4):511–26.

126. Gowers SG, Jones JC, Kiana S, North CD, Price DA. Family functioning: a correlate of diabetic control? *J Child Psychol Psychiatry* 1995;36(6):993–1001.

127. Dashiff CJ. Parents' perceptions of diabetes in adolescent daughters and its impact on the family. *J Pediatr Nurs* 1993;8(6):361–9.

128. Anderson BJ, Auslander WF, Jung KC, Miller JP, Santiago JV. Assessing family sharing of diabetes responsibilities. *J Pediatr Psychol* 1990;15(14):477–92.

129. La Greca AM. Children with diabetes and their families: coping and disease management. In: Field TM, McCabe PM, Schneiderman N, editors. *Stress and Coping Across Development*. Hillsdale, NJ: Erlbaum, 1988:139–59.

130. Bobrow ES, Avruskin TW, Siller J. Mother-daughter interaction and adherence to diabetes regimens. *Diabetes Care* 1985;8(2):146–51.

131. Hauser ST, Jacobson AM, Lavori P, et al. Adherence among children and adolescents with insulin-dependent diabetes mellitus over a 4-year longitudinal follow-up: II. Immediate and long-term linkages with the family milieu. *J Pediatr Psychol* 1990;15(4):527–42.

132. Satin W, La Greca AM, Zigo MA, Skyler JS. Diabetes in adolescence: effects of multifamily group intervention and parent simulation of diabetes. *J Pediatr Psychol* 1989;14(2):259–75.

133. Albrecht T, Edelman M. *Communicating Social Support*. Beverly Hills, CA: Sage Publications, 1987.

134. Daley B. Sponsorship for adolescents with diabetes. *Health Soc Work* 1992;17(3):173–82.

135. La Greca AM. Peer influences in pediatric chronic illness: an update. *J Pediatr Psychol* 1992;17(6):775–84.

136. Lessing DN, Swift PG, Metcalfe MA, Baum JD. Newly diagnosed diabetes: a study of parental satisfaction. *Arch Dis Child* 1992;67(8):1011–3.

137. American Diabetes Association. <http:\\www.diabetes.org/advocacy/discrimination_and_school.asp>. Last accessed: 1/12/2001.

138. Songer TJ. The socioeconomic impact of diabetes upon families with IDDM children. *Diabetes* 1991;40:(Suppl):556A.

139. Songer TJ, LaPorte RE, Lave JR, Dorman JS, Becker DJ. Health insurance and the financial impact of IDDM in families with a child with IDDM. *Diabetes Care* 1997;20(4):577–84.

140. Hanson CL, Henggeler SW, Harris MA, Mitchell KA, Carle DL, Burghen GA. Association between family members' perceptions of the health care system and the health of youths with insulin-dependent diabetes mellitus. *J Pediatr Psychol* 1988;13(4):543–54.

141. Stancin T, Link DL, Reuter JM. Binge eating and purging in young women with IDDM. *Diabetes Care* 1989;12(9):601–3.

142. Hay WW, Groothuis JR, Hayward AR, Levin MJ, editors. Adolescence. In: *Lange Medical Book. Current Pediatric Diagnosis & Treatment*. Stamford, CT: Appleton & Lange, 1997:85–128.

143. Rydall AC, Rodin GM, Olmsted MP, Devenyi RG, Daneman D. Disordered eating behavior and microvascular complications in young women with insulin-dependent diabetes mellitus. *N Engl J Med* 1997;336(26):1849–54.

144. Birk R, Spencer ML. The prevalence of anorexia nervosa, bulimia, and induced glycosuria in IDDM females. *Diabetes Educ* 1989;15(4):336–41.

145. American Psychiatric Association. *Diagnostic and Statistical Manual of Mental Disorders*. 4th ed. (DSM-IV). Washington, DC: American Psychiatric Association, 1994.

146. Hay WW, GGroothuis JR, Hayward AR, Levin MJ, editors. Psychosocial aspects of pediatrics and psychiatric disorders. In: *Lange Medical Book: Current Pediatric Diagnosis & Treatment*. Stamford, CT: Appleton & Lange, 1997:154–94.

147. Rodin GM, Johnson LE, Garfinkel PE, Daneman D, Kenshole AB. Eating disorders in female adolescents with insulin-dependent diabetes mellitus. *Int J Psychiatry Med* 1986–87;16(1):49–57.

148. Minuchin S. *Psychosomatic Families*. Cambridge, MA: Oxford University Press, 1978.

149. Jacobson AM. The psychological care of patients with IDDM. *N Engl J Med* 1996;334(19):1249–53.

150. Bruch H. *Eating Disorders: Obesity, Anorexia, and the Person Within*. New York: Basic Books, 1973.

151. Rodin GM, Craven J, Littlefield C, Murray M, Daneman D. Eating disorders and intentional insulin undertreatment in adolescent females with diabetes. *Psychosomatics* 1991;32(2):171–6.

152. Rosmark B, Berne C, Holmgren S, Lago C, Renholm G, Solberg S. Eating disorders in patients with insulin-dependent diabetes mellitus. *J Clin Psychiatry* 1986;47(11):547–50.

153. Steel JM, Young RJ, Lloyd GG, Clarke BF. Clinically apparent eating disorders in young diabetic women: associations with painful neuropathy and other complications. *Br Med J (Clin Res Ed)* 1987;294(6576):859–62.

154. Krakoff DB. Eating disorders as a special problem for persons with IDDM. *Nurs Clin North Am* 1991;26(3):707–13.

155. Steel JM. Eating disorders in young diabetic women. *Practical Diabetes, International* 1996;13:64–7.

156. Steel JM, Young RJ, Lloyd GG, MacIntyre CC. Abnormal eating attitudes in young insulin-dependent diabetics. *Br J Psychiatry* 1989;155:515–21.

157. Peveler RC, Fairburn CG, Boller IB, Dunger D. Eating disorders in adolescents with IDDM. A controlled study. *Diabetes Care* 1992;15(10):1356–60.

158. Pollock M, Kovacs M, Charron-Prochownik D. Eating disorders and maladaptive dietary/insulin management among youths with childhood-onset IDDM. *J Am Acad Child Adolesc Psychiatry* 1995;34(3):291–6.

159. Garner DM. Pathogenesis of anorexia nervosa. *Lancet* 1993;341(8861):1631–5.

160. Herzog DB, Sacks NR, Keller MB, Lavori PW, von Ranson KB, Gray HM. Patterns and predictors of recovery in anorexia nervosa and bulimia nervosa. *J Am Acad Child Adolesc Psychiatry* 1993;32(4):835–42.

CASE STUDY

Marie is 28 years old and was diagnosed with type 1 diabetes at age 9. She vividly remembers the first few years after diagnosis when she had to rely on urine testing to monitor her glucose levels and needed two insulin shots a day. This morning she does the first of six daily finger sticks to check her blood glucose and determine the settings on her insulin pump. She is thankful for the medical advances in caring for her diabetes and the access she has to these important tools, but she still has to psych herself up to do her finger sticks, change her pump settings, plan her meals and exercise, take care of her family, and do well at her job, let alone find time for herself. She wants to keep her diabetes under tight control so she can continue to be a productive wife, mother, and employee.

As she closely watches her 3-year-old daughter dart around the house, Marie is reminded of the keen interest her parents took in her diabetes and all they did as she grew up to try to protect her from the dangers of this disease. She realizes that her diabetes was expensive for the family and appreciates that her father could afford medical care. It is Marie's husband, Robert, who now shares in the daily challenges of her diabetes. Robert was very concerned about Marie and their baby during her pregnancy. He is glad that Marie received preconception counseling, had carefully planned the pregnancy, and kept an especially close watch on her blood glucose levels while she was pregnant. All these efforts were very expensive, however. Robert is a manager of a small company that does not provide insurance coverage for its employees. Marie now works as a real estate agent, and although she has some medical coverage, she has to pay a very large premium. Robert worries about the expense of diabetes management, whether their daughter will also develop diabetes, and if Marie will continue to be healthy and an active part of the family. Marie and Robert read a lot about diabetes but wish they could take more education programs to understand how to achieve even better diabetes control.

Marie works hard to keep her blood glucose well managed as she tries to balance her family life and job. It seems that the stress of her increasingly complicated daily life makes diabetes management more difficult, but her family needs her income. At a recent appointment, her physician told her that she has some signs of background retinopathy and that her blood pressure is slightly elevated. The physician also counseled Marie about the advisability of having more children. The doctor put her on an ACE inhibitor to control her blood pressure and protect her kidneys and told her that the eye problems were not too serious, but she would continue to closely monitor them. The medicines seem so expensive, but Marie knows how important it is for her to continue good care. Marie hopes for advances in diabetes treatment and progress toward a cure so that her child will not lose her mother prematurely or face getting diabetes herself one day.

4

THE REPRODUCTIVE YEARS

D.L. Rowley, MD, MPH, I.A. Danel, MD, MPH, C.J. Berg, MD, MPH, F. Vinicor, MD, MPH

This chapter presents a review of the prevalence, incidence, and secular trends of diabetes in women of reproductive age. The demographic, socioeconomic (including poverty), sociocultural, and environmental context within which many women with diabetes in this age group live, work, and raise their families is described. The effects of these factors on health behaviors are discussed. Gestational diabetes and its intergenerational effects on the future burden of diabetes among women, preconception counseling, contraception, and patterns in the use of health services are described. Available data suggest that increased awareness of the specific needs of this population is needed, that public policy initiatives be designed to provide comprehensive and continuous care for women in this life stage, and that services be delivered to assure the effective use of these resources. Public health implications of the findings for reproductive-aged women address the three core functions of public health: assessment, policy development, and assurance.

The reproductive years extend from early adolescence to midlife. However, because more than 95% of U.S. women who became pregnant between 1976 and 1996 did so between the ages of 18 and 44 years, especially during their twenties,[1] this chapter will generally address issues relevant to women aged 18–44 years with diabetes. (Reproductive health and diabetes is also addressed in Chapter 3: The Adolescent Years.)

From a public health perspective, during this age span, women's general health issues include adequate maintenance and protection of good health, and often attention to reproductive needs. These are also the years when many women are continuing to develop educationally, entering the workforce, and simultaneously establishing and maintaining their own families. Related challenges during these years may include discontinuous employment, separation and divorce, and consequent loss of economic security and health care coverage. These social and economic factors may affect health directly and may also limit access to, and use of, health care services.

Further, recent studies indicate that a healthy pregnancy is not only of immediate importance to the mother and newborn but also may affect the likelihood of each developing diabetes many years in the future (i.e., there is an intergenerational effect of pregnancy). Finally, the behaviors of women in this age category and the consequent risk factors for future chronic diseases are often established during women's reproductive years. Therefore, women in this age group represent an asymptomatic cohort with extant chronic disease risk factors but little current clinical disease. Thus, to address the future devastation caused by diabetes in women older than 44 years of age, it is important to develop a better understanding of, and public health programs for, those with or at risk for diabetes in this age group.

This chapter will emphasize some of the public health issues faced by women who have or are at risk for diabetes during their reproductive years, including during pregnancy, and discuss the public health implications of associated challenges.

4.1 Prevalence, Incidence, and Trends

Compared with female children and adolescents, reproductive-aged women have a decreased risk of developing type 1 diabetes and an increased risk of developing type 2 diabetes and gestational diabetes mellitus (GDM).[2] Thus, type 2 diabetes accounts for the majority of cases of diabetes identified during this life stage.

Prevalence

On the basis of data from the Third National Health and Nutrition Examination Survey (NHANES III, 1988–1994) of a representative sample of the noninstitutionalized population, the total prevalence (previously diagnosed plus undiagnosed) of diabetes was 1.7% among women aged 20–39 years and 6% among those aged 40–49 years (Figure 4-1).[3] As expected, women of minority racial and ethnic origins were 2–3 times more likely than non-Hispanic white women to have diabetes (Figure 4-2). Among younger women, the total prevalence was 3.3% for non-Hispanic blacks,

2.7% for Mexican Americans, and 1.3% for non-Hispanic whites; among women older than age 39, estimates were 10.4%, 14.1%, and 4.8%, respectively.

In NHANES III, the prevalence of previously diagnosed diabetes increased fourfold, from 1.1% among women aged 20–39 years to 4.4% among those aged 40–49 years (Figure 4-1). Women of minority racial and ethnic origin were more likely to have a previous diagnosis of diabetes (Figure 4-2). At younger ages (less than 40 years), prevalence was 20%–60% higher among non-Hispanic black (1.6%) and Mexican American (1.2%) women than among non-Hispanic white women (0.9%). By age 40, the disparity in diagnosed diabetes increased more than twofold: the prevalence was 6.7% for non-Hispanic black women, 9.2% for Mexican American women, and 3.5% for non-Hispanic white women. These data from NHANES III are consistent with the findings from several other surveys (Table 4-1)[4-11] and indicate the early vulnerability of minority women to diabetes.

Figure 4-1. Prevalence of diagnosed and undiagnosed diabetes among U.S. adults, by age and sex—NHANES III,* 1988–94

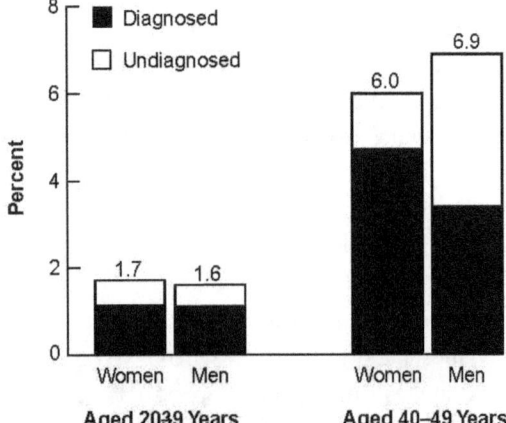

*NHANES III = Third National Health and Nutrition Examination Survey.

Source: Reference 3.

Figure 4-2. Prevalence of diagnosed and undiagnosed diabetes among U.S. women, by age and race/Hispanic origin—NHANES III,* 1988–94

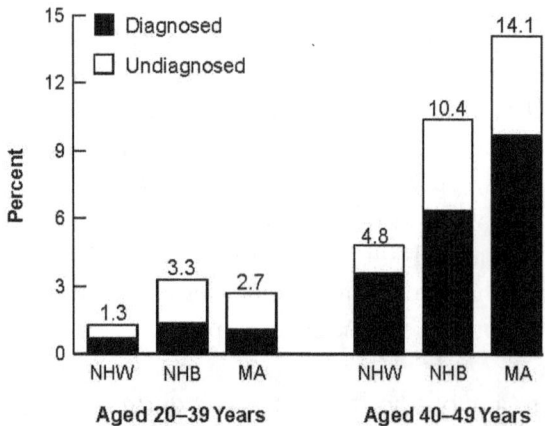

*NHANES III = Third National Health and Nutrition Examination Survey; NHW = non-Hispanic white; NHB = non-Hispanic black; MA = Mexican American.

Source: Reference 3.

Table 4-1. Prevalence of diagnosed diabetes among reproductive-aged women, by race/Hispanic origin– United States, 1965-97

Population	Year	Age group (years)	Prevalence (%)
Alaska Natives			
Alaska Area Native Health Service	1993	15–24	0.9
		25–34	1.7
		35–44	7.6
American Indians			
Navajo			
Teec Nos Pos, Arizona	1990	20–44	5.5
Navajo Health and Nutrition Survey	1991–92	20–44	10.4
Pima	1965–75	25–34	14.5
		35–44	35.1
Indian Health Service	1996	20–44	3.8
Hispanics			
Hispanic Health and Nutrition Examination Survey	1982–84	20–44	
Mexican American			2.3
Cuban			1.8
Puerto Rican			2.5
Behavioral Risk Factor Surveillance System	1994–97	18–44	2.7

Sources: References 7–12.

Using the diagnostic criteria of the American Diabetes Association (fasting plasma glucose ≥126 mg/dL),[?] NHANES III also found that 0.6% of women aged 20–39 years and 1.6% of those aged 40–49 years had diabetes that was undiagnosed (Figure 4-1).[3] Despite their higher prevalence of diagnosed diabetes, non-Hispanic black and Mexican American women were also at least 3 times as likely as non-Hispanic white women to have diabetes that was undiagnosed (Figure 4-2). Among women aged 20–29 years, undiagnosed diabetes was present in 1.7% of non-Hispanic blacks, 1.5% of Mexican Americans, and 0.4% of non-Hispanic whites; by age 40, prevalence rose to 3.7%, 4.9%, and 1.6%, respectively.

Thus, among reproductive-aged women with diabetes, about one-third (35.4%) of women younger than 40 years and about one-quarter (26.7%) of those aged 40 years or older did not know that they had the disease. When NHANES III estimates are

applied to the 1995 intercensal population,[12] nearly 1.85 million reproductive-aged women have diabetes; in approximately 500,000 of them, the disease is unrecognized.

Unlike estimates for children and adolescents, estimates of the prevalence of type 1 diabetes among U.S. adults are not routinely available by sex.[13] In addition, there are no estimates at all for young adults aged 20–29 years. The very limited data available for reproductive-aged women are based on self-reported data from the Second National Health and Nutrition Examination Survey (NHANES II, 1976–1980).[13,14] Persons diagnosed at age 30 or older were considered to have type 1 diabetes if they met the following three criteria: duration of at least 3 years, continuous insulin use since diagnosis, and current weight at 125% or less of desirable weight. Among women aged 30–49 years, the prevalence was 0.1%.

Incidence

Data from the 1990–1992 National Health Interview Surveys (NHIS) show that among women aged 25–44 years, the 3-year average annual incidence rate of diagnosed diabetes was 2.8 per 1,000.[15] When this rate is applied to the 1995 population, approximately 115,000 new cases of diabetes are diagnosed annually in reproductive-aged women.

Few studies of the incidence of diabetes have been conducted in minority populations, but regardless of how diabetes was defined, incidence rates were consistently higher among minority groups compared with the white population.[15-18] In the 16-year (1971–1987) First National Health and Nutrition Examination Survey Epidemiologic Follow-Up Study, the incidence rate of diabetes among black women aged 25–44 years was about 2–2.5 times that of their white counterparts.[15,16] In the San Antonio Heart Study, diabetes developed earlier and the incidence rate was approximately 3 times higher among Mexican American than non-Hispanic white women.[17] Among participants recruited during 1979–1982, the 8-year incidence rate of diabetes for Mexican American women was 4.5% for those aged 25–34 years and 5.2% for those aged 35–44 years. Comparable rates for non-Hispanic white women were 0% and 1.8%, respectively, or approximately one-fourth and one-third the rates for Mexican American women.[17] Age-specific annual incidence rates for Pima Indian women were similar to rates for Mexican American women: 45.2 per 1,000 at ages 25–34 (4.5%) and 56.4 per 1,000 at ages 35–44 years (5.6%).[18]

Incidence of type 1 diabetes peaks around puberty and decreases sharply in late adolescence;[2,19] therefore, many reproductive-aged women with type 1 diabetes enter this life stage with diabetes already diagnosed. No reliable incidence data are available for reproductive-aged women.

Trends

The prevalence of diabetes has been increasing in all demographic groups for several decades.[15,20-25]

Overall, between 1980 and 1996, the prevalence among females younger than 45 years of age remained steady until 1989, then increased by 27%, from 7.3 per 1,000 in 1989 to 9.3 per 1,000 in 1996.[20] An approximate 70% increase in diabetes prevalence among women aged 30–39 years has been noted between 1990 and 1998.[23] Because the majority of females younger than 45 years with diagnosed diabetes are aged 20–44 years, these data primarily reflect the secular trend among reproductive-aged women (unpublished data, CDC, Diabetes Surveillance).

Aging of the population, increased survival, an increase in the rate at which new cases develop (true incidence), and increased or improved identification of cases are factors that may, singly or in combination, contribute to secular increases in prevalence. In young adulthood, aging and mortality make relatively little contribution to the secular trend observed.[21,26] However, data from several large population-based studies indicate that since the 1960s, a rising temporal trend in incidence of type 2 diabetes has been occurring in all age, sex, and racial/ethnic groups.[22,24,25] The steepest rise has occurred among younger adults. Consequently, at this stage of life, incidence is making the greatest contribution to the increasing prevalence observed among young women.

Overweight,[27] weight gain,[28] and lack of physical activity[29] are major risk factors for developing diabetes. These factors have become increasingly common among adolescents and young adults since the 1960s, with the greatest increase taking place during the 1980s.[30-33] One population-based study of women aged 18–30 years found that over the 7 years from 1985–1986 to 1992–1993,[33] average daily energy intake increased while physical activity and physical fitness decreased; these changes occurred concurrently with increasing body mass.[33] Weight gain was strongly associated with decreased physical fitness.[33]

The rapid changes in these risk factors among reproductive-aged women suggest a populationwide impact of social and environmental factors. Moreover, they also suggest that increasing numbers of women, especially nonwhite women, are now at risk of having pregnancies complicated by diabetes.

Gestational Diabetes

As defined by the Fourth International Workshop-Conference on Gestational Diabetes Mellitus, GDM is the presence of carbohydrate intolerance of varying degrees of severity with onset or first recognition during pregnancy.[34] This definition includes all diabetes in pregnancy whether or not the condition was treated with insulin, persisted after pregnancy, or was provoked by or preceded the index pregnancy.[34]

GDM is significant because it is associated with both immediate and long-term implications for the health of the woman[35-37] and her offspring.[38-40] Women with GDM have a 25%–45% higher risk for recurrence in the next pregnancy[37] and a future risk of nongestational diabetes (primarily type 2) ranging from 17% to 63% during the 5 to 16 years following the index pregnancy.[36,38]

The prevalence of GDM is highly variable within and between populations throughout the world.[41] In the United States, estimates of overall prevalence of GDM range from 2.5% to 4% of pregnancies that result in live births.[42-44] Generally, prevalence of GDM is based on data from universal screening of pregnant women.[45-48] Variation in estimates of frequency of GDM may arise from differences in screening[45] and diagnostic[34] protocols, case ascertainment criteria,[42,43,49,50] distributions of risk factors,[41,46,47] and background level of type 2 diabetes.[41]

Women are more likely to develop GDM if they are older; have high prepregnancy weight, high body mass index, or weight gain in young adulthood; have high parity or a history of a previous adverse pregnancy; or have preexisting hypertension or a family history of diabetes.[36,38,47,51] Of interest, these predictive characteristics are also similar to traditional risk factors for type 2 diabetes.

As with type 2 diabetes, the prevalence of GDM varies by race and ethnicity.[41,43-48] Estimates for all women who had single live births during 1993–1995 show considerable variation within and between groups of mothers in the United States.[43,44] For example, among Hispanics, the age-adjusted prevalence of GDM is lowest in Cuban (2.3%), highest in Puerto Rican (3.9%), and intermediate for Mexican (2.8%) and South American (2.4%) mothers (Table 4-2).[43] Some groups of American Indian women have prevalence rates of GDM considerably higher than the national average.[49,51] Among Zuni Indian mothers, reported prevalence is 15.1%; among Navajo Indian women, prevalence was 7.8% and 10.4% at ages 20–29 and 30–39 years, respectively.

4.2 Sociodemographic Characteristics

Age, Race, and Ethnicity

In the reproductive years, women with type 1 diabetes are more likely than women with type 2 diabetes to be diagnosed before adulthood (mean ages, 15.7 years versus 29.3 years). The age distributions of the two groups are therefore very different—8 of 10 women with type 1 diabetes are aged 18–44 years, compared with approximately 1 of 10 women with type 2 diabetes.[52]

No data are available on the racial and ethnic distribution of women with diabetes in this age group. However, in the 1989 NHIS, it was observed that 20.2% of persons with diabetes are non-Hispanic black, 4.8% are Mexican American, and 5.4% are of other races.[52]

Marital Status/Living Arrangements

The 1989 NHIS found that women aged 18–44 years with type 2 diabetes were more likely than their nondiabetic counterparts to report that they were married, divorced, or separated and less likely to report that they had never married (Table 4-3).[52] These differences in marital status between diabetic and nondiabetic women were more pronounced among black than white women. Furthermore, among women with diabetes, black women were less likely than white women to be married (59.9% versus 70.4%) and more likely to be divorced or separated (21.8% versus 13.6%). In addition, black women with diabetes were almost twice as likely as their white counterparts to live alone (9.3% versus 5.7%) and also more likely to live in larger households (59.2% versus 37.3%).

Education/Income/Employment

Reproductive-aged women with type 2 diabetes have fewer years of education, lower incomes, and are less likely than women without diabetes to be in the labor force (Table 4-3).[52] Among women aged 18–44 years, the percentage of those with diabetes who reported that they had completed more than 12 years (30.8%) of education was substantially lower than that of women without diabetes (45.6%); the percentage who had completed at

least 16 years was about half that of their nondiabetic peers (12.8% versus 20.0%). Second, more than half (52.9%) of all women with type 2 diabetes reported a family income less than $20,000. Indeed, for almost half of these women with diabetes, income was less than $10,000. In contrast, the percentages for women without diabetes were 30.7% and 12.2%, respectively. Third, women with diabetes (52.1%) were less likely than those without diabetes (70.8%) to report that they were employed and more likely to report that they were not in the labor force (38.9% versus 25.7%). As expected, in this age group, most women who were not working reported that keeping house was their usual activity in the past 12 months.

These differences were magnified in terms of race and ethnicity. Regardless of diabetes status, black

Table 4-2. Crude and age-adjusted* prevalence† of diabetes during pregnancy, by race/Hispanic origin- United States, 1993- 95

Race or Hispanic origin	Number of women	Prevalence (%)	
		Crude	Age-adjusted
Non-Hispanic			
White	6,996,046	25.3	24.3
Black	1,770,102	22.6	27.5
Hispanic			
Mexican	1,331,361	22.8	27.5
Puerto Rican	161,065	31.6	38.7
Cuban	35,148	24.9	22.7
Central/South American	271,639	25.4	24.3
American Indian/Alaska Native	108,982	43.9	52.4
Asian/Pacific Islander			
Chinese	77,359	39.1	27.3
Japanese	25,885	26.8	21.6
Hawaiian	16,982	28.9	32.6
Filipino	88,487	39.8	32.0
Asian Indian‡	31,574	56.1	44.3
Korean‡	24,918	19.3	16.1
Samoan‡	4,855	25.7	28.7
Vietnamese‡	34,140	24.3	19.5
Total	**11,384,926**	**25.3**	–

* Per 1,000 singleton live-born infants.

† Standard population = aggregate of all races and Hispanic origin.

‡ Data available for seven states only.

Source: Reference 43.

women had fewer years of education, lower incomes, and were less likely to be employed than white women (Table 4-3).[52] Black diabetic women were less likely than their white counterparts to have completed more than 12 years of education (30.2% versus 34.6%) and even less likely to have completed 16 or more years (4.8% versus 17.3%). Among black women with diabetes, more than three-fourths (77.4%) reported family incomes less than $20,000, and although approximately 37% were employed, almost half (49.0%) were not in

the labor force. Comparable percentages for white women were 44.0%, 56.2%, and 34.9%, respectively. These racial disparities in education, income, and employment were more pronounced among women with diabetes than among those without diabetes.

Reproductive-aged women with diabetes also have fewer years of education, lower incomes, and are less likely to be in the labor force than their male counterparts.[52] Further, these sex differences are

Table 4-3. Prevalence (%) of sociodemographic characteristics of women aged 18-44 years with and without type 2 diabetes, by race/Hispanic origin- United States, 1989

Characteristic	Non-Hispanic white		Non-Hispanic black		Total	
	Diabetes	No diabetes	Diabetes	No diabetes	Diabetes	No diabetes
Marital status						
Married	70.4	67.2	59.9	37.0	65.6	62.7
Widowed	1.0	0.6	3.6	1.5	2.1	0.7
Divorced or separated	13.6	10.5	21.8	17.7	19.0	11.4
Never married	15.0	22.2	14.7	43.8	13.2	25.2
Living arrangements						
Alone	5.7	8.7	9.3	8.2	6.1	8.3
Nonrelative only	1.4	3.4	2.4	0.9	1.9	2.9
Spouse	69.7	66.7	59.9	35.1	65.3	61.8
Other relative only	23.2	21.2	28.5	55.8	26.8	27.0
Household size (no. of persons)						
1	7.0	12.1	11.7	9.2	8.0	11.3
2	24.6	20.8	23.1	20.6	22.4	20.2
3	31.0	24.3	6.1	23.4	25.9	23.9
≥4	37.3	42.8	59.2	46.7	43.8	44.6
Education (years)						
<9	2.6	1.8	6.3	3.0	6.9	3.6
9–12	62.9	49.7	63.5	61.3	62.3	50.8
>12	34.6	48.4	30.2	35.7	30.8	45.6
≥16	17.3	22.3	4.8	10.8	12.8	20.0
Annual family income ($thousands)						
<10	21.0	8.7	30.5	28.6	25.7	12.2
10 – <20	23.0	16.8	46.9	24.9	27.2	18.5
20 – <40	36.2	37.7	8.6	31.5	29.6	36.5
≥40	19.9	36.8	14.1	15.0	17.5	32.8
Employment status						
Employed	56.2	73.3	37.4	65.1	52.1	70.8
Unemployed	8.9	3.0	13.6	6.9	9.0	3.5
Not in labor force	34.9	23.7	49.0	28.0	38.9	25.7

Source: Reference 52.

greater among persons with diabetes than in the nondiabetic population. Education, income, and employment are commonly used indicators of socioeconomic status (SES). The findings from the 1989 NHIS suggest that among reproductive-aged women, diabetes amplifies the racial and sex disparities in SES found in the general population. Moreover, the gap in SES between women with and without diabetes appears to have worsened over time.[53] For example, data from the 1979–1981 NHIS showed that 37.1% of women without diabetes were in the highest income group (≥$25,000), compared with 32.7% of women with diabetes. By 1989, 32.8% of women without diabetes were in the highest income group (≥$40,000) compared with only 17.5% of women with diabetes. Further, whereas the percentage of employed nondiabetic women increased from 62.7% in 1979–1981 to 70.8% in 1989, the percentage of employed diabetic women increased only slightly, from 49.8% during 1979–1981 to 52.1% in 1989.

Presently, no data on sociodemographic characteristics among women with diabetes of other ethnic origins are available, nor are they available for reproductive-aged women with type 1 diabetes.[52]

4.3. Impact of Diabetes on Health Status

Death Rates

Diabetes mellitus is a leading cause of death among American women of reproductive age.[54] In 1996, diabetes ranked ninth overall, ninth among white and Hispanic women, and seventh among black women aged 25–44 years. However, because diabetes is not recorded anywhere on more than 60% of the death certificates of decedents with diabetes,[55] data derived from death certificates significantly underestimate the actual contribution of diabetes to total mortality in the U.S. population as well as the mortality risk for people with diabetes.

Many clinical and epidemiologic studies of selected populations have shown consistently that people with diabetes have higher mortality rates than those without diabetes.[10,26,55-65] Most of these studies

recruited middle-aged subjects and provided summary age-adjusted measures; consequently, few data on mortality exist for diabetic women younger than 45 years of age.

The First National Health and Nutrition Examination Survey (NHANES I, 1971–1975) included a representative sample of the noninstitutionalized U.S. population aged 25–74 years. Participants with and without diabetes at baseline examination were followed through 1992–1993.[63] Vital status was ascertained for 97.9% of persons with diabetes and 96.1% of those without. In all age, sex, and non-Hispanic racial groups, death rates were higher for people with diabetes than for those without diabetes.

Among those aged 25–44 years, the overall death rate for women with diabetes was more than 3 times the rate for women without diabetes (9.3 per 1,000 person-years versus 2.9 per 1,000 person-years).[63] Excess mortality among women with diabetes was present in both white and black groups, but the magnitude of the excess in black women (2.6) was smaller than that in white women (4.0).

Figure 4-3. All-cause mortality rates for U.S. adults aged 25-44 years, by diabetes status, sex, and race/ Hispanic origin, 1971-93

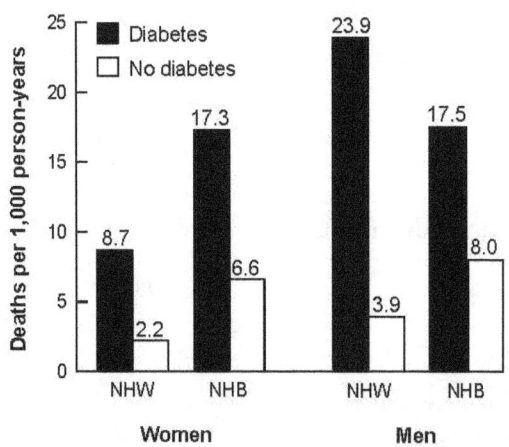

NHW = non-Hispanic white; NHB = non-Hispanic black.

Source: Reference 63.

This racial difference may be due, in part, to the higher death rates experienced by nondiabetic black women than by nondiabetic white women (Figure 4-3).

Among women with diabetes, the death rate among black women was twice the rate of white women (17.3 per 1,000 person-years versus 8.7 per 1,000 person-years) (Figure 4-3). The sex differential in mortality seen in the general population is also found in the diabetic population (i.e., the death rate among diabetic women is lower than the rate among diabetic men). However, the NHANES I Follow-Up Study found that whereas the death rate among diabetic white reproductive-aged women was approximately one-third the rate of their male counterparts (8.7 per 1,000 person-years versus 23.9 per 1,000 person years), in this age group no sex differential in mortality was seen among diabetic blacks in this age group.[63]

Data from the NHANES I Follow-Up Study represent the experience of adults primarily with type 2 diabetes; only 49 persons were thought to have type 1 diabetes.[63] The Diabetes Epidemiology Research International (DERI) Mortality Study followed persons in Allegheny County, Pennsylvania, who were diagnosed with type 1 diabetes before the age of 18 years.[64] Estimated death rates for women with diabetes were 2.6 per 1,000 at ages 20–24 years, 7.7 per 1,000 at ages 25–29 years, and 16.6 per 1,000 at 30–39 years. Follow-up data for the period through 1990 also suggest that the racial disparity in mortality present in persons with type 2 diabetes is also present among persons with type 1.[65] In the DERI cohort, black women died at almost 4 times the rate of white women (15.9 per 1,000 person-years versus 4.0 per 1,000 person-years). Although the numbers of events were small, the data also suggest that among persons with type 1 diabetes, the burden of mortality among younger black women is markedly higher than that among black men of similar age.[65] Of interest, there was no sex difference in mortality among whites in this age group.

Complications

All people with diabetes, including reproductive-aged women, have higher risks of morbidity than those without diabetes. Common medical complications associated with diabetes include microvascular disease (retinopathy, nephropathy, and neuropathy) that is specific to diabetes and manifestations of atherosclerotic macrovascular disease (coronary heart disease, stroke, and peripheral vascular disorders). These complications, especially microvascular diseases, are strongly related to the duration of exposure to the altered metabolic state associated with diabetes. Consequently, most data available for younger adults are derived from studies of persons who developed diabetes before adulthood.

Retinopathy. Diabetic retinopathy is caused by alterations in the small blood vessels in the retina in response to hyperglycemia and hypertension.[66] Diabetic retinopathy is classified as either nonproliferative or proliferative diabetic retinopathy (PDR).

Retinopathy is associated with the duration of diabetes.[66] Seven years after the diagnosis of type 1 diabetes, 50% of patients will have some degree of retinopathy; 20 years after diagnosis, more than 90% are affected. In the Wisconsin Epidemiologic Study of Diabetic Retinopathy (WESDR), 3 years after diagnosis among people with the onset of diabetes after age 30 who were not taking insulin, 23% had retinopathy and 2% had PDR. After 20 years, 60% in this group had retinopathy and 5% had PDR.

In the WESDR, there were no significant differences in the 4- or 10-year incidence or progression of diabetic retinopathy between the sexes for people with either younger-onset (less than 30 years of age) or older-onset diabetes.[66] It is therefore important to realize that women who develop retinopathy during their reproductive years are most likely to have been diagnosed before adulthood (i.e., they probably have type 1 diabetes). In addition, pregnancy is a risk factor for the progression of retinopathy among women with type 1 diabetes.[67] In one case-control study, pregnant women were twice as likely to progress to PDR as nonpregnant women (7.3% versus 3.7%). This finding remained statistically significant even after controlling for glycated hemoglobin (HbA$_{1c}$).[68]

Nephropathy. Diabetic nephropathy is the most common single cause of end-stage renal disease (ESRD) in the U.S. population (about 40% of new cases of ESRD are due to diabetes) and is the diabetic complication associated with increased cardiovascular disease morbidity and mortality.[69] Among people with diabetes for 15 or more years, nephropathy develops in 35%–40% of patients with type 1 diabetes and less than 20% of those with type 2 diabetes.[70] However, because type 2 diabetes is much more common than type 1, the majority of cases of ESRD due to diabetes are in persons with type 2 diabetes.[70] In the reproductive years, diabetic nephropathy may be diagnosed somewhat earlier in women than men because as many as 25% of all cases of diabetic nephropathy among women can be diagnosed during pregnancy. In early pregnancy, women with preexisting diabetic nephropathy may have a marked increase in protein excretion because of the rise in glomerular filtration rate that normally occurs in pregnancy.[70] This phenomenon may increase the likelihood of earlier detection of diabetic nephropathy.

Pregnancy does not seem to adversely affect the course of early diabetic renal disease.[70,71] However, pregnancy hastens the onset of end-stage renal disease in women who have more severe impairment as manifested by hypertension and decreased renal function.

Cardiovascular disease. Diabetes is a major risk factor for cardiovascular disease (CVD), primarily atherosclerotic coronary heart disease (CHD), and stroke.[72] CHD is the most common cause of mortality and morbidity among people with diabetes. CHD is also the most costly of the long-term chronic complications of diabetes because of the

frequency of events and the need for hospitalization and use of technological devices.[73,74] However, CHD is uncommon before 30 years of age, even when diabetes is diagnosed in childhood.[73] In addition, the data from most population-based studies are derived from middle-aged participants. Thus, data are sparse on the frequency of CHD among reproductive-aged women; the most reliable data are from studies of persons with type 1 diabetes.

The EURODIAB IDDM complications study of 3,250 adults with type 1 diabetes included men (51%) and women (49%) with similar mean age (33 years) and duration of diabetes (14.6 years).[75] Among women, the overall prevalence of total CVD was 10%, including myocardial infarction (1.5%), angina (1.8%), and stroke (0.9%). There was no sex difference in prevalence of CVD. Within the reproductive age range, estimates for the prevalence of CVD were 6% and 8% for women aged 15–29 and 30–44 years, respectively. The prevalence of CVD was associated strongly with duration of diabetes in both sexes. For duration of less than 15 years, the prevalence was somewhat greater among women than men (for 1–7 years, 9% versus 6%; for 8–14 years, 7% versus 5%, respectively).[76] These data suggest that the protection from CVD found in nondiabetic women is lost in the presence of diabetes, even at these younger ages.[77]

Other population-based studies provide additional information regarding CVD in reproductive-aged women with diabetes. According to the 1989 NHIS, among adults aged 18–44 years with diabetes, the overall prevalence of self-reported angina was 3.9%.[73] In this age group, angina was twice as likely to be reported among those with type 2 diabetes as those with type 1 diabetes (1.9%). Insulin users were more likely to report angina (4.9%) than those who did not use insulin (3.8%). Perhaps most impressively, compared with persons without diabetes, those with diabetes reported a 10-fold higher prevalence of self-reported ischemic heart disease (2.7% versus 0.2%).[73] Unfortunately, these NHIS data were not stratified by sex.

In the Nurses' Health Study, a cohort of women recruited at ages 30–55 years and followed for the 8-year period 1976 to 1984, the risk of developing CHD and stroke among women with diabetes was 6.7 and 4.1 times that among women without diabetes, respectively.[58] Women who were diagnosed with diabetes before age 30 years had greater incidence of cardiovascular disease: the relative risks (RR) were at least 10 times those of their nondiabetic counterparts (CHD, RR=12.2; stroke, RR=10.0).[58]

Because of 1) the magnitude of the problem of CVD in persons with diabetes, including women,[77,78] 2) evidence of efficacious interventions involving lipid and blood pressure reduction in diabetic women in this age category,[79,80] 3) the need to target high-risk diabetic persons,[81] and 4) gaps in the application of these efficacious prevention programs in actual practice, improved delivery of effective clinical interventions is needed.

However, to maximize efforts to reduce the burden of diabetes for women at this stage of life (as well as future generations),[82,83] one must move beyond a clinical view of diabetes.[84] For example, reproductive-aged women with diabetes—even in the absence of clinically apparent diabetes complications—often have risk factors leading to later development of cardiovascular disease, renal disease, retinopathy, and other chronic conditions. Reproductive-aged women with diabetes are silently "cardio-toxic" and poised to display the consequences of these diabetes-associated risk factors. How should these diabetic women who have yet to develop typical clinical manifestations of diabetes be identified? What are the risks and benefits of such screening programs? Should this large cohort of reproductive-aged women with diabetes but no apparent clinical disease be the target of interventions before they develop CVD? If CVD does develop, what is the impact on the family (since the woman is most often the family caregiver and manager as well as a contributor to the economic security of the family)? These important public health

issues relevant to reproductive-aged women with diabetes must be considered.

Intensive Therapy and Its Effects on Quality of Life

In determining the burden of a disease, clinical medicine and public health have traditionally monitored mortality rates. This singular criterion for disease burden reflects the dominance of acute, infectious diseases in the first half of the 20th century. With the emergence of chronic diseases during the latter half of the 20th century, other indicators—morbidity, disability, economic impact, and especially health-related quality of life (HRQOL)—have been used as measures of disease burden. HRQOL captures aspects of self-perceived well-being affected by the presence or treatment of disease[85,86] and focuses on outcomes within the context of patient expectations.[86-88] As a result of increasing attention to "tight diabetes regulation,"[89,90] HRQOL measurements are being used. In the Diabetes Control and Complications Trial (DCCT), multiple indices of quality of life (one specific to diabetes and two more general measures) examined the effect of intensive therapy compared with conventional glucose control for type 1 diabetes.[91] Despite the increased demands of intensive therapy, no deterioration was noted in quality of life except among patients who experienced repeated, severe hypoglycemic episodes.[91] No differences were noted between sexes. However, these patients had access to a multidisciplinary team of professionals, and time, effort, and resources were directed to patients receiving intensive therapy.[92] The United Kingdom Prospective Diabetes Study, which examined the impact of improved glucose and blood pressure control in persons with type 2 diabetes, also measured HRQOL and could detect no significant differences in quality of life measurements between intensive and control treatment strategies, or between women and men.[93] Indeed, studies suggest that with improved glycemic—and perhaps blood pressure—control, perceived quality of life is better among patients, including reproductive-aged women.[88,94,95]

However, the complexities of HRQOL need greater study, including analyses of such factors as type of therapy, sex, education level, cultural factors, race and ethnicity, and professional or social support among reproductive-aged women.[88,96] Although measurement of HRQOL for chronic conditions such as diabetes is a useful indicator of disease burden, present assays still focus almost exclusively on the individual woman with diabetes. Poor quality of life due to diabetes or its treatment, however, has a considerably broader impact on groups of people and society at large. If the HRQOL of an individual reproductive-aged woman is low, the family, community, and society also experience a lower HRQOL. For example, diminished job performance, productivity, and income associated with low HRQOL of an individual woman with diabetes also affects the family income and perhaps business productivity.[95] Further, with improved diabetes control, not only does the individual experience a higher HRQOL, but also society at large benefits in terms of employment and productivity.[95] Thus, even as the diabetes community moves toward measurements of quality of life as an important indicator of disease control, a broader societal view of this dimension should be considered as part of a public health approach to diabetes among reproductive-aged women.

Hospitalizations

Data on hospitalization rates for women with diabetes are available from the National Hospital Discharge Survey (NHDS). However, NHDS data are limited by a lack of personal identifiers and hence offer no way to distinguish people with multiple annual hospitalizations. Using NHDS data, a U-shaped trend was noted between 1980 and 1994 in hospital discharge rates among women aged 20–44 years with diabetes as the primary, or first-listed, diagnosis. These rates decreased from 14 per 10,000 population in 1980 to 8.4 in 1990 and then increased to 11.2 in 1994.[97] Women with diabetes aged 20–44 had higher hospitalization rates than men in the same age group in the early 1980s, but these hospitalization rates decreased during the 1990s. White women aged 20–44 with diabetes as a primary diagnosis had lower hospitalization rates

than all women; however, the same U-shaped trend curve was noted: rates were 10.9 per 10,000 population in 1980, 5.7 in 1990, and 7.4 in 1994.[97] Because of small numbers, no reliable information is available on hospitalization rates among black women with diabetes as a first diagnosis.

Among people aged 20–44 years, hospitalization discharge rates for diabetes as any listed diagnosis (per 10,000 population) are slightly higher for women than for men. Between 1980 and 1994, rates for men showed a tendency to increase from 24.8 to 32.0 discharges per 10,000 population, while those for women fluctuated between 33 and 42 with no clear trend. Black people had higher discharge rates for diabetes than white people, and black women had the highest rates of all, fluctuating between 57 and 74 discharges per 10,000 population.

Among persons aged 44 years or younger with diabetes, hospitalization rates with diabetes listed as the primary diagnosis decreased during this time period from 162 per 1,000 diabetic population to 110.[97] Rates were slightly higher for men than for women but decreased for both sexes. Rates for white women with diabetes as a primary diagnosis were lower than for women as a whole, suggesting that black women with diabetes had a higher discharge rate. However, results were not reported separately for black women.

Hospital discharge rates among people aged 44 years or younger with diabetes as any listed diagnosis also decreased between 1980 and 1994, from 325 per 1,000 diabetic population to 283. Rates decreased for both sexes and were slightly higher for women than for men. Hospitalization rates for white men and women with diabetes tended to decrease between 1980 and 1994 but remained unchanged for black men and women. Between 1990 and 1994, hospitalization rates with diabetes as any listed diagnosis were 300–360 per 1,000 diabetic population for black women and 195–235 per 1,000 diabetic population for white women.[97] The higher hospital discharge rates for black women with diabetes than for white women with diabetes suggest that black women may receive less adequate or appropriate ambulatory care and thus require more hospitalizations for complications.

Data from the 1994–1997 NHIS are consistent with the findings presented above. Approximately 21% of women aged 18–44 years with diabetes reported at least one hospitalization in the previous year (excluding any hospitalizations for childbirth), compared with only 6% of women without diabetes.

Hyperglycemia During Pregnancy

An initial recognition of hyperglycemia occurs in pregnancy either because of prepregnancy diabetes or because of GDM. Earlier studies of hyperglycemia during pregnancy focused primarily on the health of the infant because of higher rates of perinatal morbidity, particularly when GDM is not treated or when preexisting diabetes is not well controlled.[34,35] Mothers with diabetes or GDM also deserve attention because they are at greater risk than nondiabetic pregnant women for pregnancy complications including preeclampsia, caesarean section, and infections.[34,35,84]

However, in addition to these clinical reasons for attention to hyperglycemia during pregnancy, the future of the reproductive-aged woman with GDM as well as the future of her offspring are two important public health issues that are receiving increasing recognition. For women, GDM is a risk factor for the recurrence of GDM in future pregnancies and also for the subsequent future development of type 2 diabetes.[35-37] Recurrence rates for progression to subsequent type 2 diabetes increase with the age of the mother and for women with other risk factors for developing type 2 diabetes, especially ethnicity, prepregnancy and postpregnancy weight and weight gain, parity, family history of type 2 diabetes, and level of physical activity after pregnancy.[35-37]

Several important public health issues require additional study, such as what should be the screening recommendations for GDM, including cut-off points as well as evidence to decide whether screening should be routinely performed for all women.[34,98,99] For example, it is possible that considerable harm could occur when a woman is told that she has GDM in the absence of solid evidence that adverse outcomes will occur in all women.[99] Also, what should be the clinical practice recommendations for women with either prepregnancy diabetes or GDM? Should all women with either of these conditions receive only specialty care? Is overuse of services (such as universal screenings and C-sections[100]) now occurring, which from a societal perspective is as harmful as underuse of services for the individual woman? Finally, considering the evidence documenting the progression of GDM to type 2 diabetes, especially in minority populations, what should be the guidelines for follow-up to detect type 2 diabetes early? Even more importantly, are primary prevention programs, especially behavioral strategies, likely to either prevent or at least delay this progression, as has been demonstrated with the use of medication in high-risk populations?[101]

Recent studies have identified other important consequences of maternal hyperglycemia—the impact on offspring beyond the immediate peripartum period. This intergenerational effect of hyperglycemia during pregnancy has long-term effects on the metabolism and health of the offspring of that pregnancy. Children of diabetic mothers have up to a 10-fold increased risk of becoming obese during childhood and adolescence, as well as developing glucose intolerance in puberty.[39,102-104] Further, it has been observed that the likelihood of a person developing type 2 diabetes is 70% greater if the mother has type 2 diabetes than if the father has diabetes,[105] suggesting that the intrauterine environment, in addition to genetics, contributes to the subsequent development of diabetes in the offspring of diabetic mothers.

Additional studies have extensive documentation of the effects of the intrauterine environment on the subsequent development of many chronic diseases, even in the offspring of women without hyper-glycemia during pregnancy. Initial studies in the United Kingdom have indicated that the develop-ment of components of the insulin resistance syn-drome (IRS)—hypertension, central adiposity, dys-lipidemia, insulin resistance, and hyperglycemia—was inversely correlated with the size of the baby at birth (i.e., the smaller the baby, the more likely that newborn will develop components of the IRS 20–40 years later).[39,106-110] This relationship, with some variation (e.g., U-shaped relationship between fetal/newborn size and subsequent IRS),[39] has now been observed in different populations throughout the world.[110,111] These findings suggest that changes in the growth and development of the fetus in utero that are secondary to nutritional disturbances are associated with permanent metabolic alterations in the offspring that will result in chronic condi-tions like impaired glucose tolerance, type 2 dia-betes, CVD, and hypertension. Although a specific pathophysiologic mechanism for the effect of improper in utero nutrition has yet to be identified, the concept of "fetal programming" may be rele-vant.[112,113] Impaired beta cell function or peripheral insulin resistance secondary to impaired fetal matu-rity associated with maternal hyperglycemia[114] may contribute, along with obesity and inadequate phys-ical activity, to type 2 diabetes in youth.[115-117]

Several important public health issues emerge from the preceding metabolic and epidemiologic observa-tions of reproductive-aged women, especially if hyperglycemia is present. Considering 1) the dia-betes epidemic in the United States and throughout the world,[118-120] 2) recognition of the importance of primary prevention (in addition to improved dia-betes care) to control the emerging burden of dia-betes,[121] and 3) initial evidence that the progression of GDM or impaired glucose tolerance to type 2 diabetes can be reduced,[101,122] decisions need to be made about screening for GDM, as well as offering effective nutrition and physical activity programs for those at higher risk of developing diabetes (e.g., reproductive-aged women).

4.4 Health-Related Behaviors

Risk Behaviors and Risk Factors

Although several immutable factors are associated with an increased risk of developing type 2 diabetes (e.g., genetics, age, race/ethnicity),[6,123,124] personal patterns of behavior also contribute to a greater incidence of diabetes. Thus, nutritional patterns that increase the risk for elevated body mass index (BMI) or weight gain after age 18, lack of physical activity, and cigarette smoking are behavioral risk factors associated with the development of type 2 diabetes and its complications.

Obesity. Population-based data from several studies document an increase in overweight (BMI ≥ 25 kg/m^2) and obesity (BMI ≥ 30 kg/m^2) in the United States over the last decade.[125,126] A 47% increase in the percentage of women who were obese among those aged 18 years or older was noted between 1991 and 1998.[126] Overweight, weight gain, and obesity are associated with consequent impaired glucose tolerance and type 2 diabetes.[27,28,127] For example, NHANES II data indicate that diabetes is 2.9 times more prevalent among overweight people than those of normal weight status.[28] Thus, increased obesity in the United States may be con-tributing to the increase in the prevalence of dia-betes. Between the National Health Examination Survey (NHES, 1963–1965) and NHANES II (1976–1980), the prevalence of obesity among girls aged 12 to 17 years increased by 108% among whites and 151% among blacks.[128] Obesity is also greater among black than white women, and the percentage of women of both races who are over-weight increases with age up to age 70.[126] Data from NHANES II showed that 9% of white women and 24% of black women aged 20–24 years were over-weight as were 25% of white women and 41% of black women aged 35–44 years—a prevalence 65% higher among black women.[28]

In recent studies documenting a disturbing increase in diabetes in the United States,[23,120] a statistical association between weight and increasing prevalence of diabetes in both black and white women has been confirmed. Among women aged 30–55 years in the Nurses' Health Study, the risk for diagnosed diabetes increased almost exponentially with increases in BMI:[27,127] women with a BMI of 23–23.9 kg/m² had a risk of developing diabetes 3.6 times higher than women with a BMI of less than 22 kg/m². The risk of developing diabetes for women with a BMI of 29–30.9 kg/m² was 20 times higher, and for women with a BMI of 35 kg/m² or more, it was 61 times higher. A separate analysis of data from the Nurses' Health Study showed that attributable risk for body weight to the incidence of type 2 diabetes also increased with BMI. Among women with a BMI of more than 33 kg/m², 98% of the diagnoses of diabetes were attributable to obesity. Further, weight gain after age 18 years was a major determinant of risk. Finally, the Nurses' Health Study found that in addition to BMI, waist-to-hip ratio (WHR) and waist circumference were also independent predictors of subsequent development of diabetes,[27,127] suggesting that useful, accessible, and simple tools to determine the risk of developing diabetes are available.

The impact of pregnancy on subsequent weight gain over time and with increasing age is a unique challenge to women and increases their chances of developing diabetes.[129-132] For example, over a 5-year period, women who had previously given birth at least once gained 2 kg–3 kg and had a greater increase in WHR, independent of weight gain, than did women who were giving birth for the first time.[129,130] Further, black women had greater increases in adiposity at each level of parity than did white women.[130] Although not all studies have confirmed this impact of pregnancy on subsequent weight gain in reproductive-aged women,[131] about 15%–20% of women experience substantial weight gain after delivery,[132] thereby acquiring a greater risk of developing type 2 diabetes. The interaction of this weight gain after pregnancy with the presence of GDM may be a major factor in progression to type 2 diabetes, especially in women from minority populations.[35,37,46,48]

Physical inactivity. The interrelationships between weight gain and physical inactivity in the development of type 2 diabetes are complex. In a prospective 7-year study of residents of urban areas aged 18–30 years, a strong association between weight gain and decrease in physical fitness was noted.[33,133] Further, the association of weight gain with decreased physical fitness was greatest among those who were overweight at baseline. Finally, black women weighed more and reported significantly less physical activity at baseline than white women and had a higher percent increase in overweight.[133]

Several recent publications have examined relationships between physical activity and the subsequent development of diabetes in high-risk populations, including women aged 18–44.[29,33,122,134] In general, women who engage in more physical activity over a longer period of time have a decreased likelihood of developing type 2 diabetes. In terms of differences in amount, type, or duration of physical activity between women with and without diabetes, among women aged 18–44 years, rates of physical activity and exertion of 2,000 kcal/wk or more did not vary by diabetic status. Although women with diabetes were more likely than women without this condition to engage in walking, they were less likely to report other regular physical activity.[135]

Improving physical activity behaviors among reproductive-aged women is clearly a relevant intervention for preventing type 2 diabetes.[121,136]

Cigarette smoking. The prevalence of cigarette smoking among persons with or at risk for diabetes is not very different than in persons without diabetes.[137] In addition to the likely greater incidence of diabetes complications in diabetic persons who smoke,[138,139] more recent studies suggest that cigarette consumption is associated with a greater incidence of type 2 diabetes in an independent and dose-dependent fashion,[140,141] perhaps due to increased insulin resistance in association with cigarette use.[142] Thus, an increased risk for the development of diabetes may be another complication of smoking.

Health-Promoting Behaviors

Despite the association between four risk factors—nutrition behaviors (and resultant weight or weight gain), physical inactivity, smoking, and maternal health prior to and during pregnancy—and the subsequent development of type 2 diabetes, is there also evidence that improving behaviors in each of these areas will reduce the risk of diabetes to the woman or her offspring? Further, what are the public health implications of this evidence?

Weight/nutrition. Although longitudinal studies have established the association between weight, weight gain, nutrition, and diabetes incidence,[33,125-127,143] few investigations have scientifically examined the impact of planned changes in behaviors that affect these factors and diabetes incidence. Further, few have examined the impact of improved nutrition alone (i.e., separate from concomitant changes in physical activity). Among overweight persons with established diabetes, intentional weight loss was associated with substantial reductions in all-cause mortality as well as CVD mortality.[144] Preliminary investigations on the impact of intentional weight loss in preventing the onset of diabetes also suggest a clear effect in women, including reproductive-aged women.[145] Finally, in the Da Qing study, weight control itself resulted in an approximately one-third decrease in the conversion of impaired glucose tolerance (IGT) to diabetes in both women and men.[134] Additional information will soon be forthcoming from two primary prevention trials to provide further support for the benefits of weight management itself in preventing type 2 diabetes.[146,147] In the meantime, there is reason for optimism that weight control can be achieved, particularly in youth,[148] and that the onset of type 2 diabetes can be prevented, if not substantially delayed.

Physical activity. As with weight management, several studies of varied design have linked higher levels of physical activity with a decreased risk of developing type 2 diabetes in women.[29,133,134,148,149] One randomized controlled trial examined the effect of physical activity alone in reducing the conversion of

IGT to type 2 diabetes, resulting in about a one-third decrease in the incidence of diabetes.[134] Other studies wherein weight control and increased physical activity were combined in a randomized control study design have demonstrated an approximate 50% reduction in the incidence of diabetes over a 5-year follow-up period.[122] While recent investigations in men indicate the beneficial effects of exercise-induced weight loss,[149] similar studies in reproductive-aged women are pending. Results from the important randomized controlled trial—the Diabetes Prevention Program[147]—will provide additional support for the benefits of physical activity (along with weight management) in the efficacy and cost-effectiveness of preventing type 2 diabetes in several populations, including reproductive-aged women. Other benefits of physical activity among reproductive-aged women with type 2 diabetes include improved physical and social functioning and mental health.[150] In this regard, physical activity, because of its psychological benefits, may be especially advantageous to women with diabetes, whose quality of life scores are lower than those of men with diabetes.[150] At present, given the increasing evidence of the benefits of physical activity for persons at risk for or with diabetes, many lifestyle guidelines are available. The challenge will be increasingly directed toward implementing and sustaining both weight control and physical activity patterns to prevent several chronic diseases, not to determine if such programs will work.[151]

Smoking cessation. For people with established diabetes, smoking cessation for both men and women is ultimately beneficial in terms of mortality.[136] However, the risk for mortality remains higher for several years in persons with diabetes who once smoked compared with diabetic persons who never smoked. Further, the longer duration of smoking among persons with diabetes significantly lessens the benefit of quitting smoking.[139,140] For persons without diabetes who smoke, the impact of cigarette use on the incidence of diabetes appears to decrease over time but may take a decade to return to nonsmoking levels.[140]

Family planning. Healthy behaviors are very relevant to several aspects of family planning, including planning for pregnancy, metabolic control prior to and during pregnancy, and postpregnancy status and follow-up of the mother and her offspring.

Because a woman with diabetes can have a normal, healthy pregnancy and delivery, it is important that conception and subsequent pregnancies be carefully planned.[152] Should pregnancy not be desired, proper contraception is an important consideration.[153] Diabetes affects the preferred method of contraception. Because intrauterine devices (IUDs) have been associated with an increased risk for pelvic infection, use among women with diabetes has previously been limited. However, several controlled studies using newer IUDs have shown them to be safe and effective in reproductive-aged women with diabetes.[154]

Low-dose combination oral contraceptives can also be used for contraception by women with diabetes. However, selection of the proper progestin and estrogen dosages for diabetic women to minimize potential adverse effects on glucose, lipid, and blood pressure should be considered.[153,154]

Preconception care. Previous epidemiologic and clinical studies have confirmed that women with type 1 or 2 diabetes have a higher incidence of spontaneous abortions, maternal complications during pregnancy, and fetal and neonatal mortality and morbidity.[153,154] These devastating complications are related to the level of glycemic regulation at the time of conception and in the first weeks of pregnancy, and with good metabolic control, can be reduced to rates almost comparable to those of women without diabetes.[155-159] Further, evidence indicates that these interventions are actually cost saving.[155,160]

Given these scientific and economic data, public health responsibilities are to ensure that the benefits of this knowledge are applied to all reproductive-aged women so that proper health systems are available and used widely. One approach has been to establish registries of persons with diabetes, especially of reproductive-aged women, to ensure proper planning, counseling, and care prior to and during pregnancy.[161] Further, such registries can also facilitate careful follow-up of women with GDM to minimize subsequent conversion to IGT or type 2 diabetes.

Among prepregnancy counseling issues, decisions about risks for diabetes in offspring should be considered. A parental history of diabetes has been a major exposure in several epidemiologic investigations of the development of diabetes in offspring.[162] Of particular interest is the fact that both the sex of the parent with diabetes and the type of diabetes have a differential effect on diabetes developing in the offspring. Paternal type 1 diabetes is more likely to "transmit" type 1 diabetes to the offspring than type 1 diabetes in the mother.[163,164] In contrast, the presence of type 2 diabetes in the mother is associated with a greater likelihood of type 2 diabetes ultimately developing in the offspring than if the father has type 2 diabetes.[165,166] These observations regarding maternal transmission of type 2 diabetes may be a consequence of the environmental impact of maternal hyperglycemia during pregnancy (i.e., a component of fetal programming).[107,114]

Lactation. Women with type 1 diabetes choose to breast-feed at the same rate as mothers from the general hospital population;[167] however, mothers with type 1 diabetes are more likely to add formula supplements within several weeks of delivery.[167,168] In addition, the onset of copious milk production is delayed among women with type 1 diabetes. The extent of the delay in lactogenesis correlates directly with adequacy of maternal glycemic control.[169]

Once lactation is established, the breast milk of women with type 1 diabetes does not differ in lactose, protein, lipid, or calcium content, but it may contain higher levels of glucose and sodium and lower concentrations of long-chain polyunsaturated fatty acids. Data on any effects of these qualitative differences in breast milk are not presently available.

An emerging issue that may have an impact on lactation counseling for women with and without diabetes is the possible association of cow's milk during the newborn period with the subsequent development of type 1 or 2 diabetes.[170-176] However, results of studies and recommendations have been controversial. A recent study documented high insulin concentrations in breast milk.[177] Thus, with formula/cow's milk use, an increased incidence of type 1 diabetes could reflect an absence of a toleragen, such as maternal insulin, and not the presence of an immunogenetic substance in cow's milk. Better designed studies are presently ongoing that should provide more definitive information in the near future.[178]

Behaviors in the postpartum period may well influence the likelihood of developing subsequent type 2 diabetes in both the mother and the newborn. As previously discussed, a very high percentage of reproductive-aged women who have GDM progress to type 2 diabetes.[37] Although an initial study has demonstrated an impressive effect of an insulin-sensitizing agent in reducing the progression from GDM to diabetes in a high-risk population,[101] evidence that weight management by the mother during the postpartum period and beyond reduces the incidence of type 2 diabetes requires confirmation. Certainly, results from studies in nonpregnant women[134,136] indicate such activities would be expected to be beneficial for women with previous GDM, but confirmation is required.

Similarly, given the evidence supporting fetal programming[107-114] and the additional impact of weight gain in early youth on the subsequent development of insulin resistance and type 2 diabetes,[148] ensuring proper nutrition and physical activity in the early years of life would be a reasonable risk-reduction strategy, if not yet firmly proven.

Adherence and Self-Management

Because of the increasing awareness in the diabetes community that individual and organizational behaviors can be positive or negative in terms of the impact of diabetes on reproductive-aged women, investigations in this important domain of behavior have become very relevant to a public health perspective on diabetes. Adherence is one term used to describe the extent to which patients engage in health-promoting behaviors recommended by health professionals.[179] The results of nonadherence in terms of adverse health and economic consequences are substantial, whether the condition is infectious,[180] acute,[181] chronic,[182] or reflective of appropriate use of health care systems.[183,184] Initially, a lack of adherence was assumed to be due to a lack of information.[185] More recent conceptual frameworks recognize that adherence is influenced by individual beliefs and attitudes; the influence of family, community, and other forms of social support; physician characteristics; and the home, work, and practice care settings.[179,185,186] Few studies have specifically addressed adherence among women aged 18–44 years; however, women who have multiple family roles that place high demands on them could experience difficulties with requirements of diabetes control.[179]

Studies on compliance and adherence approaches have been criticized because they imply that problems of patient management are due solely to the patient's individual and conscious behavior.[179,185,187] These studies confirm both the complexity of human behavior as well as the need to incorporate multiple approaches to improving the behaviors of patients, health care providers, and health systems alike.[188] Certainly, there is ample evidence that scientifically and economically validated diabetes preventive care practices are not used as widely as desired (i.e., a gap exists between what should be and what is happening in diabetes care).[189,190] Although the factors accounting for this gap are numerous and complex (e.g., type of diabetes, education level, social support, age, insurance coverage, employment status[191]), and although assignment of the gap to any one of these many factors is difficult,[186,187] the ability of a person with diabetes to understand, agree to, and follow a diabetes treatment plan is likely to be important.

A framework for understanding choices about daily diabetes self-management can include two major domains: 1) knowledge about diabetes as provided primarily by comprehensive diabetes patient education, and 2) psychosocial skills (discussed in section 4.5) that can significantly influence the success of a diabetes self-care plan.[192]

Patient education. From a public health perspective on diabetes education, four important dimensions must be recognized. First, validity of the benefits of diabetes patient education in terms of improved health outcomes is currently limited yet is necessary to more broadly ensure the availability of such programs.[185,193,194] In large part, this challenge may reflect an inappropriate evaluation framework for validating more broadly based population/community-focused interventions.[195] Second, frameworks for more broadly considering how to understand and improve patient education programs for persons with diabetes, including reproductive-aged women, have been developed.[185,186,195,196] Third, policy decisions by government, as well as legal processes, including not only content but also reimbursement strategies and efforts to ensure that all persons with diabetes have access to at least some education, can be very influential in making diabetes education available.[04,197-199] Finally, only a few studies at present have directly examined diabetes patient education programs for reproductive-aged women, but these investigations have confirmed the importance of cultural factors in patient adherence.[200-202]

4.5 Psychosocial Determinants of Health Behaviors and Health Outcomes

Four aspects of psychosocial determinants, each with a public health dimension, deserve further discussion: 1) social environment, 2) nondisease-related stress, 3) personal disposition, and 4) relationships with the health care system.[185,186]

Social Environment
A chronic disease like diabetes is managed within an interpersonal milieu.[203] A woman's social environment consists of the network of persons who provide her with various types of support and the social context in which this support is provided.[185] A major (but not the only) part of a woman's network is her family. In 1995, approximately 7% of women aged 20–44 lived alone, 51% lived with a spouse, 32% lived with other relatives only, and 10% lived with nonrelatives only.[204] The family, defined broadly as a group of people living together or in close geographic proximity with strong emotional bonds and with a history and future,[151] may provide a helpful context for understanding management challenges of diabetes, especially a complex medical regimen, over a long period of time.[151,203] Within the family construct (and indeed, beyond the family itself and including such factors as community and work),[151] cultural differences among reproductive-aged women may work synergistically or independently to influence the family network.[205-209] For example, in Hispanic communities and families, health needs may be viewed as a lower priority than work; joint family meals may be difficult; and relevancy of education programs can be problematic.[206] Similarly, black women may face multiple barriers to diabetes management based on family support, including availability of healthy food, level of family support, and perceptions of a healthy body image that may include being overweight.[200,207,209] Finally, the importance of extended family concepts, such as friends and the faith community, are examples of how different cultures may influence diabetes management of a reproductive-aged woman with diabetes.[151] The relevance and importance of the social environment to the development and management of diabetes among women in the reproductive years needs further systematic investigation.

During the past several years, there has been increased recognition of the importance of the social and cultural environment wherein a person lives, works, or plays, because it significantly influences the present and future health of that person.[210-212] The term "social capital" is typically defined as "an instantiated informal norm that promotes cooperation between two or more individuals."[213] In essence, social capital is a reflection of the degree of cooperative interaction among people and is based on a sense of trust, common interests, and willingness to work together.[214]

Indicators of social capital (e.g., trust, income or educational disparities, participation in civic organizations) have been studied in terms of defining and quantifying community or society cooperation.[215,216] Further, initial investigations have explored the relationships between various indicators of positive or negative social capital and clinical health outcomes such as perceived quality of life and mortality[217,218] Although more investigations will be necessary to both confirm the concepts inherent in social capital as well as determine if and how social capital can be intentionally altered,[219] initial studies strongly suggest that individual behaviors are largely influenced by social class, social capital, and the characteristics of a community. Thus, in considering management of diabetes among women in their reproductive years, it is very important to reflect on the social environment, which can strongly influence individual behaviors and choices, and the importance of life stress and personal disposition, as discussed in the following paragraphs.

Life Stress

Women of reproductive age with diabetes face both biological and behavioral components of stress.[220] Studies of biological stress focus on the physiologic adaptation of the body to life circumstances, whereas behavioral stress research addresses emotional responses to environmental and various psychosocial situations.[221] A limited number of studies have examined relationships between stress and glycemic control in diabetic reproductive-aged women.[222-224] However, broader views of stress must be incorporated into studies. For example, relationships between stress and use of health care services by persons with diabetes deserve additional investigation.[225] Other public health perspectives of stress and diabetes include relationships between environmental experiences (e.g., work, church) and both biological and behavioral components of stress.[225]

Personal Disposition

Personal disposition refers to long-standing emotional and psychological characteristics of an individual that may intervene in the pathway from stress to health outcomes. Personal disposition is often measured by examining coping styles, perceived control, and mastery/self-efficacy.[226] A common measure of perceived control is the use of locus of control—external versus internal—to measure ability to control events. Studies using this approach have yielded contradictory results regarding diabetes control and other diabetes-related health outcomes.[227-229] In contrast, concepts such as self-efficacy, defined as the belief in one's ability to maintain behavior change in the face of situational challenges, are considered better predictors of adherence to medical treatment and health-promotion regimens because they are associated with better adherence to complex diabetes regimens.[229]

Interactions with the Health Care System

Several aspects of women's interactions with the health care system deserve attention from the public health community. Reproductive-aged women, not only during pregnancy (for possible GDM), may need to be screened for undiagnosed diabetes. As recently reviewed, however, general screening for undiagnosed diabetes (except in the case of pregnant women) must be considered within the larger context of long-term diabetes management and economics.[230] Cost-effective screening for unrecognized diabetes would be better targeted at persons younger than 45 years of age, including women of reproductive age, and in those groups (such as younger women from minority racial and ethnic groups) with a high incidence of preventable diabetes complications.[230]

Regarding actual diabetes care and women of reproductive age, convincing clinical and economic evidence suggests that both secondary prevention (improved glycemic, lipid, and blood pressure control) and tertiary prevention (improved complication detection and treatment) are efficacious and cost-effective.[231,232] Public health response to the scientific evidence would focus on two aspects: 1) ensuring that all people with diabetes receive at least some benefit, and 2) establishing health systems that both recognize and accommodate the particular characteristics of reproductive-aged women with diabetes.

With respect to equity and availability of efficacious secondary and tertiary care, several factors are disturbing: 1) millions of Americans, including women in their reproductive years, do not have health insurance and thus must pay directly if they are to receive these scientifically justified preventive programs,[233] 2) policies often require ideal standards and objectives, without considering the reality of limits in terms of financial or health professional resources or availability (i.e., some people may get very good care, but others will get nothing),[233-235] and 3) scientific data on the benefits of glucose and blood pressure control demonstrate that any improvement in metabolic indices results in improvement in outcomes, and the greatest absolute benefit is obtained by improvement among persons with the highest levels of blood glucose and blood pressure.[236-238] Thus, if the public health community has a responsibility of assurance,[239] it must assure that all women of reproductive age have access to secondary and tertiary care.

In terms of the nature of the interaction between women who have diabetes in their reproductive years and the health care system, managed care organizations are becoming the main source of health care services for persons with diabetes.[240] Although various managed care plans function with different rules, regulations, and policies, fragmentation of care may be particularly challenging for women of reproductive age because of the many other roles and responsibilities they face—such as work, family, home, children.[241,242] In addition to access to quality care, women with or at risk for diabetes may also be concerned about the appropriateness or the nature of their interactions with the health care system. New definitions of comprehensive care, particularly relevant to reproductive-aged

women with diabetes, have been proposed that include interpersonal care (provider partnership-building behavior and a participatory decision-making style) as well as clinical care.[243,244] This movement toward collaborative care may have important implications for the care of women with diabetes. The public health challenge in response to these newer models for diabetes care for reproductive-aged women is to work with the health care system to facilitate the availability and use of these models.

4.6 Concurrent Illness as a Determinant of Health Behaviors and Health Outcomes

Diabetes mellitus does not make an individual immune to health conditions that are not related to the metabolic abnormalities of diabetes. These concurrent illnesses, however, may significantly compromise efforts to achieve metabolic control. Indeed, given the complexities and demands of diabetes, these conditions, especially psychological conditions, may significantly attenuate the effects of proper diabetes management.

Eating Disorders
Although the onset of eating disorders among women with type 1 diabetes usually occurs in adolescence (see chapter 3), persistence of these conditions into adulthood as well as the presence of subclinical eating disorders during the reproductive years are of concern.[245-247] Less information is available on eating disturbances among women with type 2 diabetes, particularly among women aged 18–44 years. Unlike women with type 1 diabetes, however, a majority of reproductive-aged women with type 2 diabetes report that eating disorders preceded the onset of their diabetes and that binge eating more accurately describes the nature of their eating disorder.[245,248]

Depression
The prevalence of depression is 3–4 times greater among people with diabetes (15%–20%) than among the general population (5%–8%).[249] Women

with diabetes are considered to be at increased risk for depression because of both their sex and their disease,[250] but very few population-based studies have examined rates of depression among men and women with and without diabetes between the ages of 18 and 44 years.[251] The higher prevalence of depression among women with diabetes remains unexplained, but the concurrence of these two disorders may have harmful interactions, with resulting poor metabolic control and increased requirements for diabetes regulation.[250,252,253] Despite the increased prevalence among people with diabetes, depression is diagnosed and treated in fewer than one-third of patients, perhaps in part because managing diabetes is very time-consuming. Further, some of the symptoms—fatigue, changes in appetite, and sleep disturbances—are seen in both disorders. Thus, diagnosing the coexistence of diabetes and depression is unlikely. Structured psychiatric interviews and validated survey instruments can distinguish the two disorders, however.[250-253]

In considering the studies regarding diabetes and various psychosocial issues (e.g., life stress, associated psychological conditions) among diabetic women of reproductive age, several caveats are important: 1) most reports emanate from tertiary academic institutions, and thus given inevitable referral bias, issues of generalizability to the entire population need to be considered, 2) perspectives on the various psychosocial issues are often limited to a clinical viewpoint and only consider what is happening in the person's life *at that moment.* Regarding the former, it is very possible that a lower social class designation or low social capital could cause both in the development of diabetes and impaired psychological function (i.e., depression and diabetes may not be directly related at all).[254]

Similarly, recent studies indicate that experiencing childhood abuse may be associated with not only impaired psychological function but also a considerably greater likelihood of developing a chronic disease like diabetes among women of reproductive age.[255] Further, there is reason to consider whether

lower social capital or a lower social class with less income and education would result in both a greater number of cases of diabetes among women of reproductive age, as well as greater difficulty in diabetes care among these same individuals.[256]

Public health challenges concerning mental health disorders in diabetic women of reproductive age are 1) to improve surveillance efforts to more clearly define the extent and nature of the coexistence of these conditions, 2) to encourage better etiologic research including measurement of social capital and early life events detection to understand the pathophysiologic reasons for the co-occurrence of these conditions, 3) to obtain population-based data on mental health disorders and diabetes, and 4) to ensure health care systems will permit and facilitate both the identification and appropriate treatment of the mental disorders commonly seen in diabetic women of reproductive age.

4.7 Public Health Implications

Surveillance and epidemiologic data presently suggest that the prevalence of diabetes, especially type 2, is increasing most dramatically among reproductive-aged women—an increase most noteworthy in women from communities of color.

- Better surveillance information is required to confirm these initial observations and should focus on minority populations where additional confirmatory data about the prevalence of diabetes and associated complications among diabetic women of reproductive age would enhance our ability to target intervention efforts.

- Improved epidemiologic and health services data are required to understand environmental and behavioral factors (e.g., weight gain, physical inactivity, community exercise facilities) and genetic-environmental interactions that may account for the increasing trends in incidence of type 2 diabetes among women in their reproductive years.

Population-based studies confirm the intergenerational effects of fetal nutrition status during pregnancy as well as the relationship of early life experiences on subsequent risk for chronic disease in adulthood. The degree to which this effect contributes to the increase in the prevalence of diabetes among persons younger than 45 years of age should be investigated.

- Improved epidemiologic information is needed to confirm this intergenerational effect and to clarify the exact factors that account for its existence. Primary prevention of type 2 diabetes needs to systematically address pregnancy—not only to ensure a healthy mother and baby, but also to decrease the likelihood of subsequent diabetes in the mother and offspring.

- Additional information about GDM is required, including basic epidemiologic data on screening policies, possible preventive strategies among women at risk for GDM, and appropriate treatment strategies once GDM is diagnosed. In addition, the postpartum period for women with GDM needs attention both to better document the high rate of progression from GDM to type 2 diabetes, as well as to identify interventions during the months and years following delivery that would prevent or delay the onset of diabetes.

In women of reproductive age with diabetes, it is necessary to systematically identify the presence of risk factors for the development of microvascular and macrovascular complications. Such information will help in the development of risk reduction programs to reduce the occurrence of these complications in midlife.

- Various health care systems must be structured and must function in a manner that will facilitate improved detection of risk factors and, when appropriate, management of these risk factors so that the appearance of common complications of diabetes will be reduced in women after age 44 years.

- The interaction between reproductive-aged women with diabetes and the health care system needs to be collaborative in nature.

- Policies at the federal, state, and local levels must ensure that all women with diabetes during the reproductive years have access to appropriate preventive strategies for diabetes and associated conditions, including various mental health disorders.

- Attention to the various and critical environmental factors is needed to move beyond the important but limiting individual view of health and behavior. Research is needed to gain insight into the effects of community-level characteristics, such as social capital and equity, on diabetes prevention and control.

References

1. Ventura SJ, Mosher WD, Curtin SC, Abma JC, Henshaw S. Trends in pregnancies and pregnancy rates by outcome: estimates for the United States, 1976–96. *Vital Health Stat* 2000;21(56):1–47.

2. Harris MI. Classification, diagnostic criteria, and screening for diabetes. In: National Diabetes Data Group, editors. *Diabetes in America*. 2nd ed. Bethesda, MD: National Institutes of Health, 1995:15–36. (NIH Publication No. 95-1468)

3. Harris MI, Flegal KM, Cowie CC, et al. Prevalence of diabetes, impaired fasting glucose, and impaired glucose tolerance in U.S. adults. The Third National Health and Nutrition Examination Survey, 1988–1994. *Diabetes Care* 1998;21(4):518–24.

4. Day JC. *Population Projections of the United States by Age, Sex, Race, and Hispanic Origin: 1995 to 2050*. U.S. Bureau of the Census, Current Population Reports, P25-1130. Washington, DC: U.S. Government Printing Office, 1996.

5. American Diabetes Association. Report of the Expert Committee on the Diagnosis and Classification of Diabetes Mellitus. *Diabetes Care* 1997;20(7):1183–97.

6. Carter JS, Pugh JA, Monterrosa A. Non–insulin-dependent diabetes mellitus in minorities in the United States. *Ann Intern Med* 1996;125(3):221–32.

7. Ellis JL, Campos-Outcalt D. Cardiovascular disease risk factors in Native Americans: a literature review. *Am J Prev Med* 1994;10(5):295–307.

8. Will JC, Strauss KF, Mendlein JM, Ballew C, White LL, Peter DG. Diabetes mellitus among Navajo Indians: findings from the Navajo Health and Nutrition Survey. *J Nutr* 1997;127(10 Suppl):2106S–2113S.

9. CDC. Prevalence of diagnosed diabetes among American Indians/Alaskan Natives—United States, 1996. *MMWR* 1998;47(42):901–4.

10. Schraer CD, Adler AI, Mayer AM, Halderson KR, Trimble BA. Diabetes complications and mortality among Alaska Natives: 8 years of observation. *Diabetes Care* 1997;20(3):314–21.

11. Flegal KM, Ezzati TM, Harris MI, et al. Prevalence of diabetes in Mexican Americans, Cubans, and Puerto Ricans from the Hispanic Health and Nutrition Examination Survey, 1982–1984. *Diabetes Care* 1991;14(Suppl 3):628–38.

12. CDC. Self-reported prevalence of diabetes among Hispanics—United States, 1994–1997. *MMWR* 1999;48(1):8–12.

13. LaPorte RE, Matsushima M, Chang Y-F. Prevalence and incidence of insulin-dependent diabetes. In: National Diabetes Data Group, editors. *Diabetes in America*. 2nd ed. Bethesda, MD: National Institutes of Health, 1995:37–46. (NIH Publication No. 95-1468)

14. Harris MI, Robbins DC. Prevalence of adult-onset IDDM in the U.S. population. *Diabetes Care* 1994; 17(11):1337–40.

15. Kenny SJ, Aubert RE, Geiss LS. Prevalence and incidence of non–insulin-dependent diabetes. In: National Diabetes Data Group, editors. *Diabetes in America*. 2nd ed. Bethesda, MD: National Institutes of Health, 1995:47–67. (NIH Publication No. 95-1468)

16. Lipton RB, Liao Y, Cao G, Cooper RS, McGee D. Determinants of incident non–insulin-dependent diabetes mellitus among blacks and whites in a national sample. The NHANES I Epidemiologic Follow-up Study. *Am J Epidemiol* 1993;138(10):826–39.

17. Haffner SM, Hazuda HP, Mitchell BD, Patterson JK, Stern MP. Increased incidence of type II diabetes mellitus in Mexican Americans. *Diabetes Care* 1991;14(2): 102–8.

18. Knowler WC, Bennett PH, Hamman RF, Miller M. Diabetes incidence and prevalence in Pima Indians: a 19-fold greater incidence than in Rochester, Minnesota. *Am J Epidemiol* 1978;108(6):497–505.

19. Libman I, Songer T, LaPorte R. How many people in the U.S. have IDDM? *Diabetes Care* 1993;16(5):841–2.

20. CDC. <http://www.cdc.gov/diabetes/statistics/survl99/2chap2/table10.html>. Last revised March 20, 2000.

21. CDC. Trends in the prevalence and incidence of self-reported diabetes mellitus—United States, 1980–1994. *MMWR* 1997;46(43):1014–8.

22. Leibson CL, O'Brien PC, Atkinson E, Palumbo PJ, Melton LJ 3rd. Relative contributions of incidence and survival to increasing prevalence of adult-onset diabetes mellitus: a population-based study. *Am J Epidemiol* 1997;146(1):12–22.

23. Mokdad AH, Ford ES, Bowman BA, et al. Diabetes trends in the U.S.: 1990–1998. *Diabetes Care* 2000; 23(9):1278–83.

24. Burke JP, Williams K, Gaskill SP, Hazuda HP, Haffner SM, Stern MP. Rapid rise in the incidence of type 2 diabetes from 1987 to 1996: results from the San Antonio Heart Study. *Arch Intern Med* 1999;159(13):1450–6.

25. Knowler WC, Saad MF, Pettitt DJ, Nelson RG, Bennett PH. Determinants of diabetes mellitus in the Pima Indians. *Diabetes Care* 1993;16(1):216–27.

26. Gu K, Cowie CC, Harris MI. Diabetes and decline in heart disease mortality in U.S. adults. *JAMA* 1999; 281(14):1291–7.

27. Colditz GA, Willett WC, Stampfer MJ, et al. Weight as a risk factor for clinical diabetes in women. *Am J Epidemiol* 1990;132(3):501–13.

28. Ford ES, Williamson DF, Liu S. Weight change and diabetes incidence: findings from a national cohort of U.S. adults. *Am J Epidemiol* 1997;146(3):214–22.

29. Manson JE, Rimm EB, Stampfer MJ, et al. Physical activity and incidence of non–insulin-dependent diabetes mellitus in women. *Lancet* 1991;338(8770): 774–8.

30. Freedman DS, Srinivasan SR, Valdez RA, Williamson DF, Berenson GS. Secular increases in relative weight and adiposity among children over two decades: the Bogalusa Heart Study. *Pediatrics* 1997;99(3):420–6.

31. Flegal KM, Carroll MD, Kuczmarski RJ, Johnson CL. Overweight and obesity in the United States: prevalence and trends, 1960–1994. *Int J Obes Relat Disord* 1998; 22(1):39–47.

32. Crespo CJ, Keteyian SJ, Heath GW, Sempos CT. Leisure-time physical activity among U.S. adults: results from the Third National Health and Nutrition Examination Survey. *Arch Intern Med* 1996;156(1): 93–8.

33. Lewis CE, Smith DE, Wallace DD, Williams OD, Bild DE, Jacobs DR Jr. Seven-year trends in body weight and associations with lifestyle and behavioral characteristics in black and white young adults: the CARDIA Study. *Am J Public Health* 1997;87(4):635–42.

34. Metzger BE, Coustan DR, the Organizing Committee. Summary and recommendations of the Fourth International Workshop-Conference on Gestational Diabetes Mellitus. *Diabetes Care* 1998;21(Suppl 2): B161–B167.

35. Kjos SL, Buchanan TA. Gestational diabetes mellitus. *N Engl J Med* 1999;341(23):1749–56.

36. Moses RG. The recurrence rate of gestational diabetes in subsequent pregnancies. *Diabetes Care* 1996;19(12): 1348–50.

37. Dornhorst A, Rossi M. Risk and prevention of type 2 diabetes in women with gestational diabetes. *Diabetes Care* 1998;21(Suppl 2):B43–B49.

38. Persson B, Hanson U. Neonatal morbidities in gestational diabetes mellitus. *Diabetes Care* 1998;21(Suppl 2):B79–B84.

39. Pettitt DJ, Knowler WC. Long-term effects of the intrauterine environment, birth weight, and breast-feeding in Pima Indians. *Diabetes Care* 1998;21(Suppl 2):B138–B141.

40. Silverman BL, Rizzo TA, Cho NH, Metzger BE. Long-term effects of the intrauterine environment. The Northwestern University Diabetes in Pregnancy Center. *Diabetes Care* 1998;21(Suppl 2):B142–B149.

41. King H. Epidemiology of glucose intolerance and gestational diabetes in women of childbearing age. *Diabetes Care* 1998;21(Suppl 2):B9–B13.

42. Engelgau MM, Herman WH, Smith PJ, German RR, Aubert RE. The epidemiology of diabetes and pregnancy in the U.S., 1988. *Diabetes Care* 1995;18(7):1029–33.

43. CDC. Diabetes during pregnancy—United States, 1993–1995. *MMWR* 1998;47(20):408–14.

44. Kieffer EC, Martin JA, Herman WH. Impact of maternal nativity on the prevalence of diabetes during pregnancy among U.S. ethnic groups. *Diabetes Care* 1999;22(5):729–35.

45. Nahum GG, Huffaker BJ. Racial differences in oral glucose screening test results: establishing race-specific criteria for abnormality in pregnancy. *Obstet Gynecol* 1993; 81(4):517–22.

46. Berkowitz GS, Lapinski RH, Wein R, Lee D. Race/ ethnicity and other risk factors for gestational diabetes. *Am J Epidemiol* 1992;135(9):965–73.

47. Green JR, Pawson IG, Schumacher LB, Perry J, Kretchmer N. Glucose tolerance in pregnancy: ethnic variation and influence of body habitus. *Am J Obstet Gynecol* 1990;163:86–92.

48. Dornhost A, Paterson CM, Nicholls JS, et al. High prevalence of gestational diabetes in women from ethnic minority groups. *Diabet Med* 1992;9(9):820–5.

49. Benjamin E, Winters D, Mayfield J, Gohdes D. Diabetes in pregnancy in Zuni Indian women. Prevalence and subsequent development of clinical diabetes after gestational diabetes. *Diabetes Care* 1993; 16(9):1231–5.

50. Solomon CG, Willett WC, Carey VJ, et al. A prospective study of pregravid determinants of gestational diabetes mellitus. *JAMA* 1997;278(13):1078–83.

51. Strauss KF, Mokdad A, Ballew C, et al. The health of Navajo women: findings from the Navajo Health and Nutrition Survey, 1991–1992. *J Nutr* 1997;127(10 Suppl):2128S–2133S.

52. Cowie CC, Eberhardt MS. Sociodemographic characteristics of persons with diabetes. In: National Diabetes Data Group, editors. *Diabetes in America*. 2nd ed. Bethesda, MD: National Institutes of Health, 1995:85–116. (NIH Publication No. 95-1468)

53. Drury TF, Danchik KM, Harris MI. Sociodemographic characteristics of adult diabetics. In: National Diabetes Data Group, editors. *Diabetes in America*. 1st ed. Bethesda, MD: National Institutes of Health; 1985:VII-1–VII-37. (NIH Publication No. 85-1468)

54. Peters KD, Kochanek KD, Murphy SL. Deaths: final data for 1996. *Natl Vital Stat Rep* 1998;47(9):1–100.

55. Bild DE, Stevenson JM. Frequency of recording of diabetes on U.S. death certificates: analysis of the 1986 National Mortality Followback Survey. *J Clin Epidemiol* 1992;45(3):275–81.

56. Geiss LS, Herman WH, Smith PJ. Mortality in non–insulin-dependent diabetes. In: National Diabetes Data Group, editors. *Diabetes in America*. 2nd ed. Bethesda, MD: National Institutes of Health, 1995:233–57. (NIH Publication No. 95-1468)

57. Garcia MJ, McNamara PM, Gordon T, Kannel WB. Morbidity and mortality in diabetics in the Framingham population. Sixteen-year follow-up study. *Diabetes* 1974; 23:105–11.

58. Manson JE, Colditz GA, Stampfer MJ, et al. A prospective study of maturity-onset diabetes mellitus and risk of coronary heart disease and stroke in women. *Arch Intern Med* 1991;151(2):1141–7.

59. Moss SE, Klein R, Klein BE. Cause-specific mortality in a population-based study of diabetes. *Am J Public Health* 1991;81(9):1158–62.

60. Stamler J, Vaccaro O, Neaton JD, Wentworth D. Diabetes, other risk factors, and 12-yr cardiovascular mortality for men screened in the Multiple Risk Factor Intervention Trial. *Diabetes Care* 1993;16(2):434–44.

61. Sievers ML, Nelson RG, Knowler WC, Bennett PH. Impact of NIDDM on mortality and causes of death in Pima Indians. *Diabetes Care* 1992;15(11):1541–9.

62. Wei M, Gaskill SP, Haffner SM, Stern MP. Effects of diabetes and level of glycemia on all-cause and cardiovascular mortality. The San Antonio Heart Study. *Diabetes Care* 1998;21(7):1167–72.

63. Gu K, Cowie CC, Harris MI. Mortality in adults with and without diabetes in a national cohort of the U.S. population, 1971–1993. *Diabetes Care* 1998;21(7): 1138–45.

64. International analysis of insulin-dependent diabetes mellitus mortality: a preventable mortality perspective. The Diabetes Epidemiology Research International (DERI) Study. *Am J Epidemiol* 1995;142(6):612–8.

65. Tull ES, Barinas E. A twofold excess mortality among black compared with white IDDM patients in Allegheny County, Pennsylvania. Pittsburgh DERI Mortality Study Group. *Diabetes Care* 1996;19(12):1344–7.

66. Klein R, Klein BE. Vision disorders in diabetes. In: National Diabetes Data Group, editors. *Diabetes in America*. 2nd ed. Bethesda, MD: National Institutes of Health, 1995:293–338. (NIH Publication No. 95-1468)

67. Hemachandra A, Ellis D, Lloyd CE, Orchard TJ. The influence of pregnancy on IDDM complications. *Diabetes Care* 1995;18(7):950–4.

68. Chew EY, Mills JL, Metzger BE, et al. Metabolic control and progression of retinopathy. The Diabetes in Early Pregnancy Study. National Institute of Child Health and Human Development Diabetes in Early Pregnancy Study. *Diabetes Care* 1995;18(5):631–7.

69 American Diabetes Association. Diabetic nephropathy. *Diabetes Care* 1999;22(Suppl 1):S66–S69.

70. Nelson RG, Knowler WC, Pettitt DJ, Bennett PH. Kidney diseases in diabetes. In: National Diabetes Data Group, editors. *Diabetes in America*. 2nd ed. Bethesda, MD: National Institutes of Health, 1995:349–400. (NIH Publication No. 95-1468)

71. Klein BE, Moss SE, Klein R. Effect of pregnancy on progression of diabetic nephropathy. *Diabetes Care* 1990;13(1):34–40.

72. Grundy SM, Benjamin IJ, Burke GL, et al. Diabetes and cardiovascular disease: a statement for health care professionals from the American Heart Association. *Circulation* 1999;100(10):1134–46.

73. Wingard DL, Barrett-Connor E. Heart disease and diabetes. In: National Diabetes Data Group, editors. *Diabetes in America*. 2nd ed. Bethesda, MD: National Institutes of Health, 1995:429–48. (NIH Publication No. 95-1468)

74. Selby JV, Ray GT, Zhang D, Colby CJ. Excess costs of medical care for patients with diabetes in a managed care population. *Diabetes Care* 1997;20(9):1396–1402.

75. Koivisto VA, Stevens LK, Mattock M, et al. Cardiovascular disease and its risk factors in IDDM in Europe. EURODIAB IDDM Complications Study Group. *Diabetes Care* 1996;19(7):689–97.

76. Lloyd CE, Kuller LH, Ellis D, Becker DJ, Wing RR, Orchard TJ. Coronary artery disease in IDDM. Gender differences in risk factors but not risk. *Arterioscler Thromb Vasc Biol* 1996;16(6):720–6.

77. Sowers J. Diabetes mellitus and cardiovascular disease in women. *Arch Intern Med* 1998;158(6):617–21.

78. American Diabetes Association; National Heart, Lung, and Blood Institute; Juvenile Diabetes Foundation International; National Institute of Diabetes and Digestive and Kidney Disease; American Heart Association. Diabetes mellitus: a major risk factor for cardiovascular disease. *Circulation* 1999;1000:1132–3.

79. Haffner SM. Management of dyslipidemia in adults with diabetes. *Diabetes Care* 1998;21(1):160–78.

80. American Diabetes Association. Implications of the United Kingdom Prospective Diabetes Study. *Diabetes Care* 1999;22(Suppl 1):27S–31S.

81. Yudkin JS, Chaturvedi N. Developing risk stratification charts for diabetic and nondiabetic subjects. *Diabet Med* 1999;16(3):219–27.

82. Vinicor F. The public health burden of diabetes and the reality of limits. *Diabetes Care* 1998;21(Suppl 3): C15–C18.

83. Glasgow RE, Wagner EH, Kaplan RM, Vinicor F, Smith L, Norman J. If diabetes is a public health problem, why not treat it as one? A population-based approach to chronic illness. *Ann Behav Med* 1999; 21(2):159–70.

84. Lunt H. Women and diabetes. *Diabet Med* 1996;13: 1009–16.

85. Glasgow R, Toobert D, Riddle M, Donnelly J, Mitchell D, Calder D. Diabetes-specific social learning variables and self-care behaviors among persons with type 2 diabetes. *Health Psychol* 1989;8(3):285–303.

86. Garay-Sevilla ME, Nava LE, Malacara JM, Huerta R, et al. Adherence to treatment and social support in patients with non–insulin-dependent diabetes mellitus. *J Diabetes Complications* 1995;9(2):81–6.

87. Larsson D, Lager I, Nilsson PM. Socioeconomic characteristics and quality of life in diabetes mellitus—relation to metabolic control. *Scand J Public Health* 1999;27(2): 101–5.

88. Rubin RR, Peyrot M. Quality of life and diabetes. *Diabetes Metab Res Rev* 1999;15(3):205–18.

89. Clark CM Jr. The National Diabetes Education Program: changing the way diabetes is treated. *Ann Intern Med* 1999;130:324–6.

90. The Diabetes Control and Complications Trial Research Group. The effect of intensive treatment of diabetes on the development and progression of long-term complications in insulin-dependent diabetes mellitus. *N Engl J Med* 1993;329(14):977–86.

91. Diabetes Control and Complications Trial Research Group. Influence of intensive diabetes treatment on quality-of-life outcomes in the Diabetes Control and Complications Trial. *Diabetes Care* 1996;19(3):195–203.

92. Diabetes Control and Complications Trial Research Group. Implementation of treatment protocols in the Diabetes Control and Complications Trial. *Diabetes Care* 1995;18(3):361–76.

93. UK Prospective Diabetes Study (UKPDS) Group. Quality of life in type 2 diabetic patients is affected by complications but not by intensive policies to improve blood glucose or blood pressure control (UKPDS 37). *Diabetes Care* 1999;22(7):1125–36.

94. Wikblad K, Leksell J, Wibell L. Health-related quality of life in relation to metabolic control and late complications in patients with insulin-dependent diabetes mellitus. *Qual Life Res* 1996;5(1):123–30.

95. Testa MA, Simonson DC. Health economic benefits and quality of life during improved glycemic control in patients with type 2 diabetes mellitus: a randomized, controlled, double-blind trial. *JAMA* 1998;280(17):1490–6.

96. Glasgow RE, Ruggiero L, Eakin EG, Dryfoos J, Chobanian L. Quality of life and associated characteristics in a large national sample of adults with diabetes. *Diabetes Care* 1997;20(4):562–7.

97. Centers for Disease Control and Prevention. *Diabetes Surveillance 1997*. Atlanta: U.S. Department of Health and Human Services, 1997.

98. Kerbel D, Glazier R, Holzapfel S, Yeung M, Lofsky S. Adverse effects of screening for gestational diabetes: a prospective cohort study in Toronto, Canada. *J Med Screen* 1997;4(3):128–32.

99. Dornhorst A, Chan SP. The elusive diagnosis of gestational diabetes. *Diabet Med* 1998;15(1):7–10.

100. Naylor CD, Sermer M, Chen E, Sykora K. Cesarean delivery in relation to birth weight and gestational glucose tolerance: pathophysiology or practice style? *JAMA* 1996;275(15):1165–70.

101. Azen SP, Peters RK, Berkowitz K, Kjos S, Xiang A, Buchanan TA. TRIPOD (TRoglitazone In the Prevention Of Diabetes): a randomized, placebo-controlled trial of troglitazone in women with prior gestational diabetes mellitus. *Control Clin Trials* 1998; 19(2):217–31.

102. Pettitt DJ, Baird HR, Aleck KA, Bennett PH, Knowler WC. Excessive obesity in offspring of Pima Indian women with diabetes during pregnancy. *N Engl J Med* 1983;308(5):242–5.

103. Silverman BL, Rizzo T, Green OC, et al. Long-term prospective evaluation of offspring of diabetic mothers. *Diabetes* 1991;40(Suppl 2):121–5.

104. Pettitt DJ, Aleck KA, Baird HR, Bennett PH, Knowler WC. Congenital susceptibility to NIDDM. Role of intrauterine environment. *Diabetes* 1988;37(5):622–8.

105. Karter AJ, Rowell SE, Ackerson LM, Ferrara A. Excess maternal transmission of type 2 diabetes across all races: the Northern California Kaiser Permanente Diabetes Registry. *Diabetes* 1998;47(Suppl 2):25A.

106. Reaven G. Insulin resistance and human disease: a short history. *J Basic Clin Physiol Pharmacol* 1998;9(2–4):387–406.

107. Barker DJ. The fetal origins of type 2 diabetes mellitus. *Ann Intern Med* 1999;130:322–4.

108. Valdez R, Athens MA, Thompson GH, Bradshaw BS, Stern MP. Birth-weight and adult health outcomes in a biethnic population in the USA. *Diabetologia* 1994;37:624–31.

109. McCance DR, Pettitt DJ, Hanson RL, Jacobson LT, Knowler WC, Bennett PH. Birth weight and non–insulin-dependent diabetes: thrifty genotype, thrifty phenotype, or surviving small baby genotype? *BMJ* 1994;308(6934):942–5.

110. Egeland GM, Skjaerven R, Irgens L. Birth characteristics of women who develop gestational diabetes: population based study. *BMJ* 2000;321(7260):546–7.

111. Rich-Edwards JW, Colditz GA, Stampfer MJ, et al. Birth-weight and the risk for type 2 diabetes mellitus in adult women. *Ann Intern Med* 1999;130:278–84.

112. Dabelea D, Knowler WC, Pettitt DJ. Effects of diabetes in pregnancy on offspring: follow-up research in the Pima Indians. *J Matern Fetal Med* 2000;9(1):83–8.

113. Lucas A, Fewtrell MS, Cole TJ. Fetal origins of adult disease—the hypothesis revisited. *BMJ* 1999;319(7204): 245–9.

114. Dabelea D, Hanson RL, Lindsay RS, et al. Intrauterine exposure to diabetes conveys risks for type 2 diabetes and obesity: study of discordant sibships. *Diabetes* 2000;49(12):2208–11.

115. Fagot-Campagna A, Pettitt DJ, Engelgau MM, et al. Type 2 diabetes among North American children and adolescents: an epidemiologic review and a public health perspective. *J Pediatr* 2000;136(5):664–72.

116. Rosenbloom AL, Young RS, Joe JR, Winter WE. Emerging epidemic of type 2 diabetes in youth. *Diabetes Care* 1999;22(2):345–54.

117. Bavdekar A, Yajnik CS, Fall CH, et al. Insulin resistance syndrome in 8-year-old Indian children: small at birth, big at 8 years, or both? *Diabetes* 1999;48(12):2422–9.

118. Seidell JC. Obesity, insulin resistence, and diabetes—a worldwide epidemic. *Br J Nutr* 2000;83(Suppl 1): S5–S8.

119. International Diabetes Federation. *Diabetes Atlas 2000.* Brussels, Belgium: International Diabetes Federation, 2000.

120. King H, Aubert RE, Herman WH. Global burden of diabetes, 1995–2025: prevalence, numerical estimates, and projections. *Diabetes Care* 1998;21(9):1414–31.

121. Mann J. Stemming the tide of diabetes mellitus. *Lancet* 2000;356(9240):1454–5.

122. Tuomilehto J, Lindstrom J, Ericksson JG, et al. Prevention of type 2 diabetes mellitus by lifestyle changes among subjects with impaired glucose tolerance. *N Engl J Med* 2001;344(18):1343–50.

123. So WY, Ng MC, Lee SC, Sanke T, Lee HK, Chan JC. Genetics of type 2 diabetes mellitus. *Hong Kong Med J* 2000;6:69–76.

124. Black SA, Ray LA, Markides KS. The prevalence and health burden of self-reported diabetes in older Mexican Americans: findings from the Hispanic established populations for epidemiologic studies of the elderly. *Am J Public Health* 1999;89(4):546–52.

125. Must A, Spadano J, Coakley EH, Field AE, Colditz G, Dietz WH. The disease burden associated with overweight and obesity. *JAMA* 1999;282(16):1523–9.

126. Mokdad AH, Serdula MK, Dietz WH, Bowman BA, Marks JS, Koplan JP. The spread of the obesity epidemic in the United States, 1991–1998. *JAMA* 1999;282(16): 1519–22.

127. Colditz GA, Willett WC, Rotnitzky A, Manson JE. Weight gain as a risk factor for clinical diabetes mellitus in women. *Ann Intern Med* 1995;122(7):481–6.

128. CDC. <http://www.cdc.gov/nchs/products/pubs/pubd/ hus/tables/2000/00hus069.pdf> Last accessed March 20, 2001.

129. Smith DE, Lewis CE, Caveny JL, Perkins LL, Burke GL, Bild DE. Longitudinal changes in adiposity associated with pregnancy. The CARDIA Study. Coronary Artery Risk Development in Young Adults Study. *JAMA* 1994;271(22):1747–51.

130. Manson JE, Colditz GA, Stampfer MJ. Parity, ponderosity, and the paradox of a weight-preoccupied society. *JAMA* 1994;271(22):1788–90.

131. Williamson DF, Madans J, Pamuk E, Flegal KM, Kendrick JS, Serdula MK. A prospective study of childbearing and 10-year weight gain in U.S. white women 25 to 45 years of age. *Int J Obes Relat Metab Disord* 1994;18(8):561–9.

132. Gunderson EP, Abrams B. Epidemiology of gestational weight gain and body weight changes after pregnancy. *Epidemiol Rev* 1999;21(2):261–75.

133. Schmitz KH, Jacobs DR Jr, Leon AS, Schreiner PJ, Sternfeld B. Physical activity and body weight: associations over ten years in the CARDIA study. Coronary Artery Risk Development in Young Adults. *Int J Obes Relat Metab Disord* 2000;24(11):1475–87.

134. Pan XR, Li GW, Hu YH, et al. Effects of diet and exercise in preventing NIDDM in people with impaired glucose tolerance. The Da Qing IGT and Diabetes Study. *Diabetes Care* 1997;20(4):537–44.

135. Ford ES, Herman WH. Leisure-time physical activity patterns in the U.S. diabetic population. Findings from the 1990 National Health Interview Survey—Health Promotion and Disease Prevention Supplement. *Diabetes Care* 1995;18(1):27–33.

136. Harris SB, Zinman B. Primary prevention of type 2 diabetes in high-risk populations. *Diabetes Care* 2000; 23(7):879–81.

137. Haire-Joshu D, Glasgow RE, Tibbs TL. Smoking and diabetes. *Diabetes Care* 1999;22(11):1887–98.

138. Nicholl ID, Bucala R. Advanced glycation endproducts and cigarette smoking. *Cell Mol Biol* 1998;44(7): 1025–33.

139. Goldberg RB. Cardiovascular disease in diabetic patients. *Med Clin North Am* 2000;84(1):81–93.

140. Rimm EB, Manson JE, Stampfer MJ, et al. Cigarette smoking and the risk of diabetes in women. *Am J Public Health* 1993;83(2):211–4.

141. Will JC, Galuska DA, Ford ES, Mokdad AH, Calle EE. Cigarette smoking and diabetes mellitus: evidence of a positive association from a large prospective cohort study. *Int J Epidemiol* 2001;30(3):540–6.

142. Targher G, Alberiche M, Zenere MB, Bonadonna RC, Muggero M, Bonora E. Cigarette smoking and insulin resistance in patients with non–insulin-dependent diabetes mellitus. *J Clin Endocrinol Metab* 1997;82(11): 3619–24.

143. Salmeron J, Manson JE, Stampfer MJ, Colditz GA, Wing AL, Willett WC. Dietary fiber, glycemic load, and risk of non–insulin-dependent diabetes mellitus in women. *JAMA* 1997;277(6):472–7.

144. Williamson DF, Thompson TJ, Thun M, Flanders D, Pamuk E, Byers T. Intentional weight loss and mortality among overweight individuals with diabetes. *Diabetes Care* 2000;23(10):1499–1504.

145. Will JC, Williamson DF, Ford ES, et al. Averting the U.S. diabetes epidemic: does weight loss help? *Diabetologia* 2000;43(Suppl 1):A4.

146. Chaisson JL, Gomis R, Hanefeld M, Josse RG, Karasik A, Laakso M. The STOP-NIDDM Trial: an international study on the efficacy of an alpha-glucosidase inhibitor to prevent type 2 diabetes in a population with impaired glucose tolerance: rationale, design, and preliminary screening data. Study to Prevent Non–Insulin-Dependent Diabetes Mellitus. *Diabetes Care* 1998; 21(10):1720–5.

147. DPP Study Group. The Diabetes Prevention Program. Design and methods for a clinical trial in the prevention of type 2 diabetes. *Diabetes Care* 1999;22(4):623–34.

148. Baranowski T, Mendlein J, Resnicow K, et al. Physical activity and nutrition in children and youth: an overview of obesity prevention. *Prev Med* 2000; 31(Suppl 1):S1–S10.

149. Helmrich SP, Ragland DR, Paffenbarger RS Jr. Prevention of non–insulin-dependent diabetes mellitus with physical activity. *Med Sci Sports Exerc* 1994; 26(7):824–30.

150. Ross R, Dagnone D, Jones PJ, et al. Reduction in obesity and related comorbid conditions after diet-induced weight loss or exercise-induced weight loss in men. A randomized, controlled trial. *Ann Intern Med* 2000; 133(2):92–103.

151. Fisher L, Chesla CA, Bartz RJ, et al. The family and type 2 diabetes: a framework for intervention. *Diabetes Educ* 1998;24(5):599–607.

152. Bennett PH. Primary prevention of NIDDM: a practical reality. *Diabetes Metab Rev* 1997;13:(2)105–11.

153. American Diabetes Association. *Medical Management of Pregnancy Complicated by Diabetes.* 2nd ed. Alexandria, VA: American Diabetes Association, 1995.

154. Ryan EA. Pregnancy in diabetes. *Med Clin North Am* 1998;82(4):823–45.

155. Herman WH, Janz NK, Becker MP, Charron-Prochownik D. Diabetes and pregnancy. Preconception care, pregnancy outcomes, resource utilization, and costs. *J Reprod Med* 1999;44(1):33–8.

156. McElvy SS, Miodovnik M, Rosenn B, et al. A focused preconceptional and early pregnancy program in women with type 1 diabetes reduces perinatal mortality and malformation rates to general population levels. *J Matern Fetal Med* 2000;9(1):14–20.

157. Wiznitzer A, Reece EA. Assessment and management of pregnancy complicated by pregestational diabetes mellitus. *Pediatr Ann* 1999;28(9):605–13.

158. Jovanovic L. Role of diet and insulin treatment of diabetes in pregnancy. *Clin Obstet Gynecol* 2000;43(1): 46–55.

159. Hadden DR, McCance DR. Advances in management of type 1 diabetes and pregnancy. *Curr Opin Obstet Gynecol* 1999;11(6):557–62.

160. Kitzmiller J. Cost analysis of diagnosis and treatment of gestational diabetes mellitus. *Clin Obstet Gynecol* 2000;43(1):140–53.

161. Weiss SR, Cooke CE, Bradley LR, Manson JM. Pharmacist's guide to pregnancy registry studies. *J Am Pharm Assoc (Wash)* 1999;39(6):830–4.

162. Carlsson S, Persson PG, Alvarsson M, et al. Low birth weight, family history of diabetes, and glucose intolerance in Swedish middle-aged men. *Diabetes Care* 1999; 22(7):1043–7.

163. El-Hashimy M, Angelico MC, Martin BC, Krolewski AS, Warram JH. Factors modifying the risk of IDDM in offspring of an IDDM parent. *Diabetes* 1995;44(3): 295–9.

164. Lorenzen T, Pociot F, Stilgren L, et al. Predictors of IDDM recurrence risk in offspring of Danish IDDM patients. Danish IDDM Epidemiology and Genetics Group. *Diabetologia* 1998;41(6):666–73.

165. Klein BE, Klein R, Moss SE, Cruickshanks KJ. Parental history of diabetes in a population-based study. *Diabetes Care* 1996;19(8):827–30.

166. Groop L, Forsblom C, Lehtovirta M, et al. Metabolic consequences of a family history of NIDDM (the Botnia study): evidence for sex-specific parental effects. *Diabetes* 1996;45(11):1585–93.

167. Kjos SL. Postpartum care of the woman with diabetes. *Clin Obstet Gynecol* 2000;43(1):75–86.

168. Murtaugh MA, Ferris AM, Capacchione CM, Reece EA. Energy intake and glycemia in lactating women with type 1 diabetes. *J Am Diet Assoc* 1998;98(6):642–8.

169. Preparing pregnant women with diabetes for special breast-feeding challenges. *J Am Diet Assoc* 1998;98(6): 648.

170. Harrison LC, Honeyman MC. Cow's milk and type 1 diabetes: the real debate is about mucosal immune function. *Diabetes* 1999;48(8):1501–7.

171. Scott FW, Norris JM, Kolb H. Milk and type 1 diabetes. *Diabetes Care* 1996;19(4):379–83.

172. Vaarala O, Knip M, Paronen J, et al. Cow's milk formula feeding induces primary immunization to insulin in infants at genetic risk for type 1 diabetes. *Diabetes* 1999; 48(7):1389–94.

173. Karjalainen J, Martin JM, Knip M, et al. A bovine albumin peptide as a possible trigger of insulin-dependent diabetes mellitus. *N Engl J Med* 1992;327(5):302–7.

174. Hammond-McKibben D, Dosch HM. Cow's milk, bovine serum albumin, and IDDM: can we settle the controversies? *Diabetes Care* 1997;20(5):897–901.

175. Pettitt DJ, Forman MR, Hanson RL, Knowler WC, Bennett PH. Breastfeeding and incidence of non–insulin-dependent diabetes mellitus in Pima Indians. *Lancet* 1997;350(9072):166–8.

176. Schrezenmeir J, Jagla A. Milk and diabetes. *J Am Coll Nutr* 2000;19(Suppl 2):176S–190S.

177. Shedadeh N, Gelertner L, Blazer S, Perlman R, Solovachik L, Etzioni A. Insulin content in infant diet: suggestion for a new infant formula. *Diabetologia* 2001; 43(Suppl 1):A3.

178. Hamalainen AM, Ronkainen MS, Akerblom HK, et al. Postnatal elimination of transplacentally acquired disease-associated antibodies in infants born to families with type 1 diabetes. *J Clin Endocrinol Metab* 2000;85:4249–53.

179. Anderson B, Funnell M, editors. *The Art of Empowerment: Stories and Strategies for Diabetes Educators.* Alexandria, VA: American Diabetes Association, 2000.

180. Weis SE, Foresman B, Matty KJ, et al. Treatment costs of directly observed therapy and traditional therapy for *Mycobacterium tuberculosis:* a comparative analysis. *Int J Tuberc Lung Dis* 1999;3(11):976–84.

181. Leslie WS, Urie A, Hooper J, Morrison CE. Delay in calling for help during myocardial infarction: reasons for the delay and subsequent pattern of accessing care. *Heart* 2000;84(2):137–41.

182. Rizzo JA, Simons WR. Variations in compliance among hypertensive patients by drug class: implications for health care costs. *Clin Ther* 1997;19(6):1424–5, 1446–57.

183. Fries JF, Koop CE, Sokolov J, Beadle CE, Wright D. Beyond health promotion: reducing need and demand for medical care. *Health Aff (Millwood)* 1998; 17(2):70–84.

184. Horner RD. Patients' sociodemographics characteristics and utilization of health care: looking beyond appearances at last. *Med Care* 1999;37(1):3–4.

185. Jack L Jr, Liburd L, Vinicor F, Brody G, Murry VM. Influence of the environmental context on diabetes self-management: a rationale for developing a new research paradigm in diabetes education. *Diabetes Educ* 1999;25(5):775–80, 782.

186. Glasgow RE, Fisher EB, Anderson BJ, et al. Behavioral science in diabetes. Contributions and opportunities. *Diabetes Care* 1999; 22(5):832–43.

187. Glasgow RE, Anderson RM. In diabetes care, moving from compliance to adherence is not enough. *Diabetes Care* 1999;22(12):2090–2.

188. Nolan TW. Understanding medical systems. *Ann Intern Med* 1998;128(4):293–8.

189. CDC. Levels of diabetes-related preventive-care practices—United States, 1997–1999. *MMWR* 2000;49(42):954–8.

190. Beckles GLA, Engelgau MM, Narayan KM, Herman WH, Aubert RE, Williamson DF. Population-based assessment of the level of care among adults with diabetes in the U.S. *Diabetes Care* 1998;21(9):1432–8.

191. Narayan KM, Gregg EW, Engelgau MM, et al. Translation research for chronic disease: the case of diabetes. *Diabetes Care* 2000;23(12):1794–8.

192. Lutfey KE, Wishner WJ. Beyond "compliance" is "adherence." Improving the prospect of diabetes care. *Diabetes Care* 1999;22(4):635–9.

193. Brown SA. Studies of educational interventions and outcomes in diabetic adults: a meta-analysis revisited. *Patient Educ Couns* 1990;16(3):189–215.

194. Norris SL, Engelgau MM, Narayan KM. Effectiveness of self-management training in type 2 diabetes: a systematic review of randomized controlled trials. *Diabetes Care* 2001;24(3):561–87.

195. Glasgow RE, Vogt TM, Boles SM. Evaluating the public health impact of health promotion interventions: the RE-AIM framework. *Am J Public Health* 1999;89(9):1322–7.

196. American Association of Diabetes Educators. Diabetes Educational and Behavioral Research Summit. *Diabetes Educ* 1999;25(Suppl):1–88.

197. Special considerations for the education and management of older adults with diabetes. American Association of Diabetes Educators. *Diabetes Educ* 2000; 26(1):37–9.

198. Mensing C, Boucher J, Cypress M, et al. National standards for diabetes self-management education. Task Force to Review and Revise the National Standards for Diabetes Self-Management Education Programs. *Diabetes Care* 2000;23(5):682–9.

199. Gostin LO. Public health law in a new century: part II: public health powers and limits. *JAMA* 2000;283(22): 2979–84.

200. Anderson RM, Barr PA, Edwards GJ, Funnel MM, Fitzgerald JT, Wisdom K. Using focus groups to identify psychosocial issues of urban black individuals with diabetes. *Diabetes Educ* 1996;22(1):28–33.

201. Anderson JM, Wiggins S, Rajwani R, Holbrook A, Blue C, Ng M. Living with a chronic illness: Chinese-Canadian and Euro-Canadian women with diabetes—exploring factors that influence management. *Soc Sci Med* 1995;41(2):181–95.

202. Glasgow RE, Hampton SE, Strycker LA, Ruggiero L. Personal-model beliefs and social-environmental barriers related to diabetes self-management. *Diabetes Care* 1997;20(4):556–61.

203. Wysocki T, Harris MA, Greco P, et al. Social validity of support group and behavior therapy interventions for families of adolescents with insulin-dependent diabetes mellitus. *J Pediatr Psychol* 1997;22(5):635–49.

204. U.S. Bureau of the Census. *Statistical Abstract of the United States: 1996.* 116th ed. Washington, DC: Government Printing Office, 1996.

205. Hennessy CH, John R, Anderson LA. Diabetes education needs of family members caring for American Indian elders. *Diabetes Educ* 1999;25(5):747–54.

206. Anderson RM, Goddard CE, Garcia R, Guzman JR, Vazquez F. Using focus groups to identify diabetes care and education issues for Latinos with diabetes. *Diabetes Educ* 1998;24(5):618–25.

207. El-Kebbi IM, Bacha GA, Ziemer DC, et al. Diabetes in urban African Americans. V. Use of discussion groups to identify barriers to dietary therapy among low-income individuals with non–insulin-dependent diabetes mellitus. *Diabetes Educ* 1996;22(5):488–92.

208. Maillet NA, D'Eramo Melkus G, Spollett G. Using focus groups to characterize the health beliefs and practices of black women with non–insulin-dependent diabetes. *Diabetes Educ* 1996;22(1):39–46.

209. Liburd LC, Anderson LA, Edgar T, Jack L Jr. Body size and body shape: perceptions of black women with diabetes. *Diabetes Educ* 1999;25(3):382–8.

210. Baum FE. Social capital, economic capital and power: further issues for a public health agenda. *J Epidemiol Community Health* 2000;54(6):409–10.

211. Lynch JW, Due P, Muntaner C, Smith GD. Social capital—is it a good investment strategy for public health? *J Epidemiol Community Health* 2000;54(6):404–8.

212. Baum FE, Bush RA, Modra CC, et al. Epidemiology of participation: an Australian community study. *J Epidemiol Community Health* 2000;54(6):414–23.

213. Fukuyama F. *Social capital and civil society.* IMF Institute. Working Paper WP/00/74. International Monetary Fund, 2000.

214. Leeder S, Dominello A. Social capital and its relevance to health and family policy. *Aust N Z J Public Health* 1999;23(4):424–9.

215. Burdine JN, Felix MR, Wallerstein N, et al. Measurement of social capital. *Ann N Y Acad Sci* 1999; 896:393–5.

216. Lomas J. Social capital and health: implications for public health and epidemiology. *Soc Sci Med* 1998;47(9): 1181–8.

217. Lantz PM, Lynch JW, House JS, et al. Socioeconomic disparities in health change in a longitudinal study of US adults: the role of health-risk behaviors. *Soc Sci Med* 2001;53(1):29–40.

218. Kawachi I, Kennedy BP. Income inequality and health: pathways and mechanisms. *Health Serv Res* 1999;34: 215–27.

219. Kawachi I. Social capital and community effects on population and individual health. *Ann N Y Acad Sci* 1999; 896:120-30.

220. Peyrot M, McMurry JF Jr, Kruger DF. A biopsychosocial model of glycemic control in diabetes: stress, coping, and regimen adherence. *J Health Soc Behav* 1999;40(2):141–58.

221. Lloyd CE, Dyer PH, Lancashire RJ, Harris T, Daniels JE, Barnett AH. Association between stress and glycemic control in adults with type 1 (insulin-dependent) diabetes. *Diabetes Care* 1999;22(8):1278–83.

222. Capes SE, Hunt D, Malmberg K, Gerstein HC. Stress hyperglycaemia and increased risk of death after myocardial infarction in patients with and without diabetes: a systematic overview. *Lancet* 2000;355(9206):773–8.

223. Kelly GS. Insulin resistance: lifestyle and nutritional interventions. *Altern Med Rev* 2000;5(2):109–32.

224. Shehadeh N, On A, Kessel I, et al. Stress hyperglycemia and the risk for the development of type 1 diabetes. *J Pediatr Endocrinol Metab* 1997;10(3):283–6.

225. Manning MR, Fusilier MR. The relationship between stress and health care use: an investigation of the buffering roles of personality, social support, and exercise. *J Psychosom Res* 1999;47(2):159–73.

226. Elder JP, Ayala GX, Harris S. Theories and intervention approaches to health-behavior change in primary care. *Am J Prev Med* 1999;17(4):275–84.

227. Hunt LM, Valenzuela MA, Pugh JA. Porque me toco a mi? Mexican American diabetes patients' causal stories and their relationship to treatment behaviors. *Soc Sci Med* 1998;46(8):959–69.

228. Peyrot M, Rubin RR. Structure and correlates of diabetes-specific locus of control. *Diabetes Care* 1994;17(9): 994–1001.

229. Tillotson LM, Smith MS. Locus of control, social support, and adherence to the diabetes regimen. *Diabetes Educ* 1996;22(2):133–9.

230. Engelgau MM, Narayan KM, Herman WH. Screening for type 2 diabetes. *Diabetes Care* 2000;23(10):1563–80.

231. Keen H. Therapeutic objectives and their practical achievement in type 2 diabetes. *J Diabetes Complications* 2000;14(4):180–4.

232. Dalen JE. Health care in America: the good, the bad, and the ugly. *Arch Intern Med* 2000;160(17):2573–6.

233. Mariner WK. Rationing health care and the need for credible scarcity: why Americans can't say no. *Am J Public Health* 1995;85(10):1439–45.

234. McKinlay JB, Marceau LD. To boldly go…. *Am J Public Health* 2000;90(1):25–33.

235. Ubel PA, Goold SD. "Rationing" health care. Not all definitions are created equal. *Arch Intern Med* 1998; 158(3):209–14.

236. Diabetes Control and Complications Trial Study Group. The absence of a glycemic threshold for the development of long-term complications: the perspective of the Diabetes Control and Complications Trial. *Diabetes* 1996;45(10):1289–98.

237. Stratton IM, Adler AI, Neil HA, et al. Association of glycaemia with macrovascular and microvascular complications of type 2 diabetes (UKPDS 35): prospective observational study. *BMJ* 2000;321(7258):405–12.

238. Adler AI, Stratton IM, Neil HA, et al. Association of systolic blood pressure with macrovascular and microvascular complications of type 2 diabetes (UKPDS 36): prospective observational study. *BMJ* 2000;321(7258): 412–19.

239. Brennan TA. The Institute of Medicine report on medical errors—could it do harm? *N Engl J Med* 2000; 342(15):1123–5.

240. Robinson JC. The future of managed care organizations. *Health Aff* 1999;18:7–24.

241. Pavalko EK, Woodbury S. Social roles as process: caregiving careers and women's health. *J Health Soc Behav* 2000;41(1):91–105.

242. Khlat M, Sermet C, Le Pape A. Women's health in relation with their family and work roles: France in the early 1990s. *Soc Sci Med* 2000;50(12):1807–25.

243. Walowitz PA, Jellen BC, Hanold K, Lee GF, Ropp AL, Lucas VA. Desperately seeking synergy: the journey to systems integration of women's health services. *Womens Health Issues* 2000;10(4):161–77.

244. Kirchner JT. Women's health issues. Introducing a new series with an underlying emphasis on comprehensive care. *Postgrad Med* 2000;107(1):15–16, 19.

245. Herpertz S, Albus C, Wagener R, et al. Comorbidity of diabetes and eating disorders. Does diabetes control reflect disturbed eating behavior? *Diabetes Care* 1998; 21(7):1110–16.

246. Affenito SG, Backstrand JR, Welch GW, Lammi-Keefe CJ, Rodriguez NR, Adams CH. Subclinical and clinical eating disorders in IDDM negatively affect metabolic control. *Diabetes Care* 1997;20(2):182–4.

247. Affenito SG, Lammi-Keefe CJ, Vogel S, Backstrand JR, Welch GW, Adams CH. Women with insulin-dependent diabetes mellitus (IDDM) complicated by eating disorders are at risk for exacerbated alterations in lipid metabolism. *Eur J Clin Nutr* 1997;51(7):462–6.

248. Levine MD, Marcus MD. Women, diabetes, and disordered eating. *Diabetes Spectrum* 1997;10:191–5.

249. Gavard JA, Lustman PJ, Clouse RE. Prevalence of depression in adults with diabetes. An epidemiological evaluation. *Diabetes Care* 1993;16(8):1167–78.

250. Peyrot M, Rubin RR. Persistence of depressive symptoms in diabetic adults. *Diabetes Care* 1999;22(3): 448–52.

251. Peyrot M, Rubin RR. Levels and risks of depression and anxiety symptomatology among diabetic adults. *Diabetes Care* 1997;20(4):585–90.

252. Lustman PJ, Griffith LS, Gavard JA, Clouse RE. Depression in adults with diabetes. *Diabetes Care* 1992;15(11):1631–9.

253. Griffith LS, Lustman PJ. Depression in women with diabetes. *Diabetes Spectrum* 1997;10:216–23.

254. Taipale V. Ethics and allocation of health resources—the influence of poverty on health. *Acta Oncol* 1999;38(1): 51–5.

255. Fellitti VJ, Anda RF, Nordenberg D, et al. Relationship of childhood abuse and household dysfunction to many of the leading causes of death in adults. The Adverse Childhood Experiences (ACE) Study. *Am J Prev Med* 1998;14(4):245–58.

256. Lynch JW, Kaplan GA, Salonen JT. Why do poor people behave poorly? Variation in adult health behaviors and psychosocial characteristics by stages of the socioeconomic lifecourse. *Soc Sci Med* 1997;44(6):809–19.

CASE STUDY

Mrs. Rose Oliver hummed as she got ready for her clinic appointment. She was experiencing some changes that she knew were related to menopause, including hot flashes and mood swings. She would discuss how to manage these symptoms with her nurse practitioner. At her last appointment, they had also agreed to discuss the benefits and concerns of hormone replacement therapy in view of her medical history. Her blood pressure had increased a couple of points at the last visit, and the doctor asked about her diet and salt intake. Rose felt confident she and her health care team would figure out how to keep her healthy and strong for a long time to come. She knew, too, that she would continue to play the biggest role in her own health.

Straightening her dresser a little as she reached for her appointment slip, she gazed affectionately at the smiling picture of her youngest child, Jean, now 22 and about to graduate from college. Rose recalled that some of her beliefs about her own ability to protect her health dated back to the time of Jean's birth. Born after a difficult delivery the month of Rose's 29th birthday, Jean had weighed 9½ pounds. The obstetrician told Rose that she probably had undetected gestational diabetes during her pregnancy. Fortunately, Rose and Jean were fine, but when Rose took a glucose tolerance test 6 weeks after Jean's birth, she learned she had type 2 diabetes.

Rose always said she had "gotten a lot of mileage" from the steps she took after her diagnosis, and she was proud of her dedication in managing her diabetes that had allowed so many years of good health. Her physician had pointed out then that they had caught the disease early and chances were good that gradual weight loss, through a healthy diet and exercise, could help control the disease for years. Having lost a dear aunt to diabetes-related heart disease the previous year, Rose had taken the physician's advice seriously. During the year of her diagnosis, she lost 20 pounds (from 156 pounds on her 5'1" frame). Even though she was nursing, Rose kept up her walking regimen. Once her glucose had consistently dropped to less than 100 mg/dL, Rose had her hemoglobin A_{1c} checked once a year at the clinic, and it was always within the normal range.

Rose knew there was a chance her glucose readings could go up again, especially if she gained weight. She was a little bit worried about her blood pressure, but she felt she was an old hand at controlling her diabetes and that together, she and her health care team could prevent diabetes complications. She was also grateful that her husband was supportive of her efforts to exercise and to eat properly. He actually liked some of the recipes from the diabetes cookbook. Rose knew that managing diabetes by sticking to her diet, exercise, and medication regimens would go a long way to protect her from heart disease and other diabetes complications.

5

THE MIDDLE YEARS

M. Sabolsi, MD, MPH, C.G. Solomon, MD, MPH, J.E. Manson, MD, DrPH

This chapter presents a review of data for women aged 45–64 years with diabetes. Socioeconomic status, the epidemiology of the disease in this age group, and the health behaviors of middle-aged women are described. The middle years are a time of adjustment for those who are recently diagnosed, and for many who have already been diagnosed with diabetes, the emergence of macrovascular and microvascular complications or other chronic diseases is a major issue. Coupled with other personal issues such as aging parents and an increasing lack of social support, many women in this age group are concerned about issues related to improvement in their quality of life. In particular, the unique vulnerabilities of women with diabetes in this age group and the differential application of diagnostic and treatment procedures are presented. Epidemiologic evidence indicates that women with diabetes who have a heart attack are at increased risk for poorer health outcomes and death. The changes associated with menopause are also discussed. The public health implications of these findings are framed under the three core functions of public health: assessment, policy development, and assurance. Public health practitioners are urged to assure recommended care guidelines are met and to encourage translational research that involves women in this age group to improve quality of care.

Midlife is the period in which chronic diseases emerge as a major burden on the adult U.S. population. In the mid-1990s, the number of U.S. women in midlife (aged 45–64 years) was 27 million; by 2010, the number is expected to grow to 41 million.[1] Thus, a large number of women are vulnerable to major chronic diseases such as diabetes.

As women age out of their reproductive years into their middle years, they experience major shifts in their social roles. For many women these changes include the transition from childbearing to childrearing, returning to full participation in the labor force, and often coping with sole responsibility for their households. These are also the years in which women's health issues include the effects of prolonged exposure to biological and behavioral risk factors acquired in adolescence and young adulthood. Specifically, factors such as prepregnancy weight, gestational weight gain and retention, gestational diabetes, and low levels of physical activity that continue from young adulthood increase women's risk of developing diabetes in midlife. This is also the period of life when some women experience the diminution in their physical and psychological health that may be associated with the menopause.[2] Circumstances such as past discontinuity in employment, separation, divorce, and widowhood may make middle-aged women vulnerable to low family incomes and inadequate health care coverage so that they may forego needed services, including preventive care for serious diseases such as diabetes.

This review will address some of the issues faced by women with diabetes and their public health implications. Nearly all persons with diabetes aged 45 years or older have type 2 diabetes, formerly called non–insulin-dependent diabetes mellitus. Throughout this chapter, the term "diabetes" will refer to type 2 diabetes unless otherwise specified.

5.1. Prevalence, Incidence, and Trends

Prevalence

The prevalence of diabetes increases with age. Data from the Third National Health and Nutrition Examination Survey (NHANES III, 1988–1994) show that, regardless of racial or ethnic origin, the prevalence of diabetes doubles as women age out of the reproductive years into the middle years.[3] Overall, the total prevalence of diagnosed and undiagnosed diabetes was 12.4% among women aged 50–59 years compared with 6% among those a decade younger (Figure 5-1). When the NHANES III estimates are applied to the 1995 population estimates,[4] approximately 2.7 million women aged 40–59 years have diabetes.

For middle-aged women, diabetes is at least twice as common among nonwhites as among whites (Figure 5-2). Among women aged 50–59 years, the total prevalence was 23.0% for non-Hispanic blacks, 24.0% for Mexican Americans, and 9.7% for non-Hispanic whites; estimates for women aged 40–49 years were 10.4%, 14.1%, and 4.8%, respectively.

Among non-Hispanic whites and Mexican Americans, the total prevalence of diabetes is similar in both sexes; however, among non-Hispanic blacks, the total prevalence of diabetes is higher in women than in men, notably in those aged 50–59 years (23.0% versus 16.0%).[3]

In NHANES III, 6.6% of women aged 50–59 years and 4.4% of those aged 40–49 years reported that they had been diagnosed with diabetes by a physician (Figure 5-1). The racial difference in total prevalence noted above was also evident among the women with diagnosed diabetes, and this difference widened with aging. Thus, among women aged 50–59 years, non-Hispanic blacks (14.5%) and Mexican Americans (16.5%) were about 3 times as likely as non-Hispanic whites (5.3%) to report a previous diagnosis (Figure 5-2). This racial and ethnic contrast was much less marked among men of similar age.[3]

Figure 5-1. Prevalence of diagnosed and undiagnosed diabetes among U.S. adults, by age and sex-NHANES III,* 1988-94

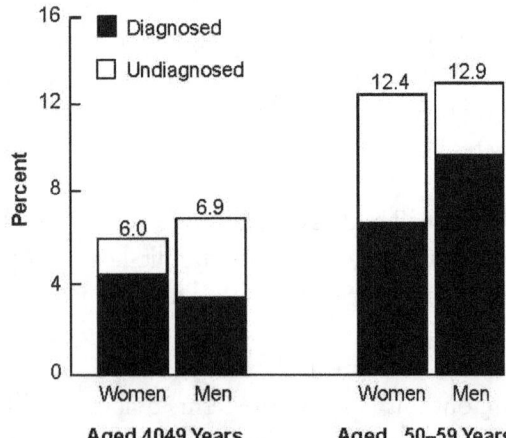

Figure 5-2. Prevalence of diagnosed and undiagnosed diabetes among U.S. women, by age and race/Hispanic origin- NHANES III,* 1988-94

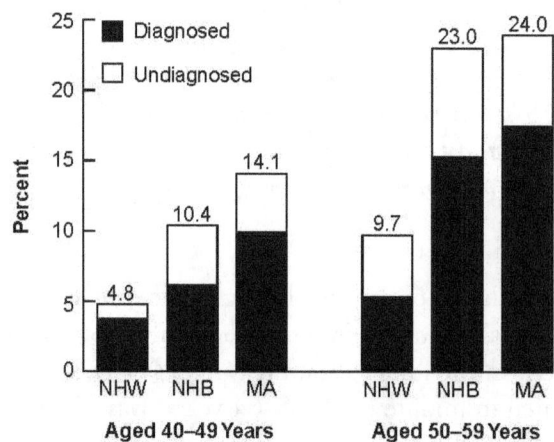

*NHANES III = Third National Health and Nutrition Examination Survey.

Source: Reference 3.

*NHANES III = Third National Health and Nutrition Examination Survey; NHW = non-Hispanic white; NHB = non-Hispanic black; MA = Mexican American.

Source: Reference 3.

Using the 1997 diagnostic criteria of the American Diabetes Association (ADA) (fasting plasma glucose 7.0 mmol/L),[5] NHANES III also found undiagnosed diabetes in 5.8% of women aged 50–59 years and 1.6% of those aged 40–49 years (Figure 5-1). Despite their higher prevalence of diagnosed diabetes, non-Hispanic black and Mexican American women also had higher rates of undiagnosed diabetes than their non-Hispanic white counterparts, with rates as much as 3 times higher among those aged 40–49 years and about 2 times higher among those aged 50–59 years (Figure 5-2). Among persons aged 50–59 years, undiagnosed diabetes was more common among women than men (5.8% versus 3.3%) and accounted for nearly half of the total prevalence in women compared with about one-quarter of the prevalence in men (46.8% versus 25.6%). Thus, in late midlife, a considerably larger number of women than men are at high risk of developing diabetes complications as a result of undiagnosed diabetes.

NHANES III estimates for diagnosed diabetes among women aged 50–59 years (6.6%, 5.3%, and 14.5% for total, non-Hispanic white, and black women, respectively) are consistent with those for women aged 45–64 years who participated each year in the National Health Interview Survey (NHIS) from 1994 through 1996. For example, in the 1996 NHIS, the annual prevalence of diabetes was approximately 6.2% overall, 5.3% among white women, and about 14% among black women.[6]

No national survey data provide stable estimates for women of other ethnic origins, but evidence from surveys of selected populations shows consistently that nonwhite U.S. women in midlife are more vulnerable to diabetes than their white counterparts (Table 5-1).[7-15] In the Strong Heart Study, which examined American Indian women aged 45–74 years in three different geographic locations, the prevalence of diabetes in women aged 55–64 years was 78% in Arizona, 47% in Oklahoma, and 51% in the Dakotas.[9] A 1974–1982 survey found that approximately 70% of Pima Indian women aged

45–64 years had diabetes as defined by World Health Organization (WHO) criteria or use of diabetic medications.[10] Estimates for Navajo women participating in the Navajo Health and Nutrition Survey (1992) were similarly high at 41% among those aged 45–64 years.[11] The wide variation in prevalence among American Indian women is also seen among Hispanics.[14] Data for middle-aged Asian Americans, a very rapidly growing segment of the U.S. population, are sparse. However, among women aged 45–74 years who participated in the Seattle Japanese American Community Diabetes Study, the prevalence of diabetes was 17%.[15]

Incidence

Based on data from the NHIS, an estimated 135,000 newly diagnosed cases of diabetes were reported by women aged 45–64 years in 1996, for an incidence rate of 4.9 per 1,000.[16] The incidence of diabetes was lower among women than men (4.9 per 1,000 versus 7.3 per 1,000).[16,17]

Data from the few population-based studies conducted show consistently that, regardless of how diabetes is defined, high-prevalence populations also have high incidence rates.[18-23] For example, in the San Antonio Heart Study, 8-year cumulative incidence rates among Mexican American women were 11.6% at ages 45–54 years and 7.5% at ages 55–64 years; comparable rates for non-Hispanic white women were 2.3% and 6.8%, respectively.[18] In the 16-year (1971–1987) First National Health and Nutrition Examination Survey (NHANES I) Epidemiologic Follow-Up Study, incident cases were identified from self-report, medical records, and death certificates.[19] Among those aged 45–54 and 55–64 years, incidence rates among black women were about 3 times the rates of their white counterparts. During 1986–1989, the Atherosclerosis Risk in Communities (ARIC) Study recruited probability samples of adults aged 45–64 years. Incident cases of diabetes were identified using the 1997 ADA diagnostic criteria, current drug treatment, and self-reported diagnosis. During 9 years of follow-up, the risk of developing diabetes was higher among African Americans than whites:

among women, incidence rates were 25.1 per 1,000 person-years and 10.4 per 1,000 person-years, respectively. African American women were about 2.5 times as likely as white women to develop diabetes even after controlling for the confounding effects of other known risk factors for diabetes.

Unlike among whites, there was no risk differential by sex among African Americans. The differences in risk between African Americans and whites were greater for women compared with men in relative terms (2.4 versus 1.5, respectively), and in absolute terms (14.7 per 1,000 person-years versus 7.5 per 1,000 person-years, respectively).

Trends

The prevalence of diabetes has been increasing steadily in all demographic groups for several decades.[6,7,24,25] Among middle-aged women, prevalence rates for diagnosed diabetes were less than 2% for women aged 45–54 years and less than 4% for those aged 55–64 years in the early 1960s; these rates increased to fairly consistent prevalence rates of 5%–6% in the 1980s and early 1990s for women aged 45–64 years. These rates have been generally comparable to those among men.[7]

The average annual rate of newly diagnosed cases for women in midlife increased steadily from the 1960s up to the mid-1980s. After the mid-1980s, however, the rate of new cases among women younger than 55 years of age showed no further change, whereas the rate for women aged 55–64 years decreased.[7]

Table 5-1. Prevalence (%) of diagnosed and undiagnosed diabetes among adults aged 45-64 years, by race/Hispanic origin- United States, 1986-97

Data source	Population	Age group (years)	Diagnosed diabetes (%) Women	Men	Undiagnosed diabetes (%) Women	Men
Navajo Health and Nutrition Survey (NHANS), 1991–92*	Navajo	45–64	30.8	20.5	10.7	15.8
The Strong Heart Study, 1988	Arizona†	45–54	56	55	9	7
		55–64	69	60	9	12
	Oklahoma‡	45–54	22	23	9	8
		55–64	35	12	12	11
	South and North Dakota§	45–54	24	10	10	9
		55–64	41	10	10	11
Indian Health Service (IHS), 1996	Non-Hispanic white American Indian/ Alaska Native	45–64	5.1	5.4	–	–
			21.1	16.7	–	–
Behavioral Risk Factor Surveillance System (BRFSS), 1994–97	Non-Hispanic white Hispanic	45–64	5.7	6.2	–	–
			11.5	12.6	–	–
King County, Washington, 1986–88	Japanese American (Nisei)	45–74	6.7	10.9	10.3	–

*WHO criteria.

†Pima, Maricopa, and Papago.

‡Apache, Caddo, Comanche, Delaware, Kiowa, and Wichita.

§Oglala, Cheyenne River, and Devils Lake Sioux.

Sources: References 9–12, 14, 15.

Aging of the population, improved identification of cases, increased survival, and an increase in the rate at which new cases develop (true incidence) are factors that may, singly or in combination, contribute to secular changes in prevalence. Aging of the population has been shown to contribute little to the increasing trends in prevalence,[25] and survival of women with diabetes in midlife was unchanged from 1971 to 1993.[26] The pattern of the national trend in the annual rate of newly diagnosed cases may reflect increased case ascertainment. However, data from several studies of selected populations indicate that since the 1960s, a rising temporal trend in true incidence of type 2 diabetes has been occurring among middle-aged adults in several ethnic groups.[20,22-24] The rate of increase has been most rapid among minority populations.[20-23] Overweight, weight gain, and lack of physical activity—major risk factors for diabetes in women[27-29]—have become increasingly common at all ages, especially among women and minority groups.[30-31] Consequently, despite the constant mortality, it is likely that increasing true incidence is making the greatest contribution to the steadily rising burden of diabetes among women in midlife. This increase in burden is estimated to continue into the middle of the 21st century.[32]

5.2. Sociodemographic Characteristics

Age, Sex, Race/Ethnicity
The age, sex, and racial/ethnic structures of the diabetic population vary markedly throughout the general population, especially among minority groups. Although sex-specific prevalence is similar, age-specific data are lacking. Adults aged 18 years or older with type 2 diabetes are more likely to be female than male (58.4% versus 41.6%) because women outnumber men in the U.S. population, especially in minority groups.[33] In the diabetic population, people of nonwhite racial and ethnic origin are overrepresented and whites are underrepresented when compared with the nondiabetic population. Among adults with diabetes, 69.6% are non-Hispanic white, 20.2% are non-Hispanic black, 4.8% are Mexican American, and 5.4% are of other races.[33]

In contrast, the percentages in the nondiabetic population are 79.3% of non-Hispanic whites, 10.7% of non-Hispanic blacks, 4.0% of Mexican Americans, and 6.0% of other races. Although this pattern was the same in both sexes, it may vary by age; however, no age-specific data are available. With the exception of the other races group, the racial/ethnic composition of the diabetic population reflects the higher prevalence of type 2 diabetes among both men and women in nonwhite racial and ethnic groups when compared with whites.

Marital Status/Living Arrangements
Overall, women aged 45–64 years with type 2 diabetes are less likely than women without diabetes to be married (58.3% versus 72.2%) and more likely to be widowed (15.6% versus 9.4%), divorced or separated (19.3% versus 14.5%), or to have never married (6.8% versus 3.9%) (Table 5-2). In contrast to women, men with and without diabetes in this age group do not differ by marital status.[33]

Among people with diabetes in this age group, women are more likely than men to be widowed (15.6% versus 2%) and less likely to be married (58.3% versus 82.3%).[33] In addition, nearly 1 in 5 middle-aged women with diabetes lives alone compared with only about 1 in 10 of their male counterparts.[33]

Education/Income/Employment
Diabetes imposes an enormous economic burden on the nation, and out-of-pocket costs for acute and ambulatory care incurred by persons with diabetes are 2–6 times the costs incurred by persons in the general population.[34,35] However, few data exist about the impact of diabetes on the socioeconomic status (SES) of women of any age. Education, income, and labor force participation, well-validated measures of SES, will be used to describe the social status of women with diabetes.

Overall, middle-aged women with type 2 diabetes have less education, have lower income, and are less likely to be in the labor force than their nondiabetic counterparts.[33] The percentage of all women with diabetes who reported that they had completed less

Table 5-2. Prevalence (%) of sociodemographic characteristics of women aged 45- 64 years with and without type 2 diabetes, by race/Hispanic origin- United States, 1989

Characteristic	Non-Hispanic white		Non-Hispanic black		Total	
	Diabetes	No diabetes	Diabetes	No diabetes	Diabetes	No diabetes
Marital status						
Married	63.0	76.1	44.3	46.9	58.3	72.2
Widowed	5.7	8.2	17.8	20.6	15.6	9.4
Divorced or separated	6.2	12.4	27.7	25.7	19.3	14.5
Never married	5.1	3.3	10.1	6.9	6.8	3.9
Living arrangements						
Alone	19.0	13.3	21.8	17.4	18.4	13.4
Nonrelative only	1.6	1.2	0.0	1.2	1.0	1.2
Spouse	63.0	75.7	43.0	44.7	57.6	71.5
Other relative only	16.4	9.9	35.2	36.7	23.0	14.0
Household size (no. of persons)						
1	20.6	14.5	21.8	18.6	19.4	14.6
2	44.1	49.7	25.0	31.1	39.0	46.4
3	20.8	20.0	21.3	16.7	20.5	20.0
≥4	14.6	15.8	31.9	33.6	21.0	19.0
Education (years)						
<9	13.8	5.6	22.7	21.8	22.7	9.7
9–12	67.7	60.9	59.5	53.6	60.4	58.6
>12	18.5	33.6	17.9	24.7	16.9	31.7
≥16	7.7	14.9	6.6	10.8	6.7	14.5
Annual family income ($thousands)						
<10	24.6	8.3	37.8	31.7	28.5	11.3
10 – <20	26.2	17.8	23.3	25.3	26.0	19.2
20 – <40	27.7	34.5	24.9	23.7	26.5	33.5
≥40	21.5	39.4	14.0	19.3	19.0	36.0
Employment status						
Employed	41.4	59.2	40.1	59.2	38.3	58.4
Unemployed	1.4	1.9	3.0	2.7	1.8	2.1
Not in labor force	57.2	38.9	56.9	38.2	59.9	39.5

Source: Reference 33.

than 9 years of education (22.7%) was twice the percentage reported by those without diabetes (9.7%) (Table 5-2); the percentage who reported that they had completed more than 12 years of education (16.9%) was half that for women without diabetes (31.7%). More than half of women with diabetes in this age group have an annual family income less than $20,000, and for 28.5% of them, such income is less than $10,000 a year, whereas the percentages for women without dia-

betes were 30.5% and 11.3%, respectively. The differences between women with and without diabetes in educational attainment and family income may reflect the findings among non-Hispanic white women only; among non-Hispanic black women, these SES characteristics showed very little variation with diabetes status (Table 5-2). Finally, nearly 60% of women with diabetes were not in the labor force compared with about 40% of those without diabetes (Table 5-2).

The low levels of education and family income among women in midlife with diabetes are even more striking among black women: 22.7% of black diabetic women had completed less than 9 years of education, and 61% lived in families with an annual income less than $20,000; percentages for white women were 13.8% and 50.8%, respectively (Table 5-2). Age-stratified data were not available for Mexican American women. However, overall estimates indicate that 69% of Mexican American women with type 2 diabetes have annual incomes below $20,000.[33]

Women with diabetes also have fewer years of education and lower family incomes than men with diabetes.[33] Only 23.6% of diabetic women aged 45–64 years reported at least some college education compared with 40.2% of diabetic men; additionally, more than half of diabetic women reported a family income less than $20,000, and only one-third of diabetic men reported such income.

These data from the 1989 NHIS suggest that in midlife, millions of women with diabetes have low SES. Their low levels of education and income combine to make them ill-equipped to deal with the self-management and financial demands of the disease. These issues are especially compelling for minority women.

5.3. Impact of Diabetes on Health Status

Death Rates

Diabetes is a leading cause of death among middle-aged American women.[36] In 1996, diabetes ranked fifth among white women, fourth among black and American Indian women, and third among Hispanic women aged 45–64 years. Death certificate data are subject to bias from underreporting of diabetes and misclassification of racial and ethnic categories.[37] Consequently, national vital statistics underestimate the contribution of diabetes to mortality in the total population as well as the magnitude of risk of mortality for people with diabetes.

Several epidemiologic studies of representative samples of the U.S. population and other groups have shown consistently that diabetes is a major risk factor for all-cause and cardiovascular disease (CVD) mortality.[26,38-47] The First National Health and Nutrition Examination Survey (NHANES I, 1971–1975) included a representative sample of the noninstitutionalized U.S. population aged 25–74 years. Participants with and without a medical history of diabetes at baseline examination were followed through 1992–1993.[26,46] Vital status was ascertained for 97.9% of persons with self-reported diabetes and 96.1% of those without. During the 22-year follow-up, in all age, sex, and racial groups, all-cause death rates were higher among people with diabetes than among those without diabetes.

At ages 45–64 years, the death rate among women with diabetes was almost 3 times the rate of women without diabetes (33.8 per 1,000 person-years versus 12.6 per 1,000 person-years).[26] The strength of the relationship between diabetes and mortality among non-Hispanic white women was similar to that for non-Hispanic black women (age-specific rate ratios = 2.5 and 2.2, respectively).[26] However,

Figure 5-3. All-cause mortality rates for U.S. adults aged 45-64 years, by diabetes status, sex, and race/ Hispanic origin, 1971-93

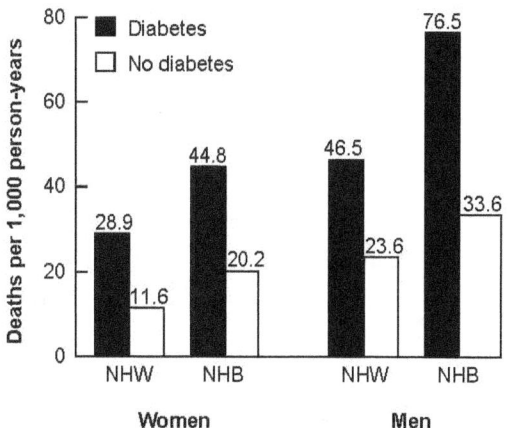

NHW = non-Hispanic white; NHB = non-Hispanic black.

Source: Reference 26.

111

in both relative and absolute terms, the impact of diabetes on mortality was greater for non-Hispanic black women than for their white counterparts (Figure 5-3). Among women with diabetes, non-Hispanic black women had a 60% higher risk for death than non-Hispanic white women after controlling for CVD risk factors; the excess mortality attributable to diabetes was 24.6 per 1,000 person-years for non-Hispanic black women compared with 17.3 per 1,000 person-years for their white counterparts.

The poorer survival experienced by persons with diabetes compared with nondiabetic persons was present throughout the follow-up period. However, among women, the diabetes-nondiabetes survival differential became progressively greater with time, being most apparent for women aged 45–54 years. Furthermore, the well-known survival advantage of women over men was much lower in the diabetic compared with the nondiabetic population, most markedly at younger ages (Figures 5-4a and 5-4b).

Among persons with diabetes, ischemic heart disease is reported to account for 40% of all deaths,

and other cardiovascular diseases for another 15% of deaths, making these conditions the leading causes of diabetes-associated deaths.[36] In a recent study, using data from NHANES I and the NHANES I Epidemiologic Follow-Up Survey, mortality rates from heart disease among women with diabetes increased 2% among those aged 55–64 years over an 8-year follow-up period. During the same period, women without diabetes of similar age experienced a 20% decrease in heart disease mortality.[46]

Hospitalizations

Across all age groups, persons with diabetes are approximately 3 times as likely to be hospitalized as persons without diabetes.[48] Among 1989 NHIS participants aged 45–64 years, 22.4% of women with diabetes reported that they had been hospitalized at least once in the past year compared with 8.8% of women without diabetes.[48] The prevalence of self-reported hospitalization did not vary by race/ethnicity or sex.[48]

Data from the 1989 NHIS indicated that patients aged 45–64 years with diabetes also had a longer

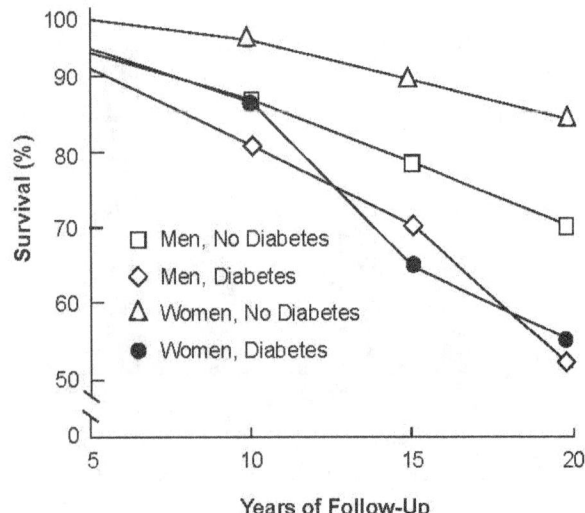

Figure 5-4a. Survival of diabetic and nondiabetic U.S. adults aged 45–54 years, by years of follow-up, 1971–93

Source: Reference 26.

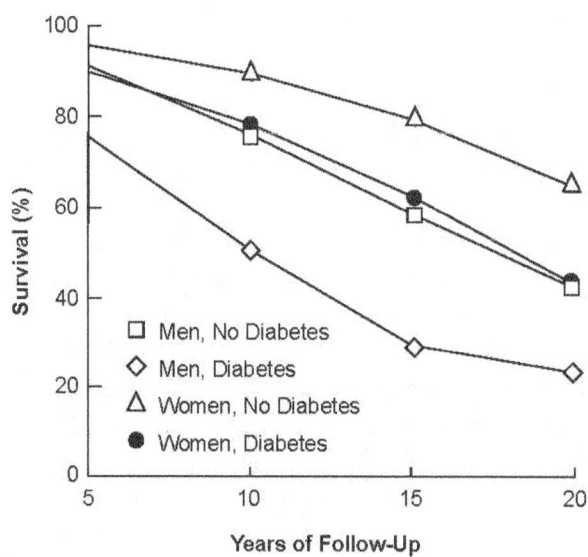

Figure 5-4b. Survival of diabetic and nondiabetic U.S. adults aged 55–64 years, by years of follow-up, 1971–93

Source: Reference 26.

average length of hospital stay (9 days) than patients without diabetes (6 days).[48] However, from 1980 to 1990, the average length of stay decreased 22% among patients with diabetes listed as any diagnosis. A North Carolina survey found that women were hospitalized for diabetes-related causes 55% more total days than men and that this sex difference increased with age; however, average hospital charges were nonetheless higher for men across all age groups.[48]

Disabilities

The public health impact and economic costs of diabetes-related disability are enormous. Data collected by 11 states and the District of Columbia for the 1998 Behavioral Risk Factor Surveillance System (BRFSS) disability module indicated that more women than men reported activity limitations.[49] The prevalence of reported activity limitations increased with age.[49]

Quality of Life

Several characteristics have been shown to affect the relationship between diabetes and quality of life. In the San Antonio Heart Study, diabetic patients with vascular complications had a higher prevalence of functional impairment (49.5%) than those without complications (31.8%).[50] In addition, among persons with diabetes in this study, increased levels of impairment were associated with a number of other factors, including age, duration of diabetes, fasting glucose level, insulin use, hypertension, and increased body mass index (BMI).[50] Finally, in a recent evaluation of two measures of quality of life among persons with diabetes, the investigators found that quality of life was reduced in persons who experienced more frequent and severe diabetic complications (unadjusted for BMI) and that separated and divorced persons experienced a lower quality of life than their married counterparts.[51] Among women aged 50–59 years in this study, 54% of those with diabetic complications had functional impairment, whereas functional impairment was found in only 30% of diabetic women without complications and 24% of women without diabetes. Among women aged 60–70 years, corresponding rates of functional impairment were 50%

among diabetic women with complications, 44% among diabetic women without complications, and 19% among women without diabetes.[51]

Studies have examined the effect of sex on perceptions of quality of life among persons with diabetes. Data from the 1989 NHIS showed that women with diabetes (4.4%) were less likely than men with diabetes (7.8%) to rate their health status as excellent, although these results were not adjusted for age. Among persons without diabetes, 31.8% of women and 38.9% of men rated their health status as excellent.[51] A better understanding is needed of the effects of gender on quality of life among persons with diabetes.

5.4. Health-Related Behaviors

Risk Behaviors and Risk Factors

A number of lifestyle factors increase a person's risk of developing type 2 diabetes and complications of type 1 or type 2 diabetes. Diet, BMI, and level of physical activity are closely interrelated and work in concert to influence a person's risk for diabetes and its complications.

An understanding of the impact of these lifestyle factors on the health of women is critical to the development of appropriate interventions to prevent diabetes and its complications. Although not all of these data regarding risk factors are limited specifically to women aged 45–64 years, these findings appear applicable to a broad population, including women in this age range.

Diet and obesity. Diet has been associated with both the development of type 2 diabetes and the onset of diabetic complications, both through its potential contribution to hyperglycemia and its relationship to other risk factors for diabetic complications. Independent of its influence on weight gain, diet composition may play an important role in the development of type 2 diabetes. Recent findings from the Nurses' Health Study suggest that women aged 38–63 years whose diets were rich in whole grain products had a significantly lower incidence of diabetes over a 10-year follow-up period.

Moreover, the relationship was stronger in overweight women (BMI > 25 kg/m²) and remained significant after adjustment for intakes of dietary fiber, magnesium, and vitamin E.[52]

The importance of dietary therapy in managing hyperglycemia and hyperlipidemia to prevent both microvascular and macrovascular complications of diabetes cannot be overemphasized.[53] The goal is to optimize glycemic control to prevent and treat both acute hypoglycemic events and chronic diabetes complications. In the 1989 NHIS, only 64% of all persons with diabetes reported following a diabetes-specific diet all or most of the time; however, 91% of persons aged 45–64 years with diabetes reported that they thought diet was very important for diabetes control.[54]

The majority of women with type 2 diabetes have additional risk factors for vascular complications of diabetes that can be controlled with dietary treatment. Approximately 52% of women aged 45–64 years with diabetes have hypertension, compared with 26% of nondiabetic women;[55] of black women with diabetes, 91.6% have hypertension compared with 57.9% of black women without diabetes. Approximately 30%–40% of women aged 45–64 years with diabetes have elevated LDL cholesterol.[55] Because abnormalities in lipid profiles and hypertension are more common among diabetic than nondiabetic women, a diet low in saturated fat, cholesterol, and sodium is essential for women with diabetes.

Among persons aged 45–64 years, BMI is higher among those with diabetes (mean BMI 28.1 kg/m²) than among those without diabetes (mean BMI 25.5 kg/m²).[55] Among persons with diabetes aged 45–64 years, the mean BMI of women exceeds that of men in all racial and ethnic groups: white women, 29.2 kg/m², and white men, 28.4 kg/m²; black women, 31.4 kg/m², and black men, 28.0 kg/m²; Mexican American women, 30.5 kg/m², and Mexican American men, 26.3 kg/m². In NHANES III, most adult participants with type 2 diabetes were overweight, and 47% of women with diabetes were obese (defined as a BMI > 30 kg/m²) com-

pared with 25% of all women.[56] This study included women with diabetes aged 45–64 years, but results were not stratified by age or sex. In data from NHANES II and the Hispanic Health and Nutrition Examination Survey (HHANES, 1982–1984), the prevalence of obesity among women with diabetes aged 45–64 was estimated to be 51% among white women, 49% among Mexican American women, and 70% among black women.[55] The mean BMI for black women with diabetes exceeded that of white women with diabetes as well. Of white women aged 45–64 years with type 2 diabetes, approximately 51% had a BMI greater than 30 kg/m², and 40% of those had a BMI greater than 35 kg/m². Among black women in the same age group with type 2 diabetes, nearly 70% had a BMI 30 kg/m² or greater; one-fifth had a BMI 35 kg/m² or greater.[55]

Controlling obesity is not only important for reducing the risk of developing type 2 diabetes but also for managing diabetes and preventing diabetes-associated complications.[57] It has been clearly shown that hyperglycemia can be controlled with dietary treatment and modest weight loss in most patients with type 2 diabetes.[58-60] Obesity, especially abdominal obesity, is also a risk factor for insulin resistance syndrome[61] and for subsequent diabetes-related macrovascular complications, including coronary heart disease and hypertension.

In a study of a weight loss intervention among women with type 2 diabetes, black women lost less weight overall and regained more weight than white women.[62] These results confirmed the observations of a previous study of nondiabetic persons that found smaller weight losses and faster weight regain among black than white women.[63] Because of the long-term ineffectiveness of weight loss interventions, prevention continues to be the most viable and effective strategy for decreasing the prevalence of obesity. Weight gain, especially in persons who are already overweight, is a strong predictor of diabetes incidence. However, in overweight adults, even modest weight loss can significantly reduce the risk of developing diabetes.[64] This study included women aged 45–64 years, but results were not stratified by age or sex. Clearly, more research is needed in the area of obesity prevention and weight reduction, especially for minority women and women with diabetes.

Physical activity. Physical activity benefits women and men with diabetes by improving glycemic control and reducing diabetes-related complications.[65] Interventions to increase physical activity in this population may significantly improve glycemic control, particularly in older, physically inactive women, who are at increased risk of developing diabetes.[66] Increased physical activity can also reduce the risk of coronary heart disease (CHD), the leading cause of death among women with diabetes. A 35%–55% reduction in risk for CHD is associated with maintaining an active lifestyle,[67] although few data are available concerning the relationship between physical activity and CHD risk specifically among women. Compared with 38% of women without diabetes, only 28% of women with type 2 diabetes participate in regular exercise despite the benefits of physical activity for weight loss, glycemic control, and prevention of CHD.[68]

Efforts to increase levels of physical activity among women, especially women with diabetes, have great potential for public health benefits. More research is needed on the relationship between physical activity and the development of type 2 diabetes and diabetes-related complications in women to guide the development of interventions.

Smoking. Evidence that cigarette smoking may impair insulin sensitivity and increase the risk for type 2 diabetes is mounting.[69] Among women in the Nurses' Health Study (NHS), those who smoked more than 25 cigarettes a day had a relative risk for type 2 diabetes of 1.42 (95% CI, 1.18 to 1.72) compared with nonsmokers.[70] Despite its associated risks, smoking has been found to be all too prevalent among persons with diabetes; according to data from the 1989 NHIS, 27% of men and 22% of women aged 45–64 years with diabetes were smokers.[55]

Smoking is also a risk factor for all of the major complications of diabetes, including CHD and stroke, that are major causes of death among women with diabetes. Among women with diabetes, smokers have a greater risk for both fatal and nonfatal coronary events than nonsmokers. In an analysis of data from NHS, the attributable risk of a coronary event among women with diabetes was 162 events per 100,000 person-years for nonsmokers and 387 events per 100,000 person-years for current smokers.[41] In addition to its effect on CHD, smoking also contributes to diabetic nephropathy, which is often a precursor of end-stage renal disease.[71] The risk of respiratory infection is also increased among diabetic patients who smoke. Because the elimination of smoking can potentially play a major role in reducing complications among women with diabetes, research is needed to determine whether intervention strategies need to be tailored specifically to meet the needs of women with diabetes.

Health-Promoting Behaviors

The four major goals of health-promoting behaviors among women with diabetes are 1) to improve metabolic control of diabetes itself, 2) to reduce the frequency and severity of microvascular complications (retinopathy, nephropathy, and neuropathy), 3) to reduce the frequency and severity of macrovascular complications (including CHD, stroke, and peripheral vascular disease), and 4) to improve quality of life. Monitoring blood glucose levels to eliminate hyperglycemia and reduce the incidence of hypoglycemia is the key to metabolic control. The cornerstone of preventing microvascular complications is maintaining serum glucose and blood pressure at normal or near-normal levels, as demonstrated among persons with type 1 diabetes in the Diabetes Control and Complications Trial (DCCT)[72] and among those with type 2 diabetes in the United Kingdom Prospective Diabetes Study (UKPDS).[73] The role of glycemic control in preventing macrovascular complications is still being defined; however, data from the UKPDS suggest that control of concomitant hypertension has a greater impact than glycemic control on preventing macrovascular complications.[73,74] The importance of assessing and managing major cardiovascular risk factors to prevent macrovascular complications of diabetes cannot be overemphasized.

Despite the importance of preventive health practices for persons with diabetes, the overall level of preventive care among patients with diabetes varies greatly. Among persons aged 25 years or older with type 2 diabetes who participated in NHANES III, most (58%) had a hemoglobin A_{1c} (HbA_{1c}) level greater than 7.0%, about 40% had uncontrolled hypertension, over one-third had microalbuminuria or clinical proteinuria, about one-quarter had undiagnosed dyslipidemia, and many had undesirable lipid levels.[56] A study using data from the Colorado BRFSS found no significant differences between men and women in levels of preventive care.[75] However, preventive care practices tended to decrease in older age groups and among those with lower levels of education. Differences were most striking for the percentage reporting that they had been monitored for HbA_{1c}: 64.5% of persons aged 30–44 years reported undergoing HbA_{1c} monitoring, compared with only 37.1% of persons aged 45–64 years and 10.6% of persons aged 65 years or older. In a study using BRFSS data from North Carolina, knowledge of HbA_{1c} decreased as age increased.[76]

In a study of data from the NHIS, only 35% of persons aged 18 years or older reported having diabetes education at some point during their disease; among those aged 40–64 years, diabetes education was reported by 52% of those with insulin-treated type 2 diabetes and 25% of those with type 2 diabetes not treated with insulin.[77] Age-stratified results were not separated by sex, but overall rates among women were similar to those among men. Although this report may have underestimated diabetes education by defining it in terms of participation in a class or program about diabetes, these studies overall suggest that diabetes education needs to be improved.

Adherence

Self-management is an important component of diabetes care.[78] Findings from several studies indicate that persons with diabetes are most likely to comply with their medication regimens and requirements for self-testing and are least likely to make lifestyle changes, such as modifying diet and exercise habits.[79,80] However, little information is presently available regarding the role of sex and age in influencing physician or patient adherence to recommendations for prevention or treatment of diabetes. Development of effective public health initiatives for women in this age group with diabetes will require further study.

5.5. Psychosocial Determinants of Health Behaviors and Health Outcomes

Social Environment

Marriage, family, and social support. Most women aged 45–64 years with diabetes are married.[33] However, almost no information is available regarding the impact of the presence of a spouse on the level or quality of diabetes care, although social context has an important influence on diabetes care and prevention goals.[81] Similarly, the role of families in the management of diabetes in adult patients is largely unexplored, and the studies that have been done show conflicting results.

A cross-sectional study of 150 insulin-requiring adults with a median age of 51.3 (34% male and 66% female) that controlled for age, duration of diabetes, and type of diabetes found that family environment may not relate to glycemic control but to psychosocial adaption.[82] When family members were supportive of recommended diabetes care practices, the person with diabetes was more satisfied with various aspects of his or her care and adaptation to the illness. Women were also found to demonstrate a higher level of satisfaction with various diabetes-related aspects of their lives. Another model[83] suggests that persons with type 1 diabetes exhibit greater psychosocial lability in glycemic control and are more responsive to psychosocial factors, while those with type 2 are affected more by variations in regimen adherence and stress. It is clear that additional research must take into consideration a multitude of factors that affect glycemic control. One must consider the type of diabetes, the social and economic environment, biologic and psychosocial factors, and the synergistic effects of these variables on the disease process in individuals.

A study of the determinants of diabetes education found that widowed patients (39%) were less likely to receive diabetes education than married patients (50%); however, this result was not controlled for age.[77] In a review of quality of life indicators, it was found that persons with diabetes who were not married were more likely to report symptoms of depression than those who were married. Men were also less likely to report symptoms of depression than women.[84] A study of persons with type 2 diabetes in Finland found that those who lived alone reported lower levels of physical functioning and psychosocial well-being than those who lived with others.[85]

A review of behavioral medicine approaches to improved diabetes care suggests that enhanced social support may be a rich resource for diabetes education and management; however, effects of gender and age should be considered.[86]

Self-help groups are one form of social support that may serve several important functions for persons with diabetes. Such functions include helping patients adapt to the diagnosis of diabetes, cope with complications, and learn to manage diabetes more effectively.[78] In a randomized trial in which patients with diabetes were assigned to either individual or group instruction, the patients in the group had greater improvements in diabetes knowledge and attitude toward diabetes than those instructed individually.[79] Community support groups provide another means of diabetes education that may be more accessible to some patients than

traditional diabetes education programs. CDC's Project DIRECT will be the first community project in the United States to apply community organization approaches to reducing the burden of diabetes by including interventions at all three levels of prevention. Project DIRECT should yield valuable information about the applicability of community organization approaches to diabetes prevention.[87]

Socioeconomic factors. On the basis of data from the 1989 NHIS, the proportion of women with diabetes aged 45–64 in the lowest quartile of educational status (fewer than 9 years of education) and in the lowest quartile of income (annual family income less than $10,000) exceeds the proportion of nondiabetic women in these quartiles for every racial group.[33] Among participants in the San Antonio Heart Study, the prevalence of diabetes and of other cardiovascular risk factors, including obesity, hypertriglyceridemia, and low high-density lipoprotein (HDL) cholesterol, fell with rising socioeconomic status (SES).[88] Previous studies looking at SES and excess prevalence of diabetes showed no correlation between these two measures.[89,90] These studies, however, did not stratify by sex. An analysis of NHANES III data that examined diabetes prevalence, SES, and other risk factors such as BMI, physical activity, and smoking among African American and non-Hispanic white men and women aged 40–74 years found that economic disadvantage may explain much of the excess prevalence of diabetes in African American women but not in African American men. The authors suggest that environmental influences such as poverty, stress, discrimination, quality of nutrition, and living conditions may affect African American men and women in different ways.[91] A recent analysis of data on 453,384 persons in the National Longitudinal Mortality Study (approximately 60,000 were black and white women aged 45–64 years) found that black women had a risk for death from diabetes nearly twice as high as white women, and 40% of this excess was explained by SES.[92] Such studies provide valuable information on the

determinants of diabetes in subpopulations. They do not, however, elucidate the relationships of these factors to morbidity among persons who have diabetes (i.e., prevalence of diabetes complications or other comorbidities). Additional studies are needed to shed more light on this issue. Differences in the determinants of morbidity and mortality between women and men would warrant the development and implementation of appropriate interventions.

In addition to increasing the risk for diabetes and mortality from diabetes, low SES has been associated with increased levels of cardiovascular risk among persons with diabetes. In a study of persons with diabetes in Scotland, the proportion of diabetic patients with three or more cardiovascular risk factors rose from 8.6% among those in the highest socioeconomic stratum to 20.2% among those in the lowest stratum.[93] For example, smoking was most prevalent among persons in the lowest socioeconomic stratum: 33% of persons with diabetes in the lowest stratum smoked, whereas only 13% in the most affluent category were smokers. However, these results were not stratified by sex and age.

Some data suggest that SES may also affect the functional status of persons with diabetes. Among 9,744 women and men aged 51–64 years sampled cross-sectionally as part of the 1992 Health and Retirement Study, SES was a significant predictor of functional status for persons with diabetes, as measured by the ability to perform several common activities of daily living, and differences in SES appeared to explain much of the worse functional status of blacks and Hispanics with diabetes compared with whites.[94] The relationship between SES and functional status may stem from the effects of SES on access to care and on a person's ability to alter the environment to improve functional status, as well as through the association of SES with other health behaviors, such as smoking and physical activity, that adversely affect health.[94] Much work remains to be done to clarify the relationships between sex, race, and SES as they affect diabetes prevention and control. Uniform definitions of SES that include household wealth as well as income are needed to enhance progress in this area. In addition, researchers need to take into account race and sex as additional variables when considering the relationship between SES and diabetes.

Social networks. A social network is a set of social ties that connects an individual with others. Analysis of social networks examines potential ties that persons may have apart from traditional sources of support such as family members or members of a particular organization such as a church. Data are lacking on the impact of social networks on women aged 45–64 years with diabetes. However, data suggesting that lack of a social network increases all-cause mortality risk among both women and men in the general population[95] indicate that such networks may have an important effect on disease outcomes. More research is needed on the effects of larger social units in communities or social networks on persons with diabetes, including women aged 45–64 years. A better understanding of social networks may be helpful in developing successful strategies for designing community-based diabetes interventions.

Community norms and acculturation. Much of behavioral research in diabetes has focused on individual behavior and family influences. The person with diabetes, however, lives in a community and invariably is influenced by the social environment within which he or she lives. No data are available on the effects of community norms and acculturation on women aged 45–64 years with diabetes. However, several studies have found that acculturation to a Western lifestyle increases a person's risk for type 2 diabetes.[96-99] In the Honolulu Heart Program, diabetes was less prevalent among Japanese American men who had retained a more traditional Japanese lifestyle than among those who had adapted to a Western lifestyle.[96] However, this study did not include women. In another study of the effects of acculturation on diabetes risk that involved both women and men (age range 17–61 years), Pima Indians residing in a rural, semi-isolated area of Mexico were compared with Pima Indians living on a reservation in Arizona. The

Pima Indians of Mexico were thinner (mean BMI 24.9 kg/m²) than those of Arizona (mean BMI 33.4 kg/m²) and had a much lower prevalence of type 2 diabetes.[99] Moreover, among both women and men, mean total cholesterol levels were significantly lower in the Mexico group than in the Arizona group. Researchers also noted that the total caloric intake of the acculturated population was substantially higher than the presumed caloric intake of Pima Indians living a traditional lifestyle.[100]

A cross-sectional study of 1,387 Mexican American women and 1,404 Mexican American men aged 25–64 years from NHANES III showed that a large waist circumference (a major risk factor for diabetes) and prevalence of abdominal obesity were strongly associated with migration and acculturation status.[101] Among women, the mean waist circumference was smallest for those born in Mexico (90.4 cm), intermediate for those who were U.S.-born English-speaking (93.6 cm), and largest for those who were U.S.-born Spanish-speaking (96.9 cm). The prevalence of abdominal obesity (waist circumference ≥ 88 cm) among U.S.-born Spanish-speaking women, U.S.-born English-speaking women, and Mexico-born women was 68.7%, 58.6%, and 55.6%, respectively. The large differences observed suggest that environmental and cultural factors may be major determinants of the diabetogenic risk profile of populations. Additional studies are needed to determine the effect of acculturation on the development of complications related to diabetes.

Acculturation and community norms are also likely to affect diabetes management in important ways, although little research has been done in this area. In a small study using focus groups of Hispanic men and women over age 40 with type 2 diabetes, participants stated that the dietary needs of the family member with diabetes were often subordinated to the dietary preferences of the rest of the family.[102] Exercise and dietary changes were difficult for members of this community, and most were unaware that increased exercise and improved diet could reduce the severity of type 2 diabetes and the

risk for complications. Another important finding of this study is that all participants reported having used some type of traditional remedy for type 2 diabetes without informing their health care providers.

In general, the beliefs of women with diabetes affect lifestyle and behavior related to nutrition, physical activity, and diabetes self-management. Acculturation is likely to affect not only a woman's chance of developing diabetes but also her way of managing the disease.

Interactions with the Health Care System
Access to care. Data from the 1990 National Health Interview Survey indicate that physician visits related to diabetes are more frequent among women than men overall and increase with age. According to that survey, diabetic women aged 45–64 years had an average of 16 outpatient physician contacts each year; this number was similar to that among men of the same age (16.3 visits annually).[103] In addition, almost all surveyed diabetic women in this age group had ongoing contact with the medical system: 95% had seen a physician in the last year, and only 2% had not had physician contact for 2 years or more; corresponding figures for men with diabetes were 92% and 2.2%, respectively. In contrast, only 78% of persons without diabetes reported a medical contact in the past year.

Nevertheless, some persons with diabetes, including women in this age group, do not have adequate access to the health care system, and barriers to access are associated with increased illness and costs. For example, in a random sample of English- and Spanish-speaking adults, perceived access to care was inversely related to hospitalization rates for diabetes, among other diseases.[104] This study included women aged 45–64 years, but results were not stratified by age or sex. We are unaware of studies of the effects of poor access to care on other markers for diabetes severity, such as hemoglobin A_{1c} levels, among women in this age group. Research that examines the role of access to care as it relates to glycemic control and the development of long-term complications of diabetes among women would be valuable in developing strategies to control diabetes and decrease its complications.

Importantly, many women who are integrated into the health care system may not necessarily be receiving recommended care for their diabetes. (See Appendix E.) For example, a national survey found that although 91% of diabetic men and women (mean age 62 years) identified one physician who provided regular care for their diabetes, only 40% of those not on insulin and 51% of those on insulin had seen an ophthalmologist in the past year. In addition, similar low rates were reported for other recommended services, including seeing a nutritionist in the past year (reported by 19% not on insulin and 24% taking insulin) and having feet checked by a health professional at least twice in the past 6 months (25% and 39%, respectively).[105] Similar findings were reported in a study in Michigan that examined the frequency with which persons with diabetes (average age 63 years and more than half women) accessed three services considered essential for diabetes management: seeing an ophthalmologist for retinopathy screening, diabetes education, and dietary counseling. Fifteen percent of the sample reported having never used any of these services, and only 33% reported having used all three services at least once in their lifetime.[106] Among presumed contributors to these low rates of accessing appropriate services were the tendency for physicians and patients to minimize the seriousness of type 2 diabetes, poor understanding and management of obesity, and the chronic multisystem nature of diabetes, which does not lend itself well to a health care system built around acute care.

Data from NHANES III also indicate that although adults with diabetes have frequent contact with health care providers, health status and outcomes are far from optimal. Glycemic control was poor, 58% had a HbA_{1c} level greater than 7%, many patients were obese (45% had a BMI > 30 kg/m^2), and among 60% of patients with known hypertension and hyperlipidimia, the blood pressure and lipid levels were not controlled at recom-

mended levels. These adverse health outcomes were distributed across all patient subgroups, but were not stratified by age and sex.[56]

Although it is certainly important to ensure that persons with diabetes have adequate access to care, it is also important to ensure that access to care includes access to preventive services necessary to optimize the health of persons with diabetes.[105] Strategies to meet these goals need to be defined for women aged 45–64 years.

Resource utilization. Data from the 1990 National Medical Care Survey indicate that women aged 45–64 years made almost 2.9 million diabetes-related office visits in 1990. Of all diabetes-related office visits by women, 35% were made by women in this age group, compared with 8% among women aged 25–44 years and 54% among women aged 65 years or older. These figures are comparable to those for men.[103]

A recent estimate of excess health care costs attributable to diabetes comes from the Kaiser Permanente database. Costs for diabetes-related treatments among the 85,209 patients with diabetes were compared with costs among age- and sex-matched controls without diabetes; excess annual expenditures associated with diabetes were estimated at $3,494 per person, or 2.4 times that of persons without diabetes.[107] Of these excess costs, 38% covered hospitalization and almost 38% covered long-term complications, primarily coronary heart disease and end-stage renal disease. Although women aged 45–64 years comprised only 21% of the entire study group and results were not stratified by sex, stratification by age indicated that excess costs for the age group 45–64 years (of whom almost half were women) were comparable to the average excess costs (i.e., $3,156 per person annually).

Because improved glycemic and blood pressure control can significantly reduce microvascular and macrovascular complications among persons with diabetes, including women aged 45–64 years,[73,74] interventions to improve glycemic and blood pressure control for women with diabetes would be expected to reduce both morbidity and costs and thus warrant broad implementation.

Patient/provider relationship. The quality of the relationship between patients with diabetes and their primary providers of diabetes care might be expected to affect the type and quality of diabetes care received. Patient/provider communication plays an important role in adherence to self-care recommendations.[108,109] However, few data are available on the association of patient/physician relationship with quality of care for women with diabetes aged 45–64 years. In a prospective cohort study of 128 patients between the ages of 18 and 79 years with diabetes, it was found that patient perception of support for autonomy from a health care provider was related to significant changes in HbA_{1c} levels at 12 months.[110] Such patients also perceived more competence in controlling their glucose levels. This study included women aged 45–64 years, but results were not stratified by age or sex. A study involving patients from general practices in England found no significant relationship between glycemic control and patient satisfaction with care received or the perceived willingness of the provider to discuss diabetes. However, certain provider characteristics did correlate directly with control, including having a special interest in diabetes and being a dietitian.[111] Only 46% of participants in this study were female, their age range was not reported, and the analyses were not stratified by sex.

Although more information on qualities of the patient/provider relationship that enhance the level of diabetes care would be useful in developing recommendations for medical training in diabetes, policy recommendations have begun to address the organizational factors that influence the delivery of diabetes care. Recommendations made at the Fifth Regenstrief Conference included universal access and payment for diabetes preventive services, comanagement of patients with diabetes by primary and specialty care providers, and special training for primary care residents in the management of type 2 diabetes.[112] These policy recommendations point out the need for changes in the structure of health care delivery and the patient/provider relationship to improve diabetes preventive care for patients with diabetes.

Personality Characteristics
Self-efficacy. The primary outcomes of effective diabetes education traditionally were improved metabolic control and patient compliance as a result of having obtained the knowledge and skills necessary to follow treatment recommendations. No research has examined the importance of self-efficacy in controlling diabetes specifically among middle-aged women. In a nonrandomized study involving 49 men and 14 women aged 32–82 years, measures of self-efficacy were highly predictive of adherence to diabetes treatment, even after adjusting for past adherence;[113] adherence was also correlated with improved glycemic control as measured by HbA_{1c} levels. A small randomized, controlled trial examined the effects of an intervention to improve self-efficacy among persons with diabetes; the average age of the study participants was 50 years, and 70% were women.[114] Although results were not stratified by age or sex, patients who received the intervention scored higher than the control group on all eight self-efficacy subscales and experienced a significantly greater reduction in HbA_{1c} levels. Thus, interventions designed to increase self-efficacy and increase patient empowerment may improve glycemic control among women with diabetes, but more research is needed.

Locus of control. Measures of locus of control, defined as a person's overriding beliefs about the causes or origins of significant events, attempt to assess personal beliefs regarding control over outcomes. In general, locus of control is divided into internal and external orientations, with two independent dimensions of externality: chance externality and powerful-other externality.[115] Several attempts have been made to develop measures of locus of control for specific diseases, including diabetes.[116,117] Using different instruments to measure locus of control, several studies have found that an internal orientation was associated with better adjustment to diabetes, better adherence to treatment,[118-120] and better glycemic control,[118,121,122] but contradictory findings have also been reported. These conflicting results may be related to the fact that locus of control involves more than one construct, each of which may have opposite effects on diabetes care practices. A recent study involving women and men separated internal locus of control into two components, autonomy and self-blame.[118] Results indicated that autonomy was generally associated with improved glycemic control and desirable self-care practices, whereas self-blame was associated with lower levels of diabetes knowledge, less frequent glucose self-monitoring, and more binge eating. In addition, high levels of chance externality were associated with poor glycemic control, low levels of exercise, and poor diabetes knowledge, while "powerful other" (specifically nonmedical) locus of control was associated with regular administration of insulin doses and infrequent binge eating. The mean age of the study participants was 47 years, and 42% were women;[118] however, results were not stratified by sex and age. These results suggest that an increased sense of autonomy and reduced self-blame may be associated with improved diabetes management in this population, but they also suggest that relying on others may not negatively affect management.

In a study that examined racial differences in locus of control among women and men with type 2 diabetes, blacks had higher levels of external locus of control than whites, as well as higher levels of stress and lower levels of family functioning, and higher levels of hemoglobin A_{1c}.[123] However, the study did not directly correlate psychosocial variables with glycemic control, and the ages of participants were not reported.

Further work in the area of locus of control should consider its interactions with other factors (e.g., sex, age, race, psychosocial factors) in predicting the ability of women to manage their own diabetes care. Findings may be relevant to the design of effective diabetes education and treatment programs for diabetic women aged 45–64 years as well as other persons with diabetes.

Traditional beliefs. Many studies have examined the relationship between psychosocial factors and successful diabetes self-management, although most of these studies have methodologic limitations.[124-126] Both the patient's internal (psychological) environment and the external social environment are of potential importance in diabetes self-management.[127-128] Barriers to diabetes self-management may arise from either the internal or external environment or interactions between the two. Personal models are part of the patient's internal environment and include representations of their illness, disease-related beliefs, diabetes knowledge, and experiences. These representations guide self-management and adherence to recommendations for treatment and preventive care.[129]

For diabetes in particular, personal beliefs about treatment effectiveness and, to a lesser extent, beliefs about disease seriousness have been shown to be predictive of behavior modifications, such as changes in diet and physical activity, that are recommended for persons with diabetes.[130] In a study that examined the relationship between personal models and diabetes self-management, the self-management activities that had the highest levels of adherence—taking diabetes medications and avoiding sweets—were highly linked to widely held traditional beliefs that diabetes management consists primarily of these two behaviors. Low-fat, low-calorie diets and increased exercise had lower levels of adherence and were rated lower in perceived effectiveness. In this study, psychosocial and behavioral factors were much stronger predictors of differences in self-management than demographic variables. In particular, personal beliefs regarding treatment effectiveness (e.g., the effectiveness of exercise in controlling diabetes and preventing complications) were highly predictive of treatment adherence.[130] This study included women aged 45–64 years, but results were not stratified by age or sex.

Focus group interviews with southern African American women aged 45–65 with type 2 diabetes revealed three consistent themes: 1) spirituality was an important factor in general health, adjustment, and coping; 2) general life stress and multiple caregiving responsibilities interfere with daily disease management; and 3) diabetes led to feelings of food deprivation and physical and emotional fatigue, worry, and fear of complications.[131] A cross-sectional study of African American and white adults from Detroit, Michigan, who had type 2 diabetes used the Diabetes Care Profile[132] to assess psychosocial factors related to diabetes. The investigators found that attitudes toward diabetes were similar for both groups, although whites who use insulin reported fewer positive attitudes and more negative attitudes toward diabetes. African Americans were less distinct in these scores. This finding suggests that insulin use may be a trigger for changes in attitudes among whites with diabetes.[132] This study included women aged 45–64 years, but results were not stratified by age or sex. Further study is needed to understand these results.

Confidence in outcome. Few data are available on the relationship between confidence in positive outcome and diabetes self-management and preventive care practices. In a small study of African American women with type 2 diabetes, confidence in positive outcomes was not related to adherence to recommended self-care practices, although self-efficacy was predictive of self-care behaviors.[133] Other studies have shown an association between confidence in treatment effectiveness and treatment-specific adherence.[130] Finally, a focus group study found that urban Caribbean Latinos with type 2 diabetes had a strong sense of fatalism regarding the course of diabetes.[102] This attitude, which may reflect an external locus of control, has been reported in other minority groups[134] and may constitute a barrier to the use of recommended diabetes self-care behaviors. Confidence in outcome appears to overlap with locus of control in predicting diabetes self-management.

More research on characteristics such as fatalism, confidence in outcome, and self-efficacy is needed to develop diabetes education strategies that are effective in producing behavioral change. In particular, an analysis of these characteristics among women and minority populations could increase our understanding of personal and social barriers to diabetes control in these vulnerable groups.

5.6. Concurrent Illnesses as Determinants of Health Behaviors and Health Outcomes

Mental Health
Eating disorders. A number of studies have examined eating disorders among women with diabetes, although all of these studies have included only women younger than age 46 with type 1 diabetes (Chapters 3 and 4). Younger women with clinical and subclinical eating disorders, as well as women who withhold insulin for weight control, have significantly worse glycemic control than women with diabetes who do not practice these behaviors. In addition, eating disorders are associated with an increase in retinopathy, as well as increased levels of serum cholesterol, triglycerides, and total lipids. Research in this area has not addressed women aged 45–64 years, a group in whom obesity and attempts at dieting are known to be frequent. Given the significant risks that may be associated with disordered eating patterns, studies should assess the prevalence of these behaviors in middle-aged women and their effects on diabetes management outcomes.

Depression. Several studies have found that the prevalence of depression is greater among men and women with diabetes than among the general population.[135-146] A review of 20 studies reported that the rate of major depression among persons with diabetes is at least 3 times greater than that of the general U.S. adult population.[135] Looking specifically at middle-aged women, a population-based study involving the Rancho Bernardo population found that among women aged 50–64 years, 14.4% of those with diagnosed diabetes but only 5.2% of those without diabetes had a Beck Depression Inventory score in the depressed range; corresponding rates in men were 7.1% and 2.0%, respectively.[136] Because these studies are cross-sectional in nature, their results cannot be used to infer a causal relationship between depression and diabetes. In fact, the prevailing clinical assumption has been that diabetes, like other chronic illnesses,[137,138] causes depression through a psychological reaction to the stress of illness or the threat of death or complications.[139-141] However, several studies have failed to show a correlation between the severity of diabetes and depressive symptoms.[142-144]

There is some evidence that depression may be a risk factor for the development of diabetes, particularly type 2. Research has suggested that diabetes and depression may have a common neuroendocrine basis, possibly mediated through depression-induced elevations in cortisol.[144-146] Results of a recent prospective 13-year follow-up study that assessed the prevalence of psychopathology among 3,481 adults suggest that major depressive disorder may increase the risk of developing type 2 diabetes (relative risk [RR] 2.2; 95% confidence interval [CI] 0.90–5.55), although the results were not statistically significant.[147] Women aged 45–64 years comprised only 16% of the group, yet they had the highest incidence of diabetes of any subgroup. Sex was not a significant predictor of diabetes in this study population, and major depression appeared predictive of diabetes even after adjusting for age, sex, and body weight. Major depressive disorder typically has its onset in the early adult years,[148] before the onset of type 2 diabetes, and is characterized by repeated episodes of depression.

No research has addressed the correlation between the number or severity of depressive episodes and the development of diabetes or the influence of antidepressive therapy on the subsequent development of diabetes among women in this age group. Whether depression represents a modifiable risk factor for the development of type 2 diabetes in this population requires further study. Moreover, since women are at greater risk for the development of

both depression and type 2 diabetes, prospective studies that address the relationship between diabetes and depression in women and control for confounding by such factors as obesity and socioeconomic status would be of great potential benefit for treating women with type 2 diabetes. In addition to the potential role of depression in the development of diabetes, the public health impact of depression in persons with diabetes needs to be assessed.

Physical Disability and Complications

Coronary heart disease. Coronary heart disease (CHD) is not only the major cause of death but also an important cause of illness among persons with diabetes. Because the risks for both type 2 diabetes and CHD are high in the middle years, a thorough understanding of the interactions between diabetes and CHD risk factors is critical for health care providers caring for women in this age group.

As noted earlier, CHD is significantly more prevalent among women with diabetes than among those without diabetes. For example, in the Nurses' Health Study, women with diabetes aged 30–55 years at study entry had a 7 times greater risk for CHD than that of their nondiabetic counterparts.[41] This increased risk may be explained in part by the increased prevalence of other recognized coronary risk factors, including obesity, hypertension, and dyslipidemia, among persons with diabetes.[149,150] However, even after adjusting for several other recognized coronary risk factors, diabetes remains a significant risk factor for CHD, with a threefold increase in risk seen among women in the NHS.[41] Furthermore, the renal disease that frequently accompanies diabetes further increases CHD risk among persons with diabetes.

Although only a small percentage of persons aged 45–64 years with diabetes have type 1 diabetes, the strikingly high CHD risk in these patients was demonstrated in a follow-up study of a Joslin Clinic cohort of patients with type 1 diabetes, 35% of whom had died of CHD-related causes by age 55; an additional 15% of these patients had clinically evident CHD.[151] As with type 2 diabetes, concomitant nephropathy increases the risk for CHD.

Effect of sex on coronary heart disease risk. Diabetes is a more powerful risk factor for CHD among women than among men and negates the overall protective effect of female sex on CHD risk, even among premenopausal women.[152-154] Numerous U.S. population-based studies have found age-adjusted mortality rates for CHD that are 3–7 times higher among women with diabetes, specifically including those aged 45–64 years, than among women without diabetes, and 2–3 times higher among men with than without diabetes.[41,152-155] Among persons with diabetes in the Framingham cohort, 7.7% of CHD among women but only 3.8% of CHD among men was attributable to diabetes.[156] Among women in the NHS, 13.8% of coronary events were attributable to diabetes.[41] The increased risk for CHD associated with diabetes in this cohort was even greater among women with other coronary risk factors such as hypertension, high cholesterol, and obesity, all of which frequently cluster with diabetes. For middle-aged and older women with diabetes, the risk posed by CHD is of special concern because the absolute risk for CHD increases with age.

The mechanisms underlying the greater risk for CHD among women than among men with diabetes are not completely understood. Contributing factors may include higher rates of hypertension and obesity among diabetic women than among men.[155,156] Lipid abnormalities also are likely to contribute to sex differences in CHD risk. Among the Rancho Bernardo study population of women and men aged 40–79 years, women with diabetes had lower HDL cholesterol levels than women without diabetes, and the difference between diabetic and nondiabetic HDL levels was greater among women than among men.[157] Furthermore, diabetes may have a greater adverse effect on LDL particle size in women than in men.[158] Diabetic women are more likely than diabetic men to have small dense LDL particles, which are considered more likely to cause atherosclerotic plaques and coronary vascular dis-

ease.[159] In all likelihood, the relationship between sex, diabetes, and CHD risk is probably influenced by several factors, including hypertension, obesity, lipid abnormalities, and hormonal (androgen/estrogen) levels.

Major coronary risk factors. The low risk for CHD among patients with diabetes in countries with low rates of CHD[160,161] supports the hypothesis that diabetes interacts with other cardiovascular risk factors to promote atherosclerotic lesions.[162] Although the basic biology that underlies the relationship between diabetes and CHD needs further clarification, the major risk factors likely to play a major role in the development of CHD in middle-aged women with diabetes include glycemic control and hyperinsulinemia, obesity, dyslipidemia, hypertension, and lifestyle factors, including smoking, weight gain, and physical inactivity. These risk factors are reviewed below.

Glycemic control and hyperinsulinemia. Data are limited on the efficacy of tight glycemic control in reducing risk for CHD in women with diabetes. However, available data indicate that poor glycemic control is associated with an increased risk for CHD among persons with diabetes. For example, in a Finnish study of 133 women and men aged 45–64 years with type 2 diabetes, baseline blood sugar level was a significant predictor of death due to CHD-related causes throughout 10 years of follow-up.[163]

Although randomized studies among persons with both type 1 (DCCT)[72] and type 2 (UKPDS)[73] diabetes have shown that tight glycemic control can produce greater reductions in microvascular disease than conventional treatment, they have failed to show a correspondingly significant reduction in macrovascular disease (e.g., stroke, myocardial infarction, CHD). Nevertheless, these studies were not completely negative. The DCCT involved a younger population and therefore did not have sufficient statistical power to assess CHD risk reduction. The UKPDS, which involved patients with a mean age of 54 years at study entry (39% women), reported a 16% reduction in myocardial infarction (p = 0.052) with tight control. Results did not differ significantly by hypoglycemic agent used (insulin or different sulfonylureas). In another arm of the study,[164] metformin, a hypoglycemic agent, produced a greater reduction in CHD risk than diet modification. As a single agent, metformin appeared possibly more effective than other hypoglycemic agents in risk reduction, but this observation may have been due simply to analytic design. This study included women aged 45–64 years, but results were not stratified by age or sex.

An important observation was the absence of an adverse impact of hypoglycemic therapy on CHD risk.[73] Studies suggesting that hyperinsulinemia is an independent risk factor for CHD among men, although possibly not among women,[165] have raised concerns that both exogenous insulin therapy and sulfonylureas raise insulin levels. Furthermore, an earlier study of glycemic control among persons with diabetes[166] reported increased cardiovascular risk among those treated with sulfonylureas or the hypoglycemic agent phenformin, a compound related to metformin. Although the failure of the UKPDS to confirm these findings is reassuring, the role of tight glycemic control in reducing cardiovascular risk among women with diabetes in this age group and among other diabetic patients requires further study.

Obesity. Obesity is a particularly important CHD risk factor for women with type 2 diabetes and is most prevalent among minority women. In NHANES II, the prevalence of obesity (BMI > 30 kg/m²) among persons aged 40–64 years with type 2 diabetes was highest among black women (65%) and was higher among white women (53%) than among black (25%) or white (17%) men.[167] In data from NHANES II and HHANES, the prevalence of obesity among Mexican American diabetic women in this age group was similar to that among white women, whereas the rate among Puerto Rican diabetic women in this age group was slightly higher (55%–60%).[55] Among Oklahoman Native American women with diabetes (women of the

Seven Tribes community, including Apache, Caddo, Comanche, Delaware, Fort Sill Apache, Kiowa, and Wichita but not limited to this age group), the prevalence of obesity was over 70%.[168]

Obesity is a risk factor of critical importance because it contributes to the development of type 2 diabetes and is an independent risk factor for cardiovascular disease.[169] In the Framingham study, which involved 2,818 women and 2,252 men aged 28–62 years at study entry, obesity was a significant predictor of cardiovascular disease throughout 26 years of follow-up, particularly among women.[170] In the Nurses' Health Study, obese women had a 3 times greater risk for CHD than lean women, and women who had significant adult weight gain had a further increase in CHD risk.[171] Obesity also increased CHD risk specifically among the subset of women with type 2 diabetes.[41]

Data are lacking on the effects of intentional weight loss on cardiovascular risk among women aged 45–64 years, particularly women with diabetes, although this question is being addressed in a major clinical trial initiated in 2001 by the National Institutes of Health (NIH). Nonetheless, available data suggest a clear benefit to avoiding obesity and weight gain.[172] Furthermore, metabolic improvements consistently observed with weight reduction[57-60,172,173] support counseling obese patients to lose weight and maintain weight loss. This issue warrants further study.

Dyslipidemia. Dyslipidemia is very common among persons with type 2 diabetes. Among diabetic white women aged 40–69 years surveyed in NHANES II, 49% had high serum total cholesterol (> 240 mg/dL), 52% had high LDL cholesterol (> 160 mg/dL), 10% had low HDL cholesterol (< 35 mg/dL), and 30% had high serum triglycerides (> 250 mg/dL). Corresponding rates among nondiabetic white women were 40%, 34%, 6%, and 6%, respectively.[174] A greater proportion of diabetic black women in this age group also had low HDL cholesterol (16%) and high triglyceride concentrations (17%) than nondiabetic black women (2%

for each), but their total cholesterol levels were similar to, and their LDL cholesterol levels lower than, those of nondiabetic black women.

Overall, compared with persons without diabetes matched for age and body weight, persons with type 2 diabetes are likely to have abnormalities in HDL cholesterol and triglyceride levels, whereas their levels of total cholesterol and LDL cholesterol are slightly but not significantly higher.[175] However, in comparing lipid profiles from a large sample of African Americans with type 2 diabetes who received care at an urban outpatient diabetes clinic, investigators reported that more women than men had high-risk LDL and HDL cholesterol profiles, but women had a lower likelihood of having a serum triglyceride concentration above goal.[176] This study included women aged 45–64 years, but results were not stratified by age or sex. At every level of total cholesterol, CHD risk is 2–3 times higher for women with diabetes than for those without diabetes.[150,171] In the Nurses' Health Study, diabetic women with self-reported high cholesterol had almost twice the incidence of CHD than women with diabetes and a normal cholesterol concentration; these women had a threefold higher incidence of CHD than nondiabetic women with high cholesterol, and a 12-fold higher incidence of CHD than nondiabetic women with normal cholesterol.[41] Although data from diabetic women are limited, low HDL cholesterol and elevated triglyceride concentrations have been shown to be independent determinants of CHD risk in patients with type 2 diabetes.[177]

In addition, analyses of subgroups of persons with diabetes in randomized controlled trials have demonstrated that pharmacologic therapy can significantly reduce CHD events by reducing total and LDL cholesterol. In the Scandinavian Simvastatin Survival Study (4S), which involved 4,446 patients, treatment with simvastatin was associated with a 42% reduction in total mortality among the 202 persons with diabetes (44 women and 158 men, mean age 60 years); this reduction was even greater than the 28% reduction among nondiabetic participants. Furthermore, the participants with diabetes experienced a 35% reduction in CHD mortality with the use of simvastatin.[178] Similarly, among 586 diabetic patients included in the Cholesterol and Recurrent Events (CARE) Study, which included patients with normal total cholesterol levels and a history of myocardial infarction, pravastatin therapy resulted in a 25% reduction in CHD events overall, and an even greater reduction was noted among women (46%) than among men (20%) with diabetes.[179,180]

In 1993, the National Cholesterol Education Program recommended that patients with diabetes be considered a high-risk group with a target LDL cholesterol concentration less than 100 mg/dL, the same level recommended for persons with a history of CHD.[181] This recommendation was also

Table 5-3. Prevalence (%) of hypertension among adults aged 45-64 years with and without type 2 diabetes, by sex and race/Hispanic origin- United States, 1976-84

Race/Hispanic origin	Women		Men	
	Diabetes	No diabetes	Diabetes	No diabetes
Non-Hispanic white	41.0	22.8	46.8	18.3
Non-Hispanic black	91.6	57.9	54.1	38.4
Mexican American	41.3	18.6	26.3	17.7
All	**52.0**	**26.0**	**47.7**	**20.0**

Source: Reference 55.

endorsed by the American Diabetes Association.[162] Nonpharmacologic interventions, such as diet changes, smoking cessation, and increased physical activity, are recommended as initial treatment to reduce LDL cholesterol; pharmacologic therapy, optimally using a statin agent, should be initiated if LDL remains elevated.[162] For high triglycerides, the first-line approach is glycemic control, diet, and increased physical activity; fibric acid derivatives are indicated if triglycerides remain elevated. Evidence from clinical trials is currently insufficient to warrant using drug therapy to modify triglyceride or HDL cholesterol levels.[183] These recommendations are all applicable to diabetic women aged 45–64 years.

Hypertension. Type 1 and type 2 diabetes and impaired glucose tolerance are all associated with hypertension.[74,184-188] In the NHANES II data, the overall prevalence of hypertension among women aged 45–64 years with a medical history of diabetes was 52%, compared with a prevalence of 26% among those with no history of diabetes (Table 5-3).[55] Among women in this age group with diabetes, the prevalence of hypertension among non-Hispanic black women (91.6%) was more than twice that of their white (41.0%) and Mexican American (41.3%) counterparts. An estimated 35%–75% of diabetic complications result from hypertension.[184] Among women with diabetes in the Nurses' Health Study, the risk for CHD was 3 times higher among those with hypertension than among those without hypertension.[41] Hypertension not only contributes to increased risk for CHD in diabetic women and men, but also increases the risk for stroke,[188] nephropathy,[189] and peripheral arterial disease.[190]

Available randomized trial data also demonstrate that improved blood pressure control reduces CHD risk among persons with diabetes. Among 1,148 hypertensive women and men (mean age 56 years) participating in a substudy of the UKPDS, tight blood pressure control with either atenolol or captopril resulted in a statistically significant 44% reduction in stroke and a nonsignificant 21% reduction in myocardial infarction.[74]

Lifestyle factors. Several lifestyle factors, including smoking, poor diet and weight gain, and physical inactivity, independently influence the incidence of diabetes and the development of complications of diabetes, including CHD. Healthy lifestyle practices have been shown to confer benefits in a variety of populations, including women aged 45–64 years.

Cigarette smoking is one of the most powerful known risk factors for CHD in general populations; among women with diabetes, it has been shown to increase CHD risk above that conferred by diabetes alone.[41,69] By increasing their HDL cholesterol levels, persons with diabetes in the Framingham study who quit smoking reduced their risk for CHD by 50%.[156]

A healthy diet and weight control are important in the prevention and management of CHD in persons with diabetes because these factors contribute to improved glycemic control, decreased adiposity, changes in lipid levels, and management of hypertension. Even moderate weight loss (less than 10% of initial body weight) can improve the cardiovascular risk profiles of both diabetic and nondiabetic obese persons by reducing blood pressure, decreasing plasma LDL cholesterol and triglycerides, and increasing serum HDL cholesterol.[172]

Regular physical activity has been associated with both reduced risk of developing type 2 diabetes and reduced obesity, both of which are independent risk factors for CHD.[57,65-68,191-193] Physical activity has been shown to increase levels of HDL cholesterol and reduce levels of LDL cholesterol, triglycerides, and fibrinogen in the general population.[194-197] Similar changes in patients with diabetes would be beneficial to treating the dyslipidemia caused by diabetes and the elevated levels of fibrinogen observed in women with diabetes.[198] Data from NHANES I indicate that diabetic women and men aged 40–69 years (72%) who reported being physically active in their leisure time had a reduced risk of dying of CHD.[199] More recent data from the NHS likewise indicate a reduced risk of CHD among women with diabetes who engage in regular physical activity.[200]

Another lifestyle factor associated with CHD risk among women with type 2 diabetes is alcohol consumption. In a recent analysis from the NHS, data from a 14-year follow-up of women (average age 48–49 years at baseline) with diabetes indicated that moderate alcohol consumption was significantly associated with reduced CHD risk.[201]

Special interventions to modify CHD risk. For women aged 45–64 with diabetes, clinical interventions to modify CHD risk include use of aspirin and hormone replacement therapy. Evidence to support these interventions follows.

Aspirin treatment. Observed alterations in platelet and endothelial function among patients with type 1 and type 2 diabetes in the Early Treatment Diabetic Retinopathy Study (ETDRS), which involved 3,711 men and women aged 18–70 years, indicate a potential role for antiplatelet therapy in persons with diabetes.[202] In the ETDRS, the group randomized to daily aspirin therapy had a 28% reduction in 5-year risk for myocardial infarction compared with the group randomized to placebo. Although the reduction in 5-year risk was greater among men (26%) than among women (9%), this difference was not statistically significant.[202] Results of a meta-analysis of controlled trials of aspirin therapy among women and men with established CHD indicated that aspirin therapy reduced overall risk of vascular events by approximately 25%, and these findings were similar among patients with and without diabetes and among both women and men.[203]

The primary concern regarding the prophylactic use of aspirin by nondiabetic women is that the benefit-to-risk ratio may differ from that observed in men, because women differ from men in their risk for myocardial infarction (the primary outcome) but have a comparable risk for stroke, and aspirin may increase the risk for hemorrhagic stroke. Healthy women, especially premenopausal women, have a lower risk for myocardial infarction than men at almost every age. However, women with diabetes (especially postmenopausal women)

have a risk for myocardial infarction that is equal to or greater than that of men in all age groups and greater risks for stroke and hypertension than diabetic men, resulting in CHD as the leading cause of death among women with diabetes.

Recent recommendations from the American Diabetes Association support the use of 81 mg–325 mg of aspirin daily by diabetic women and men with evidence of macrovascular disease and no contraindications to aspirin use.[204] The ADA also recommends considering aspirin therapy for other diabetic women and men at high risk for CHD, again in the absence of contraindications. Nevertheless, estimates from NHANES III indicate that during 1988–1994, only 20% of persons with diabetes took aspirin regularly.[205]

Hormone replacement therapy. Several observational studies have shown that women who use estrogen replacement therapy (ERT) have a 40%–50% lower risk for CHD than those who do not.[206-209] Presumed contributors to this reduced risk are favorable changes in LDL and HDL cholesterol,[206] possible improvement in insulin sensitivity,[207] and improvement in vascular reactivity.[208] Because lipid abnormalities, hyperinsulinemia, and vascular reactivity all contribute to the increased risk for CHD among women with diabetes, this group of patients might well benefit from this therapy. Although observational studies have found lower rates of heart disease among postmenopausal women who take estrogen, the results from randomized clinical trials have been unable to demonstrate such a benefit. The Heart and Estrogen/progestin Replacement Study (HERS) was unable to demonstrate lower rates of heart disease among women who took estrogen and in fact found higher rates of thromboembolic events among women who took estrogen.[210]

Indeed, limited observational data have suggested associations between ERT and reduced CHD risk among women with diabetes. For example, a recent case-control study found that postmenopausal women with diabetes who currently used ERT had a nonsignificant 49% reduction in risk for myocardial infarction.[209] In addition, data from the Nurses' Health Study on the effects of hormone replacement therapy (HRT) on the risk for myocardial infarction have likewise suggested a benefit among women with diabetes comparable to that among nondiabetic women.[206]

Data on HRT as a modifier of CHD risk among women aged 45–64 years with diabetes are currently insufficient to make recommendations regarding its use. Results from the Women's Health Initiative, an ongoing randomized, controlled trial designed to assess the potential risks and benefits of hormone replacement therapy in preventing CHD, should provide data useful for developing policy recommendations regarding the use of HRT by women with diabetes.

Cerebrovascular disease. Diabetes is a major cause of stroke and other cerebrovascular disease. Moreover, other important risk factors for stroke, including elevated blood pressure and high levels of LDL cholesterol, occur with increased frequency among women and men with diabetes, particularly those with type 2.[149,150]

Among patients with diabetes, the increased risk for stroke is greater among women than men, paralleling the greater increase in CHD risk among women with diabetes. Among women in the Nurses' Health Study, the age-adjusted risk for stroke (fatal and nonfatal) was 4.1-fold greater (95% CI: 2.8–6.1) among women with diabetes than among nondiabetic women.[171] The relative risks for fatal and nonfatal strokes from the same study were 5.0 and 3.8, respectively. In addition, the risk for stroke among women with diabetes increases with evidence of other vascular disease.

In the United States, diabetes and hypertension are both more common among blacks than whites, and these differences in prevalence contribute to the elevated risk for stroke among black Americans.[188] Cigarette smoking also greatly contributes to the risk for stroke, as do other lifestyle factors that affect the development of complications from dia-

betes, including diet, weight gain, and physical inactivity, primarily through adverse effects on lipid profiles.

Because of the elevated risk for stroke and CHD among women with diabetes, the importance of controlling cardiovascular risk factors among these patients cannot be overemphasized. Control of hypertension among diabetic women, especially black women, is of primary importance in reducing stroke-related illness and death. Smoking cessation and improvement of lipid profiles should also be high priorities for clinicians who treat women with diabetes. In addition, the increased risk for stroke among women with diabetes should be considered before such women, especially those with poorly controlled hypertension, are prescribed aspirin therapy for the primary and secondary prevention of myocardial infarction.

Peripheral vascular disease. Diabetes is an important risk factor for peripheral vascular disease (PVD). Hypertension, smoking, obesity, and hyperlipidemia are associated with an increased risk for PVD, as they are for CHD and cerebrovascular disease. Neuropathy and susceptibility to infection contribute to the progression of PVD, which may result in foot ulcerations, gangrene, and ultimately, amputation. Diabetes accounts for approximately 50% of all nontraumatic amputations in the United States.[190]

The incidence of PVD is greater among men with diabetes (12.6–21.3 per 1,000 person-years) than among women with diabetes (8.4–17.6 per 1,000 person-years),[211-213] probably because of the greater prevalence of smoking among men. The incidence of PVD also increases with age, and most women with diabetes are older than age 55.

Primary prevention of PVD for women with diabetes consists of controlling cardiovascular risk factors (especially smoking) and hyperglycemia. Tight blood pressure control in a substudy of the UKPDS involving 1,148 women and men (mean age 56 years) was associated with a 49% reduction in PVD-related amputation and death. However, these findings represented small numbers of endpoints and were not statistically significant.[74] Among the entire UKPDS cohort, tight glycemic control was likewise associated with comparable but not statistically significant reductions in these endpoints.

Because the same risk factors affect all forms of diabetes-associated vascular disease, physicians caring for women with diabetes should address not only glycemic control but also, as noted for CHD, other vascular disease risk factors. In addition, attention to foot care by physicians and education regarding self-care have been shown to be insufficient[214] and need to be improved.

Renal disease. Diabetic nephropathy, defined as increased excretion of urinary protein (principally albumin) in persons with diabetes who have no other renal disease, is one of the major complications of both type 1 and type 2 diabetes, which together account for approximately 35% of all new cases of end-stage renal disease in the United States.[215] Persons with type 1 (odds ratio, 33.7) and type 2 (odds ratio, 7.0) diabetes are at significantly greater risk for end-stage renal disease than persons without diabetes.

The incidence of end-stage renal disease attributed to diabetes among white and black women, all per 10 million population, has been reported to be 473 and 2,134 at ages 45–49 years; 730 and 3,708 at ages 50–54 years; 1,123 and 5,983 at ages 55–59 years; and 1,552 and 7,638 at ages 60–64 years.[216] Clearly, the rates for black women are much higher than those for white women; women and men appear to be equally affected. Importantly, some of the same risk factors that affect vascular disease have also been implicated in the development of diabetic nephropathy; these include hypertension, hyperglycemia, and smoking. Persons with type 1 or type 2 diabetes who have renal disease are at greater risk for CHD than persons with diabetes who do not have nephropathy.[217] In addition, the cumulative incidence of nephropathy in patients with a similar duration of diabetes may be at least as high in persons with type 2 diabetes as in those with type 1.[218]

Control of hypertension and hyperglycemia are the mainstays of the primary prevention of diabetic nephropathy. Data from the UKPDS showed nonsignificant reductions in renal failure with tight glycemic control[73] and with tight blood pressure control,[74] but few endpoints were available for comparison. Angiotensin converting enzyme (ACE) inhibitors appear to have a renoprotective effect that is independent of their effect on blood pressure.[219-224] However, these agents may offer less protection for black than for white patients with diabetes, and they have not been shown to have a long-term renoprotective benefit for persons with type 2 diabetes. More research into the role of ACE inhibitors in preventing the onset of diabetic nephropathy, especially in persons with type 2 diabetes, is needed. Because nephropathy increases with the duration of diabetes, clinicians responsible for the care of women aged 45–64 years with diabetes need to be vigilant in screening for renal complications, especially among patients with type 2, who may have had clinically silent diabetes for an undetermined length of time before diagnosis.

5.7. Public Health Implications

Assessment

Specific actions can be taken to assess the needs of women aged 45–64 years with diabetes. Several potent and modifiable risk factors for the development of diabetes, especially obesity and physical inactivity, are highly prevalent among women in this age group. In addition, many middle-aged women with diabetes are faced with issues such as the complications of diabetes, disability, and decrease in quality of life that complications frequently produce. In general, women of all races with diabetes are poorer and have less education than their nondiabetic female counterparts or men with diabetes. These women are faced with greater needs and more limited resources than women without diabetes in their age group. The public health implications of these conditions for women in this age group are listed as follows:

Surveillance and Research

- An intensive effort needs to be made to collect and report more information on women with diabetes in this age group. More women with diabetes need to be included in all types of traditional research, including randomized controlled trials.

- More creative strategies such as community-based participatory research and focus groups should be considered to gather better information on minority women and other underrepresented groups of women with diabetes, such as immigrants.

- More research is needed to examine the environmental, psychosocial, and economic factors that contribute to obesity, specifically targeting women aged 45–64 years with diabetes.

- Additional research to identify effective obesity treatments is needed. This research should include sufficient members of persons at high risk of developing diabetes.

- More data must be gathered on specific dietary factors that contribute to the development of diabetes in women to help determine specific dietary recommendations.

- Because diet, in general, is heavily culturally determined, more culturally specific and community-based research needs to be done to explore dietary factors that influence the development and outcomes of diabetes.

- More data are needed to identify the sociocultural and environmental factors that contribute to low levels of physical activity in women aged 45–64 years, particularly women with diabetes.

- It is important to explore the impact of socioeconomic status on the potential for self-care for women with diabetes, as well as the interaction between SES and access to professional diabetes care.[225]

- Research into methods for improving the SES of women with diabetes is needed (e.g., how to facilitate the health and wellness of women with diabetes in the labor force).

Tight glycemic control has been shown to reduce the risk for microvascular disease among persons with type 2 diabetes. However, its role in reducing macrovascular disease, specifically CHD, and disability remains less clear and requires further study. Because CHD is the leading cause of mortality among women aged 45–64 years with diabetes, specific research should be directed at elucidating its outcomes as well as other diabetes-related complications. Data are needed on

- Risk factors for CHD among women with diabetes to aid in risk stratification through program development.

- Potential CHD risk-modifying agents specifically among women with diabetes in this age group, including aspirin and hormone replacement therapy.

- How to better detect precursors of the initial clinical presentation of myocardial infarction among women with diabetes.

- Women's attitudes toward menopause, particularly among minority groups, to assist women with diabetes in making decisions regarding hormone replacement therapy.

- The amount of disability experienced by women in this age group and the extent to which complications of diabetes impair functional status and quality of life. Special attention should be paid to the interaction between minority status and the impact of disability in the lives of middle-aged women.

Policy Development

It is important to develop policies that increase the involvement of women with diabetes, including women aged 45–64 years, in clinical trials of diabetes, CHD, and other diabetes-associated complications. Special attention must be paid to cultural issues in the development of policies regarding women with diabetes. In the translation of research findings into practice, community representatives should be involved in the development of programs for minority women with diabetes. They should also be involved in the assessment of the effectiveness of these programs. Intensive outreach efforts must also be made on behalf of minority women with diagnosed and undiagnosed diabetes. Awareness of the risk of diabetes must be increased at the community level.

The NIH-sponsored Diabetes Prevention Program,[226] a multicenter randomized trial that is comparing the effectiveness of diet and exercise with that of pharmacologic (metformin) therapy or placebo in reducing the risk for type 2 diabetes among persons at high risk, will provide information critical to the management of patients at risk, including women aged 45–64 years. The results of this trial should provide information regarding the efficacy of specific interventions. More research is needed to determine the potential role of the community in identifying effective diabetes prevention strategies.

Other specific policies and guidelines that should be developed to address the needs of women with diabetes aged 45–64 include the following:

Diabetes Education
- All women with diabetes should have access to professional diabetes education services that teach skills for diabetes self-care. Recent Center for Medicare and Medicaid Services (CMS) (formerly Health Care Financing Administration [HCFA]) Medicare regulations are moving us closer to achieving this goal in elderly populations.
- Creative ways to educate women, using focus groups or community initiatives, should be encouraged and evaluated. In addition support groups should be available for women with diabetes to promote self- and peer education as well as resource sharing.

Obesity
- Because of the lack of effective therapies for the treatment of obesity, policies should encourage increased development of effective interventions for weight reduction, including strategies to facilitate diet and exercise adherence and new pharmacologic therapies.

- Policies should facilitate research that identifies effective strategies for the primary prevention of obesity beginning early in life, with a special focus on minority women.
- Guidelines need to be developed to assist health professionals in their efforts to educate women about healthy eating and exercise patterns.
- Policies should encourage providers to spend time educating women on the benefits of physical activity, and providers should be reimbursed appropriately.

Socioeconomic Status
Because the low SES of women with diabetes in this age group may negatively affect women's access to care, efforts must be specifically targeted at decreasing the barriers to care experienced by less wealthy and less educated women:

- Policies should be developed that ensure access to quality diabetes care for all women with diabetes regardless of ability to pay or insurance status.
- Policies should be developed to ensure that women with type 2 diabetes have access to necessary nutrition services and diabetes education as well as appropriate pharmacologic therapies.
- Programs should be developed and supported to assist women who have experienced a decrease in their functional status caused by diabetes complications to return to their previous level of functioning.

Assurance
Increased awareness must be generated at every level within the health care and public health systems about the burden of diabetes among minority women, especially in the middle and older age groups. Availability of recommended services for women at risk for diabetes and its complications needs to be improved. Because a third or more of all cases of diabetes among women aged 45–64 are undiagnosed, "opportunistic" glucose screening for these women should become standard in primary care practices. Once women are diagnosed with diabetes, they should be assured of all needed care,

including the availability of and access to a health care provider and other needed services. Health care regulatory agencies should be especially vigilant in ensuring access to all diabetes-related preventive services including eye exams, foot care, and blood pressure and lipid screening, as well as counseling about diet, HRT, and other diabetes preventive therapies. Mechanisms that may help ensure that women with diabetes receive appropriate care and services include

Oversight and Coordination of Care

- Integrated systems of care may facilitate comprehensive management, but provider and patient education is also needed to assure appropriate referrals and care.

- To ensure the delivery of quality diabetes care, delivery systems must continue to implement strategies to assess whether providers are meeting recommended care guidelines for diabetes (e.g., hemoglobin A_{1c} measurements, eye and foot care, nutritional counseling) and CHD risk reduction (e.g., monitoring lipids and blood pressure, initiating recommended treatment).

- Provider feedback, education, and incentives may all increase adherence with such guidelines and optimize diabetes care delivery.

Training

- Improved training on the risks of diabetes and the importance of preventive care in reducing diabetes-related complications is essential for health care professionals.

- A better understanding of the social and cultural factors that affect access to medical care and the success of self-care among persons with diabetes is important in designing effective diabetes interventions. In particular, because so many minority women are affected by diabetes, a greater awareness of sociocultural issues and the health effects of diabetes among minority women should be included in training for health care professionals.

- Health care professionals need to be trained in the assessment and documentation of functional status.

Diet

- Health care organizations should work to ensure that all women with diabetes receive dietary counseling.

- Diet is heavily influenced by culture. Nutritional data need to be collected separately for minority women, and dietary counseling should be culturally appropriate.

Physical Activity

- Sociocultural factors may influence physical activity levels. More opportunities (e.g., at workplaces, churches, schools, community centers) should be provided to ensure that minority women receive adequate education regarding the benefits of physical activity.

- Ensuring safe exercise space, increased availability of conveniently located exercise facilities, and child care while mothers exercise are important to the health of all women, and especially of minority women and women of low socioeconomic status.

Smoking

- Public health agencies should work to ensure that minority women are included in all smoking prevention and cessation efforts.

- Adequate training in smoking cessation techniques is essential for all health care providers. Federally funded programs and insurance companies need to increase reimbursement for patient education.

Disability and Complications

- Federal and state agencies should develop methods to ensure that all women with diabetes who experience diabetes-related disabilities receive adequate access to professional diabetes and rehabilitative care.

References

1. Day JC. *Population Projections of the United States by Age, Sex, Race, and Hispanic Origin: 1995 to 2050.* U.S. Bureau of the Census, Current Population Reports, P25-1130. Washington, DC: U.S. Government Printing Office, 1996.

2. Sowers MR, La Pietra MT. Menopause: its epidemiology and potential association with chronic diseases. *Epidemiol Rev* 1995;17(2):287–302.

3. Harris MI, Flegal KM, Cowie CC, et al. Prevalence of diabetes, impaired fasting glucose, and impaired glucose tolerance in U.S. adults: the Third National Health and Nutrition Examination Survey, 1988–1994. *Diabetes Care* 1998;21(4):518–24.

4. Deardoff KE, Hollmann FW, Montgomery PM. *U.S. Population Estimates by Age, Sex, Race, and Hispanic Origin: 1990–1995.* Population Paper Listings, No. 41. Washington, DC: U.S. Bureau of Census, Population Division, 1996.

5. American Diabetes Association. Report of the expert committee on the diagnosis and classification of diabetes mellitus. *Diabetes Care* 1997;20(7):1183–97.

6. CDC. <http://www.cdc.gov/diabetes/statistics/survl99/chap2/table10.htm>. Last revised March 2000.

7. Kenny SJ, Aubert RE, Geiss LS. Prevalence and incidence of non–insulin-dependent diabetes. In: National Diabetes Data Group, editors. *Diabetes in America.* 2nd ed. Bethesda, MD: National Institutes of Health, 1995: 47–67. (NIH Publication No. 95-1468)

8. Carter JS, Pugh JA, Monterrosa A. Non–insulin-dependent diabetes mellitus in minorities in the United States. *Ann Intern Med* 1996;125(3):221–32.

9. Lee ET, Howard BV, Savage PJ, et al. Diabetes and impaired glucose tolerance in three American Indian populations aged 45–74 years: the Strong Heart Study. *Diabetes Care* 1995;18(5):599–610.

10. Ellis JL, Campos-Outcalt D. Cardiovascular disease risk factors in Native Americans: a literature review. *Am J Prev Med* 1994;10(5):295–307.

11. Will JC, Strauss KF, Mendlein JM, Ballew C, White LL, Peter DG. Diabetes mellitus among Navajo Indians: findings from the Navajo Health and Nutrition Survey. *J Nutr* 1997;127(10 Suppl):2106S–2113S.

12. CDC. Prevalence of diagnosed diabetes among American Indians/Alaskan Natives—United States, 1996. *MMWR* 1998;47(42):901–4.

13. Schraer CD, Adler AI, Mayer AM, Halderson KR, Trimble BA. Diabetes complications and mortality among Alaska natives: 8 years of observation. *Diabetes Care* 1997;20(3):314–21.

14. CDC. Self-reported prevalence of diabetes among Hispanics—United States, 1994–1997. *MMWR* 1999; 48(1):8–12.

15. Fujimoto WY, Leonetti DL, Bergstrom RW, Kinyoun JL, Stolov WC, Wahl PW. Glucose intolerance and diabetic complications among Japanese-American women. *Diabetes Res Clin Pract* 1991;13(1-2):119–29. Data used with permission from publisher.

16. CDC. <http://www.cdc.gov/diabetes/statistics/survl99/chap2/table23.htm>. Last revised March 2000.

17. CDC. <http://www.cdc.gov/diabetes/statistics/survl99/chap2/table22.htm>. Last revised March 2000.

18. Haffner SM, Hazuda HP, Mitchell BD, Patterson JK, Stern MP. Increased incidence of type II diabetes mellitus in Mexican Americans. *Diabetes Care* 1991;14(2): 102–8.

19. Lipton RB, Liao Y, Cao G, Cooper RS, McGee D. Determinants of incident non–insulin-dependent diabetes mellitus among blacks and whites in a national sample. *Am J Epidemiol* 1993;138(10):826–39.

20. Brancati FL, Kao WH, Folsom AR, Watson RL, Szklo M. Incident type 2 diabetes mellitus in African American and white adults. The Atherosclerosis Risk in Communities Study. *JAMA* 2000;283(17):2253–9.

21. Knowler WC, Pettitt DJ, Saad MF, Bennett PH. Diabetes mellitus in the Pima Indians: incidence, risk factors and pathogenesis. *Diabetes Metab Rev* 1990;

22. Knowler WC, Saad MF, Pettitt DJ, Nelson RG, Bennett PH. Determinants of diabetes mellitus in the Pima Indians. *Diabetes Care* 1993;16(1):216–27.

23. Burke JP, Williams K, Gaskill SP, Hazuda HP, Haffner SM, Stern MP. Rapid rise in the incidence of type 2 diabetes from 1987 to 1996: results from the San Antonio Heart Study. *Arch Intern Med* 1999;159(13):1450–6.

24. Leibson CL, O'Brien PC, Atkinson E, Palumbo PJ, Melton LJ 3rd. Relative contributions of incidence and survival to increasing prevalence of adult-onset diabetes mellitus: a population-based survey. Am J Epidemiol 1997;146(1):12–22.

25. CDC. Trends in the prevalence and incidence of self-reported diabetes mellitus—United States, 1980–1994. *MMWR* 1997;46(43):1014–8.

26. Gu K, Cowie CC, Harris MI. Mortality in adults with and without diabetes in a national cohort of the U.S. population, 1971–1993. *Diabetes Care* 1998;21(7): 1138–45.

27. Colditz GA, Willet WC, Stampfer MJ, et al. Weight as a risk factor for clinical diabetes in women. *Am J Epidemiol* 1990;132(3):501–13.

28. Ford ES, Williamson DF, Liu S. Weight change and diabetes incidence: findings from a national cohort of U.S. adults. *Am J Epidemiol* 1997;146(3):214–22.

29. Manson JE, Rimm EB, Stampfer MJ, et al. Physical activity and incidence of non–insulin-dependent diabetes mellitus in women. *Lancet* 1991;338(8870):774–8.

30. Flegal KM, Carroll MD, Kuczmarski RJ, Johnson CL. Overweight and obesity in the United States: prevalence and trends, 1960–1994. *Int J Obes Relat Metab Disord* 1998;22(1):39–47.

31. Crespo CJ, Keteyian SJ, Heath GW, Sempos CT. Leisure-time physical activity among U.S. adults: results from the Third National Health and Nutrition Examination Survey. *Arch Intern Med* 1996;156(1): 93–8.

32. King H, Aubert RE, Herman WH. Global burden of diabetes, 1995–2025: prevalence, numerical estimates, and projections. *Diabetes Care* 1998;21(9):1414–31.

33. Cowie CC, Eberhardt MS. Sociodemographic characteristics of persons with diabetes. In: National Diabetes Data Group, editors. *Diabetes in America*. 2nd ed. Bethesda, MD: National Institutes of Health, 1995: 85–116. (NIH Publication No. 95-1468)

34. American Diabetes Association. Economic consequences of diabetes mellitus in the U.S. in 1997. American Diabetes Association. *Diabetes Care* 1998;21(2): 296–309.

35. Javits JC, Chiang Y-P. Economic impact of diabetes. In: National Diabetes Data Group, editors. *Diabetes in America*. 2nd ed. Bethesda, MD: National Institutes of Health, 1995:601–11. (NIH Publication No. 95-1468)

36. Peters KD, Kochanek KD, Murphy SL. Deaths: final data for 1996. *Natl Vital Stat Rep* 1998;47(9):1–100.

37. Bild DE, Stevenson JM. Frequency of recording of diabetes on U.S. death certificates: analysis of the 1986 National Mortality Followback Survey. *J Clin Epidemiol* 1992;45(3):275–81.

38. Will JC, Casper M. The contribution of diabetes to early deaths from ischemic heart disease: U.S. gender and racial comparisons. *Am J Public Health* 1996;86(4): 576–9.

39. Geiss L, Herman WH, Smith PJ. Mortality in non–insulin-dependent diabetes. In: National Diabetes Data Group, editors. *Diabetes in America*. 2nd ed. Bethesda, MD: National Institutes of Health, 1995: 233–57. (NIH Publication No. 95-1468)

40. Garcia MJ, McNamara PM, Gordon T, Kannel WB. Morbidity and mortality in diabetics in the Framingham population. *Diabetes* 1974;23(2):105–11.

41. Moss SE, Klein R, Klein BE. Cause-specific mortality in a population-based study of diabetes. *Am J Public Health* 1991;81(9):1158–62.

42. Manson JE, Colditz GA, Stampfer MJ, et al. A prospective study of maturity-onset diabetes mellitus and risk of coronary heart disease and stroke in women. *Arch Intern Med* 1991;151(6):1141–7.

43. Stamler J, Vaccaro O, Neaton JD, Wentworth D. Diabetes, other risk factors, and 12-y cardiovascular mortality for men screened in the Multiple Risk Factor Intervention Trial. *Diabetes Care* 1993;16(2):434–44.

44. Sievers ML, Nelson RG, Knowler WC, Bennett PH. Impact of NIDDM on mortality and causes of death in Pima Indians. *Diabetes Care* 1992;15(11):1541–9.

45. Wei M, Gaskill SP, Haffner SM, Stern MP. Effects of diabetes and level of glycemia on all-cause and cardiovascular mortality. The San Antonio Heart Study. *Diabetes Care* 1998;21(7):1167–72.

46. Gu K, Cowie CC, Harris MI. Diabetes and decline in heart disease mortality in U.S. adults. *JAMA* 1999; 281(14):1291–7.

47. Folsom AR, Szklo M, Stevens J, Liao F, Smith R, Eckfeldt JH. A prospective study of coronary heart disease in relation to fasting insulin, glucose, and diabetes: the Atherosclerosis Risk in Communities (ARIC) Study. *Diabetes Care* 1997;20(6):935–42.

48. Aubert RE, Geiss LS, Ballard DJ, et al. Diabetes-related hospitalization and hospital utilization. In: National Diabetes Data Group, editors. *Diabetes in America*. 2nd ed. Bethesda, MD: National Institutes of Health, 1995:553–70. (NIH Publication No. 95-1468)

49. CDC. State-specific prevalence of disability among adults—11 states and the District of Columbia, 1998. *MMWR* 2000;49(31):711–14.

50. Mitchell BD, Stern MP, Haffner SM, Hazuda HP, Patterson JK. Functional impairment in Mexican Americans and non-Hispanic whites with diabetes. *J Clin Epidemiol* 1990;43(4):319–27.

51. Jacobson AM, de Groot M, Samson JA. The evaluation of two measures of quality of life in patients with type I and type II diabetes. *Diabetes Care* 1994;17(4):267–74.

52. Liu S, Manson JE, Stampfer MJ, et al. A prospective study of whole-grain intake and risk of type 2 diabetes mellitus in U.S. women. *Am J Public Health* 2000;90(9): 1409–15.

53. American Diabetes Association. Nutrition recommendations and principles for people with diabetes mellitus. *Diabetes Care* 2001;24:S44–S47.

54. Fertig BJ, Simmons DA, Martin DB. Therapy for diabetes. In: National Diabetes Data Group, editors. *Diabetes in America*. 2nd ed. Bethesda, MD: National Institutes of Health, 1995:519–40. (NIH Publication No. 95-1468)

55. Cowie CC, Harris MI. Physical and metabolic characteristics of persons with diabetes. In: National Diabetes Data Group, editors. *Diabetes in America*. 2nd ed. Bethesda, MD: National Institutes of Health, 1995:117–33. (NIH Publication No. 95-1468)

56. Harris MI. Health care and health status and outcomes for patients with type 2 diabetes. *Diabetes Care* 2000; 23(6):754–8.

57. Tuomilehto J, Lindstrom J, Johan GE, et al. Prevention of type 2 diabetes mellitus by changes in lifestyle among subjects with impaired glucose tolerance. *N Engl J Med* 2001;344(18):1343–50.

58. Henry RR, Wiest-Kent TA, Scheaffer L, Kolterman OG, Olefsky JM. Metabolic consequences of very-low-calorie diet therapy in obese non–insulin-dependent diabetic and nondiabetic subjects. *Diabetes* 1986;35(2):155–64.

59. Henry RR, Gumbiner B. Benefits and limitations of very-low-calorie diet therapy in obese NIDDM. *Diabetes Care* 1991;14(9):802–23.

60. Grundy SM. Dietary therapy in diabetes mellitus: is there a single best diet? *Diabetes Care* 1991;14(9): 796–801.

61. Okosun IS, Liao Y, Rotimi CN, Prewitt TE, Cooper RS. Abdominal adiposity and clustering of multiple metabolic syndrome in white, black and Hispanic Americans. *Ann Epidemiol* 2000;10(5):263–70.

62. Wing RR, Anglin K. Effectiveness of a behavioral weight control program for blacks and whites with NIDDM. *Diabetes Care* 1996;19(5):409–13.

63. Kumanyaka SK, Obarzanek E, Stevens VJ, Herbert PR, Whelton PK. Weight-loss experience of black and white participants in NHLBI-sponsored clinical trials. *Am J Clin Nutr* 1991;53(6 Suppl):1631S–1638S.

64. Resnick HE, Valsania P, Halter JB, Lin X. Relation of weight gain and weight loss on subsequent diabetes risk in overweight adults. *J Epidemiol Community Health* 2000;54(8):596–602.

65. American Diabetes Association. Exercise and NIDDM. *Diabetes Care* 1990;13(7):785–9.

66. Wareham NJ, Wong MY, Day NE. Glucose intolerance and physical inactivity: the relative importance of low habitual energy expenditure and cardiorespiratory fitness. *Am J Epidemiol* 2000;152(2):132–9.

67. Paffenbarger RS, Lee IM. Exercise and fitness. In: Manson JE, Ridker PM, Gaziano JM, Hennekens CH, editors. *Prevention of Myocardial Infarction*. New York: Oxford University Press, 1996:193.

68. Ford ES, Herman WH. Leisure-time physical activity patterns in the U.S. diabetic population: findings from the 1990 National Health Interview Survey—Health Promotion and Disease Prevention Supplement. *Diabetes Care* 1995;18(1):27–33.

69. Haire-Joshu D, Glasgow RE, Tibbs TL. Smoking and diabetes. *Diabetes Care* 1999;22(11):1887–98.

70. Rimm EB, Manson JE, Stampfer MJ, et al. A prospective study of cigarette smoking and the risk of diabetes in women. *Am J Public Health* 1993;83(2):211–4.

71. Sawicki PT, Didjurgeit U, Muhlhauser I, Bender R, Heinemann L, Berger M. Smoking is associated with progression of diabetic nephropathy. *Diabetes Care* 1994;17(2):126–31.

72. The Diabetes Control and Complications Trial Research Group. The effect of intensive treatment of diabetes on the development and progression of long-term complications in insulin-dependent diabetes mellitus. *N Engl J Med* 1993;329(14):977–86.

73. UK Prospective Diabetes Study (UKPDS) Group. Intensive blood-glucose control with sulphonylureas or insulin compared with conventional treatment and risk of complications in patients with type 2 diabetes (UKPDS 33). *Lancet* 1998;352(9131):837–53.

74. UK Prospective Diabetes Study (UKPDS) Group. Tight blood pressure control and risk of macrovascular and microvascular complications in type 2 diabetes: UKPDS 38. *BMJ* 1998;317(7160):703–13.

75. CDC. Diabetes-specific preventive-care practices among adults in a managed care population—Colorado, Behavioral Risk Factor Surveillance System, 1995. *MMWR* 1997;46(43):1018–23.

76. CDC. Preventive-care knowledge and practices among persons with diabetes mellitus—North Carolina, Behavioral Risk Factor Surveillance System, 1994–1995. *MMWR* 1997;46(43):1023–7.

77. Coonrod BA, Betschart J, Harris MI. Frequency and determinants of diabetes patient education among adults in the U.S. population. *Diabetes Care* 1994;17(8):852–8.

78. Anderson RM. Is the problem of compliance all in our heads? *Diabetes Educ* 1985;11:31–4.

79. Ruggiero L, Glasgow R, Dryfoos JM, et al. Diabetes self-management: self-reported recommendations and patterns in a large population. *Diabetes Care* 1997;20(4):568–76.

80. Glasgow RE, Toobert DJ, Riddle M, Donnelly J, Mitchell DL, Calder D. Diabetes-specific social learning variables and self-care behaviors among persons with type II diabetes. *Health Psychol* 1989;8(3):285–303.

81. Brody GH, Jack L, McBride-Murray V, Landers-Potts M, Liburd L. Heuristic model linking conceptual and contextual processes to self-management and metabolic control of diabetes type 2 among African American adults. *Diabetes Care* 2001. In press.

82. Trief PM, Grant W, Elbert K, Weinstock RS. Family environment, glycemic control and the psychosocial adaptation of adults with diabetes. *Diabetes Care* 1998;21(2):241–5.

83. Peyrot M, McMurray JF Jr, Kruger DF. A biopsychosocial model of glycemic control in diabetes: stress, coping and regimen adherence. *J Health Soc Behav* 1999;40(2):141–58.

84. Peyrot M, Rubin RR. Levels of risk of depression and anxiety symptomatology among diabetic adults. *Diabetes Care* 1997;20(4):585–90.

85. Hanestad BR. Self-reported quality of life and the effect of different clinical and demographic characteristics in people with type 1 diabetes. *Diabetes Res Clin Pract* 1993;19(2):139–49.

86. Glasgow RE, Toobert DJ, Hampson SE, Wilson W. Behavioral research on diabetes at the Oregon Research Institute. *Ann Behav Med* 1995;17:32–40.

87. Engelgau MM, Narayan KM, Geiss LS, et al. A project to reduce the burden of diabetes in the African American Community: Project DIRECT. *J Natl Med Assoc* 1998;90(10):605–13.

88. Stern MP, Rosenthal M, Haffner SM, Hazuda HP, Franco LJ. Sex difference in the effects of sociocultural status on diabetes and cardiovascular risk factors in Mexican Americans: the San Antonio Heart Study. *Am J Epidemiol* 1984;120(6):834–51.

89. Brancati FL, Whelton PK, Kuller LH, Klag MJ. Diabetes mellitus, race, and socioeconomic status: a population-based study. *Ann Epidemiol* 1996;6(1):67–73.

90. Cowie CC, Harris M, Silverman RE, Johnson EW, Rust KF. Effect of multiple risk factors on differences between blacks and whites in the prevalence of non–insulin-dependent diabetes mellitus in the United States. *Am J Epidemiol* 1993;137(7):719–32.

91. Robbins JM, Vaccarino V, Zhang H, Kasl SV. Excess type 2 diabetes in African American women and men aged 40–74 and socioeconomic status: evidence from the Third National Health and Nutrition Examination Survey. *J Epidemiol Community Health* 2000;54(11): 839–45.

92. Howard G, Anderson RT, Russell G, Howard VJ, Burke GL. Race, socioeconomic status and cause-specific mortality. *Ann Epidemiol* 2000;10(4):214–23.

93. Connolly VM, Kesson CM. Socioeconomic status and clustering of cardiovascular disease risk factors in diabetic patients. *Diabetes Care* 1996;19(5):419–22.

94. Kington RS, Smith JP. Socioeconomic status and racial and ethnic differences in functional status associated with chronic disease. *Am J Public Health* 1997;87(5): 805–10.

95. Berkman LF, Syme SL. Social networks, host resistance, and mortality: a 9-year follow-up study of Alameda County residents. *Am J Epidemiol* 1979;109:186–204.

96. Huang B, Rodriguez BL, Burchfiel CM, Chyou PH, Curb JD, Yano K. Acculturation and prevalence of diabetes among Japanese American men in Hawaii. *Am J Epidemiol* 1996;144(7):674–81.

97. Wiedman DW. Adiposity or longevity: which factor accounts for the increase in type II diabetes mellitus when populations acculturate to an industrial technology? *Med Anthropol* 1989;11(3):237–53.

98. O'dea K. Westernization, insulin resistance and diabetes in Australian Aborigines. *Med J Aust* 1991;155(4): 258–64.

99. Ravussin E, Valencia ME, Esparza J, Bennet PH, Schulz LO. Effects of a traditional lifestyle on obesity in Pima Indians. *Diabetes Care* 1994;17(9):1067–74.

100. Boyce VL, Swinburn BA. The traditional Pima Indian diet: composition and adaptation for use in a dietary intervention study. *Diabetes Care* 1993;16(1):369–71.

101. Sundquist J, Winkleby M. Country of birth, acculturation status, and abdominal obesity in a national sample of Mexican American women and men. *Int J Epidemiol* 2000;29(3):470–7.

102. Quatromoni PA, Milbauer M, Posner BM, Carballeira NP, Brunt M, Chipkin SR. Use of focus groups to explore nutrition practices and health beliefs of urban Caribbean Latinos with diabetes. *Diabetes Care* 1994; 17(8):869–73.

103. Janes GR. Ambulatory medical care for diabetes. In: National Diabetes Data Group, editors. *Diabetes in America.* 2nd ed. Bethesda, MD: National Institutes of Health, 1995:541–52. (NIH Publication No. 95-1468)

104. Bindman AB, Grumbach K, Osmond D, et al. Preventable hospitalizations and access to health care. *JAMA* 1995;274(4):305–11.

105. Beckles GLA, Engelgau MM, Narayan KM, Herman WH, Aubert RE, Williamson DF. Population-based assessment of the level of care among adults with diabetes in the U.S. *Diabetes Care* 1998;21(9):1432–8.

106. Hiss RG. Barriers to care in non–insulin-dependent diabetes mellitus: the Michigan experience. *Ann Intern Med* 1996;124:146–8.

107. Selby JV, Ray GT, Zhang D, Colby CJ. Excess costs of medical care for patients with diabetes in a managed care population. *Diabetes Care* 1997;20(9):1396–1402.

108. Eakin EG, Glasgow RE. The physicians role in diabetes self-management: helping patients to help themselves. *Endocrinologist* 1996;6:1–10.

109. Golin CE, DiMatteo MR, Gelberg L. The role of patient participation in the doctor visit: implications for adherence to diabetes care. *Diabetes Care* 1996;19(10): 1153–64.

110. Williams GC, Freedman ZR, Deci EL. Supporting autonomy to motivate patients with diabetes for glucose control. *Diabetes Care* 1998;21(10):1644–51.

111. Pringle M, Stewart-Evans C, Coupland C, Williams I, Allison S, Sterland J. Influences on control in diabetes mellitus: patient, doctor, practice, or delivery of care? *BMJ* 1993;306(6878):630–4.

112. Hiss RG, Greenfield S. Forum three: changes in the U.S. health care system that would facilitate improved care for non–insulin-dependent diabetes mellitus. *Ann Intern Med* 1996;124:180–3.

113. Kavanagh DJ, Gooley S, Wilson PH. Prediction of adherence and control in diabetes. *J Behav Med* 1993; 16(5):509–22.

114. Anderson RM, Funnell MM, Butler PM, Arnold MS, Fitzgerald JT, Feste CC. Patient empowerment: results of a randomized controlled trial. *Diabetes Care* 1995;18(7): 943–9.

115. Wallston KA, Wallston BS, DeVellis R. Development of the multidimensional health locus of control (MHLC) scales. *Health Educ Monogr* 1978;6(2):160–70.

116. Bradley C, Brewin CR, Gamsu DS, Moses JL. Development of scales to measure perceived control of diabetes mellitus and diabetes-related health beliefs. *Diabet Med* 1984;1(3):213–8.

117. Ferraro LA, Price JH, Desmond SM, Roberts SM. Development of the diabetes locus of control scale. *Psychol Rep* 1987;61(3):763–70.

118. Peyrot M, Rubin RR. Structure and correlates of diabetes-specific locus of control. *Diabetes Care* 1994;17(9): 994–1001.

119. Schlenk EA, Hart KL. Relationship between health locus of control, health value, and social support and compliance of persons with diabetes. *Diabetes Care* 1984;7(6): 566–74.

120. Evans CL, Hughes IA. The relationship between diabetic control and individual and family characteristics. *J Psychosom Res* 1987;31(3):367–74.

121. Dobbins C, Eaddy J. Mood, health behaviors, perceived life control: excellent predictors of metabolic control. *Diabetes* 1986;35(Suppl 1):21A.

122. Peyrot M, McMurry JF Jr. Psychosocial factors in diabetes control: adjustment of insulin-treated adults. *Psychosom Med* 1985;47(6):542–57.

123. Bell RA, Summerson JH, Konen JC. Racial differences in psychosocial variables among adults with non–insulin-dependent diabetes mellitus. *Behav Med* 1995;21(2):69–73.

124. Jenkins CD. An integrated behavioral medicine approach to improving care of patients with diabetes mellitus (Review). *Behav Med* 1995;21(2):53–68.

125. Bradley C, editor. *Handbook of Psychology and Diabetes.* Berkshire, UK: Harwood Academic, 1994.

126. Glasgow RE, Anderson BJ. Future directions for research on pediatric chronic disease management: lessons from diabetes. *J Pediatr Psychol* 1995;20(4):389–402.

127. Hampson SE, Glasgow RE, Foster LS. Personal models of diabetes among older adults: relationship to self-management and other variables. *Diabetes Educ* 1995;21(4): 300–7.

128. Glasgow RE. Social-environmental factors in diabetes: barriers to diabetes self-care. In: Bradley C, editor. *Handbook of Psychology and Diabetes.* Berkshire, UK: Harwood Academic, 1994.

129. Hampson SE. Illness representations and self-management of diabetes. In: Weinman J, Petrie K, editors. *Perceptions of Illness and Treatment: Current Psychological Research and Applications.* Chur, Switzerland: Harwood Academic, 1996.

130. Glasgow RE, Hampson SE, Strycker LA, Ruggiero L. Personal-model beliefs and social-environmental barriers related to diabetes self-management. *Diabetes Care* 1997; 20(4):556–61.

131. Samuel-Hodge CD, Headen SW, Skelly AH, et al. Influences on day-to-day self-management of type 2 diabetes among African American women: spirituality, the multi-caregiver role, and other social context factors. *Diabetes Care* 2000;23(7):928–33.

132. Fitzgerald JT, Gruppen LD, Anderson RM, et al. The influence of treatment modality and ethnicity on attitudes in type 2 diabetes. *Diabetes Care* 2000;23(3): 313–8.

133. Skelly AH, Marshall JR, Haughey BP, Davis PJ, Dunford RG. Self-efficacy and confidence in outcomes as determinants of self-care practices in inner-city, African American women with non–insulin-dependent diabetes. *Diabetes Educ* 1995;21(1):38–46.

134. Jackson MY, Proulx JM, Pelican S. Obesity prevention. *Am J Clin Nutr* 1991;53(6 Suppl):1625S–1630S.

135. Gavard JA, Lustman PJ, Clouse RE. Prevalence of depression in adults with diabetes: an epidemiological evaluation. *Diabetes Care* 1993;16(8):1167–78.

136. Palinkas LA, Barrett-Connor E, Wingard DL. Type 2 diabetes and depressive symptoms in older adults: a population-based study. *Diabet Med* 1991;8(6):532–9.

137. Rodin G, Voshart K. Depression in the medically ill: an overview. *Am J Psychiatry* 1986;143(6):696–705.

138. Moldin SO, Schefner WA, Rice JP, Nelson E, Knesevich MA, Akiskal H. Association between major depressive disorder and physical illness. *Psychol Med* 1993;23(3):755–61.

139. Jacobson A. Depression and diabetes. *Diabetes Care* 1993;16(12):1621–3.

140. Leedom L, Meehan W, Procci W, Zeidler A. Symptoms of depression in patients with type II diabetes mellitus. *Psychosomatics* 1991;32(3):280–6.

141. Lloyd CE, Matthews KA, Wing RR, Orchard TJ. Psychosocial factors and complications of IDDM: the Pittsburgh Epidemiology of Diabetes Complications Study, VIII. *Diabetes Care* 1992;15(2):166–72.

142. Murawski BJ, Chazan BI, Balodimos MC, Ryan JR. Personality patterns in patients with diabetes mellitus of long duration. *Diabetes* 1970;19(4):259–63.

143. Lustman PJ, Griffith LS, Clouse RE, Cryer PE. Psychiatric illness in diabetes mellitus: relationship to symptoms and glucose control. *J Nerv Ment Dis* 1986; 174(12):736–42.

144. Geringer ES, Perlmuter LC, Stern TA, Nathan DM. Depression and diabetic neuropathy: a complex relationship. *J Geriatr Psychiatry Neurol* 1988;1(1):11–5.

145. Barglow P, Hatcher R, Edinin DV, Sloan-Rossiter D. Stress and metabolic control in diabetes: psychosomatic evidence and evaluation of methods. *Psychosom Med* 1984;46(2):127–44.

146. Geringer E. Affective disorders and diabetes mellitus. In: Holmes C, editor. *Neuropsychological and Behavioral Aspects of Diabetes*. New York: Springer-Verlag, 1990: 167–83.

147. Eaton WW, Armenian H, Gallo J, Pratt L, Ford DE. Depression and risk for onset of type II diabetes: a prospective population-based study. *Diabetes Care* 1996; 19(10):1097–102.

148. Eaton WW, Kramer M, Anthony JC, Dryman A, Shapiro S, Locke BZ. The incidence of specific DIS/DSM-III mental disorders: data from the NIMH Epidemiologic Catchment Area Program. *Acta Psychiatr Scand* 1989;79:163–78.

149. Krolewski AS, Warram JH, Christlieb AR. Onset, course, complications, and prognosis of diabetes mellitus. In: Marble A, Krall LP, Bradley RF, Christlieb AR, Soeldner JS, editors. *Joplin's Diabetes Mellitus*. Philadelphia: Lea & Febiger, 1985:251–77.

150. Kannel WB. Lipids, diabetes, and coronary heart disease: insights from the Framingham Study. *Am Heart J* 1985;110(5):1100–7.

151. Krolewski AS, Kosinski EJ, Warram JH, et al. Magnitude and determinants of coronary artery disease in juvenile-onset, insulin-dependent diabetes mellitus. *Am J Cardiol* 1987;59(8):750–5.

152. Heyden S, Heiss G, Bartel AG, Hames CG. Sex differences in coronary mortality among diabetics in Evans County, Georgia. *J Chron Dis* 1980;33(5):265–73.

153. Barrett-Connor E, Wingard DL. Sex differential in ischemic heart disease mortality in diabetics: a prospective population-based study. *Am J Epidemiol* 1983; 118(4):489–96.

154. Pan WH, Cedres LB, Liu K, et al. Relationship of clinical diabetes and asymptomatic hyperglycemia to risk of coronary heart disease mortality in men and women. *Am J Epidemiol* 1986;123(3):504–16.

155. Maggi S, Bush TL, Hale WE. Diabetes and other cardiovascular disease risk factors in an elderly population. *Age Ageing* 1990;19(3):173–8.

156. Kannel WB, McGee DL. Diabetes and cardiovascular risk factors: the Framingham study. *Circulation* 1979; 59(1):8–13.

157. Barrett-Connor E, Witzum JL, Holdbrook M. A community study of high-density lipoproteins in adult non–insulin-dependent diabetics. *Am J Epidemiol* 1983: 117(2):186–92.

158. Haffner SM, Mykkanen L, Stern MP, Paidi M, Howard BV. Greater effect of diabetes on LDL size in women than in men. *Diabetes Care* 1994;17(10):1164–71.

159. Laakso M, Barrett-Connor E. Asymptomatic hyperglycemia is associated with lipid and lipoprotein changes favoring atherosclerosis. *Arteriosclerosis* 1989;9(5): 665–72.

160. West KM, Ahujy MM, Bennett PH, et al. The role of circulating glucose and triglyceride concentrations and their interactions with other "risk factors" as determinants of arterial disease in nine diabetic population samples from the WHO multinational study. *Diabetes Care* 1983;6(4):361–9.

161. The Diabetes Drafting Group. Prevalence of small vessel and large vessel disease in diabetic patients from 14 centres : the World Health Organization Multinational Study of Vascular Disease in Diabetes. *Diabetologia* 1985;28:615–40.

162. Ruderman NB, Haudenschild C. Diabetes as an atherogenic factor. *Prog Cardiovasc Dis* 1984;26(5):373–412.

163. Laakso M. Glycemic control and the risk for coronary heart disease in patients with non–insulin-dependent diabetes mellitus: the Finnish studies. *Ann Intern Med* 1996;124:127–30.

164. United Kingdom Prospective Diabetes Study (UKPDS) Group. Effect of intensive blood-glucose control with metformin in complications in overweight patients with type 2 diabetes (UKPDS 34). *Lancet* 1998;352(9131): 854–65.

165. Haffner SM, Miettinen H. Insulin resistance implications for type 2 diabetes mellitus and coronary heart disease. *Am J Med* 1997;103(2):152–62.

166. Meinert CL, Knatterud GL, Prout TE, Klimt CR. A study of the effects of hypoglycemic agents on vascular complications in patients with adult-onset diabetes. II. Mortality results. *Diabetes* 1970;19(Suppl):789–830.

167. Harris MI. Summary. In: National Diabetes Data Group, editors. *Diabetes in America*. 2nd ed. Bethesda, MD: National Institutes of Health, 1995:1–13. (NIH Publication No. 95-1468)

168. Stahn RM, Gohdes D, Valway SE. Diabetes and its complications among selected tribes in North Dakota, South Dakota, and Nebraska. *Diabetes Care* 1993;16(1): 244–7.

169. DeFronzo RA, Ferrannini E, Koivisto V. New concepts in the pathogenesis and treatment of non–insulin-dependent diabetes mellitus. *Am J Med* 1983;74(1A): 52–81.

170. Hubert HB, Feinleib M, McNamara PM, Castelli WP. Obesity as an independent risk factor for cardiovascular disease: a 26-year follow-up of participants in the Framingham Heart Study. *Circulation* 1983;67(5): 968–77.

171. Manson JE, Colditz GA, Stampfer MJ, et al. A prospective study of obesity and risk of coronary heart disease in women. *N Engl J Med* 1990;322(15):882–9.

172. Goldstein DJ. Beneficial effects of modest weight loss. *Int J Obes Relat Metab Discord* 1992;16(6):397–415.

173. Hadden DR, Blair AL, Wilson EA, et al. Natural history of diabetes presenting age 40–69 years: a prospective study of the influence of intensive dietary therapy. *Q J Med* 1986;59(230):579–98.

174. Cowie CC, Howard BV, Harris MI. Serum lipoproteins in African Americans and whites with non–insulin-dependent diabetes in the U.S. population. *Circulation* 1994;90(3):1185–93.

175. American Diabetes Association. Detection and management of lipid disorders in diabetes. *Diabetes Care* 1993; 16(5):828–34.

176. Cook CB, Erdman DM, Ryan GJ, et al. The pattern of dyslipidemia among urban African Americans with type 2 diabetes. *Diabetes Care* 2000;23(3):319–24.

177. Pyorala K, Laakso M, Uusitupa M. Diabetes and atherosclerosis: an epidemiologic view. *Diabetes Metab Rev* 1987;3(2):463–524.

178. Pyorala K, Pederson TR, Kjekhus J, Faergeman O, Olsson AG, Thorgeirsson G. Cholesterol lowering with simvastatin improves prognosis of diabetic patients with coronary heart disease. A subgroup analysis of the Scandinavian Simvastatin Survival Study (4S). *Diabetes Care* 1997;20(4):614–20.

179. Fontbonne A, Eschwege E, Cambien F, et al. Hypertriglyceridaemia as a risk factor of coronary heart disease mortality in subjects with impaired glucose tolerance or diabetes: results from the 11-year follow-up of the Paris Prospective Study. *Diabetologia* 1989;32(5): 300–4.

180. Sacks FM, Pfeffer MA, Moye LA, et al. The effect of pravastatin on coronary events after myocardial infarction in patients with average cholesterol levels. Cholesterol and Recurrent Events Trial Investigators. *N Engl J Med* 1996;335(14):1001–9.

181. National Cholesterol Education Program. Summary of the second report of the National Cholesterol Education Program (NCEP) expert panel on detection, evaluation, and treatment of high blood cholesterol in adults (Adult Treatment Panel II). *JAMA* 1993;269(23):3015–23.

182. American Diabetes Association. Management of dyslipidemia in adults with diabetes. *Diabetes Care* 1999; 22(Suppl 1):S56–S59.

183. National Institutes of Health Consensus Conference. Triglyceride, high-density lipoprotein, and coronary heart disease. NIH consensus development panel on triglyceride, high-density lipoprotein, and coronary heart disease. *JAMA* 1993;269(4):505–10.

184. Levy D, Kannel WB. Cardiovascular risks: new insights from Framingham. *Am Heart J* 1988;116:266–72.

185. Hansson L, Zanchetti A, Carruthers SG, et al. Effects of intensive blood-pressure lowering and low-dose aspirin in patients with hypertension: principal results of the Hypertension Optimal Treatment (HOT) randomized trial. HOT Study Group. *Lancet* 1998;351(9118): 1755–62.

186. Alder AI, Stratton IM, Neil HA, et al. Association of systolic blood pressure with macrovascular and microvascular complications of type 2 diabetes (UKPDS 36): prospective observational study. *BMJ* 2000;321(7258): 412–19.

187. Heart Outcomes Prevention Evaluation (HOPE) Study Investigators. Effects of ramipril on cardiovascular and microvascular outcomes in people with diabetes mellitus: results of the HOPE study and MICRO-HOPE substudy. *Lancet* 2000;355(9200):253–9.

188. Kuller LH. Stroke and diabetes. In: National Diabetes Data Group, editors. *Diabetes in America*. 2nd ed. Bethesda, MD: National Institutes of Health, 1995:449–56. (NIH Publication No. 95-1468)

189. Nelson RL, Knowler WC, Pettitt DJ, Bennett PH. Kidney diseases in diabetes. In: National Diabetes Data Group, editors. *Diabetes in America*. 2nd ed. Bethesda, MD: National Institutes of Health, 1995:349–400. (NIH Publication No. 95-1468)

190. Palumbo PJ, Melton LJ. Peripheral vascular disease and diabetes. In: National Diabetes Data Group, editors. *Diabetes in America*. 2nd ed. Bethesda, MD: National Institutes of Health, 1995:401–8. (NIH Publication No. 95-1468)

191. Wing RR, Epstein LH, Paternostro-Bayles M, Kriska A, Norwalk MP, Gooding W. Exercise in a behavioral weight control programme for obese patients with type 2 (non–insulin-dependent) diabetes. *Diabetologia* 1988; 31(12):902–9.

192. Donahoe CP Jr, Lin DH, Kirschenbaum DS, Keesey RE. Metabolic consequences of dieting and exercise in the treatment of obesity. *J Consult Clin Psychol* 1984; 52(5):827–36.

193. Pavlou KN, Steffee WP, Lerman RH, Burrow BA. Effects of dieting and exercise on lean body mass, oxygen uptake, and strength. *Med Sci Sports Exerc* 1985; 17(4):466–71.

194. Haskell WL. Exercise-induced changes in plasma lipids and lipoproteins. *Prev Med* 1984;13(1):23–36.

195. Rauramaa R. Relationship of physical activity, glucose tolerance, and weight management. *Prev Med* 1984; 13(1):37–46.

196. Gordon DJ, Rifkind BM. High-density lipoprotein—the clinical implications of recent studies. *N Engl J Med* 1989;321(19):1311–6.

197. Ernst E. Fibrinogen. *BMJ* 1991;303(6803):596–7.

198. Kannel WB, D'Agostino RB, Wilson PW, Belanger AJ, Gagnon DR. Diabetes, fibrinogen, and risk of cardiovascular disease: the Framingham experience. *Am Heart J* 1990;120(3):672–6.

199. Ford ES, DeStefano F. Risk factors for mortality from all causes and from coronary heart disease among persons with diabetes. Findings from the National Health and Nutrition Examination Survey I Epidemiologic Follow-Up Study. *Am J Epidemiol* 1991;133(12):1220–30.

200. Hu FB, Hennekens CH, Stampfer MJ, et al. Physical activity and risk of coronary heart disease among diabetic women. *Circulation* 1998;98(Suppl 1):I-375, Abstract No. 1967.

201. Solomon CG, Hu FB, Stampfer MJ. Moderate alcohol consumption and risk of coronary heart disease among women with type 2 diabetes mellitus. *Circulation* 2000;102(5):494–9.

202. Early Treatment of Diabetic Retinopathy Study Investigators. Aspirin effects on mortality and morbidity in patients with diabetes mellitus. Early Treatment of Diabetic Retinopathy Study report 14. ETDRS Investigators. *JAMA* 1992;268(10):1292–300.

203. Antiplatelets Trialists' Collaboration Group. Overall effect on major vascular events: subgroup issues and comparison of agents. In: Jarrett RJ, editor. *Diabetes and Heart Disease*. New York: Elsevier, 1984:1–41.

204. American Diabetes Association. Aspirin therapy in diabetes. *Diabetes Care* 2001;22(Suppl 1):S60–1.

205. Rolka DB, Fagot-Campagna AM, Narayan KM. Aspirin use among adults with diabetes: estimates from the Third National Health and Nutrition Examination Survey. *Diabetes Care* 2001;24(2):197–201.

206. Stampfer MJ, Colditz GA, Willett WC, et al. Post-menopausal estrogen therapy and cardiovascular disease: ten-year follow-up from the Nurses' Health Study. *N Engl J Med* 1991;325(11):756–62.

207. Barrett-Connor E, Laakso M. Ischemic heart disease risks in postmenopausal women: effects of estrogen use on glucose and insulin levels. *Arteriosclerosis* 1990;10(4):531–4.

208. Lieberman EH, Gerhard MD, Uehata A, et al. Estrogen improves endothelium-dependent, flow-mediated vasodilation in postmenopausal women. *Ann Intern Med* 1994;121(12):936–41.

209. Kaplan RC, Heckbert SR, Weiss NS, et al. Postmenopausal estrogens and risk of myocardial infarction in diabetic women. *Diabetes Care* 1998;21(7):1117–21.

210. Hulley S, Grady D, Bush T, Furberg C, Herrington D, Riggs B, Vittinghoff E. Randomized trial of estrogen plus progestin for secondary prevention of coronary heart disease in postmenopausal women. Heart and Estrogen/progestin Replacement Study (HERS) Research Group. *JAMA* 1998;280(7):605–13.

211. Ebskov LB. Level of lower limb amputation in relation to etiology: an epidemiological study. *Prosthet Orthot Int* 1992;16(3):163–7.

212. Osmundson PJ, O'Fallon WM, Zimmerman BR, Kasmier FJ, Langworthy AL, Palumbo PJ. Course of peripheral occlusive arterial disease in diabetes. Vascular laboratory assessment. *Diabetes Care* 1990;13(2):143–52.

213. Kannel WB, Skinner JJ Jr, Schwartz MJ, Shurtleff D. Intermittent claudication. Incidence in the Framingham study. *Circulation* 1970;41(5):875–83.

214. Del Aguila MA, Reiber GE, Koepsell TO. How does provider and patient awareness of high-risk status for lower extremity amputation influence foot care practice? *Diabetes Care* 1994;17(9):1050–4.

215. Perneger TV, Brancati FL, Whelton PK, Klag MJ. End-stage renal disease attributable to diabetes mellitus. *Ann Intern Med* 1994;121(12):912–8.

216. U.S. Renal Data System. *USRDS 1994 Annual Data Report*. Bethesda, MD: National Institutes of Health, National Institute of Diabetes and Digestive and Kidney Diseases, 1994.

217. Mogensen CE, Christensen CK, Vittinghus E. The stages of diabetic renal disease, with emphasis on the stage of incipient diabetic nephropathy. *Diabetes* 1983;32(Suppl 2):64–78.

218. Kunzelman CL, Knowler WC, Pettitt DJ, Bennett PH. Incidence of proteinuria in type 2 diabetes mellitus in the Pima Indians. *Kidney Int* 1989;35(2):681–7.

219. Lacourciere Y, Nadeau A, Poirier L, Tancrede G. Comparing effects of converting enzyme inhibition and conventional therapy in hypertensive non–insulin-dependent diabetics with normal renal function. *Clin Invest Med* 1991;14(6):652–60.

220. Pedersen MM, Hansen KW, Schmitz A, Sorensen K, Christensen CK, Mogensen CE. Effects of ACE inhibition supplementary to beta blockers and diuretics in early diabetic nephropathy. *Kidney Int* 1992;41(4): 883–90.

221. Bjorck S, Mulec H, Johnsen SA, Norden G, Aurell M. Renal protective effect of enalpril in diabetic nephropathy. *BMJ* 1992;304(6823):339–43.

222. Ravid M, Savin H, Jutrin I, Bental T, Katz B, Lishner M. Long-term stabilizing effect of angiotensin-converting enzyme inhibition on plasma creatinine and on proteinuria in normotensive type II diabetic patients. *Ann Intern Med* 1993;118(8):577–81.

223. Morelli E, Loon N, Meyer T, Peters W, Myers BD. Effects of converting-enzyme inhibition on barrier function in diabetic glomerulopathy. *Diabetes* 1990;39(1): 76–82.

224. Walker WG, Hermann J, Anderson J. Racial differences in renal protective effect of enalapril vs hydrochlorothiazide in randomized doubly blinded trial in hypertensive type 2. *J Am Soc Nephron* 1993;4:310.

225. Roper NA, Bilous RW, Kelly WF, Unwin NC, Connolly VM. Excess mortality in a population with diabetes and the impact of material deprivation: longitudinal, population-based study. *BMJ* 2001;322(7299): 1389–93

226. The Diabetes Prevention Program Research Group. Design and methods for a clinical trial in the prevention of type 2 diabetes. *Diabetes Care* 1999;22(4): 623–34.

Case Study

Maxine carefully opens the "W" compartment on her yellow pill box to take her pills. The yellow box reminds her to take those pills in the morning; her blue container is for the evening pills. She carefully places them on the table and counts them, and recounts to be sure. There are seven: three pills to help control her diabetes, two for her hypertension, one for cholesterol, and one aspirin for her heart condition (she's been taking it since she had that mild heart attack last year). She used to take two insulin shots a day to control her diabetes, but her doctor replaced her daily insulin shots with the pills 2 years ago. When she was diagnosed with diabetes at age 52, she was able to control her diabetes for a few years by watching her diet and exercising regularly. Can it only be 13 years since frequent urination and an unquenchable thirst sent Maxine to her doctor in search of an answer? It seems like a much longer time, especially since she has had so many other health problems.

She feels pretty good this morning, although she's frustrated that once again she is unable to correctly operate her blood glucose monitor to check her blood sugar. She tried several times, but her eyes, hands, and memory are no longer reliable. The strip, approximately 2 inches long, is too thin for her hands that are weakened by the several small strokes she's suffered over the past year. A cataract and increasing retinal damage due to diabetes make the task of putting blood on just the right spot almost impossible most mornings. And because of the memory problems created by the strokes, she can't always remember the steps her daughter showed her to extract the blood from her finger and to correctly use the strip and monitor.

Maxine quickly finishes her breakfast and waits. She remembers the many years she spent working as a secretary and raising her four children. It wasn't always easy, but she did her best. At the time, she focused on the priority—"making ends meet." Who had time for exercising? Sure, she knew she needed to lose weight and stop smoking. Asthma eventually convinced Maxine not to smoke, but the effort to lose weight would be unending, especially since the medication to control her asthma and her diabetes increased her weight gain.

So quickly the years have passed. Now, widowed and retired, she realizes that she is only 65, but already she needs her children to care for her. With social security as her only source of income and only Medicare for her health insurance, what else can a woman her age with such health problems do? She watches the senior citizen van pull into the driveway of the home she now shares with her youngest daughter. As she hurries out to start her day at the local senior citizen center, she can't help wondering why she is the youngest person among all of her friends at the center.

6

THE OLDER YEARS

C.H. Hennessy, DrPH, MA, G.L.A. Beckles, MBBS, MSc

Diabetes prevalence, incidence, and secular trends associated with elderly adults are presented in this chapter. Demographic and socioeconomic indicators for this population are discussed. Of all women with diabetes, women in this age group are most vulnerable because of the high prevalence of activity limitations, other chronic conditions, and poverty. The effects of income insecurity, lack of social support, and other psychosocial determinants on health status and health behavior are presented. Public heath implications call for surveillance to assess and monitor diabetes and its complications in this age group, systems-level coordination of community services for the elderly with diabetes, and adequate insurance coverage for medications and preventive and curative care. The public health implications of the findings are discussed and framed by the three core functions of public health: assessment, policy development, and assurance.

Almost all elderly persons diagnosed with diabetes have type 2 diabetes mellitus, formerly called non–insulin-dependent diabetes. In this chapter, the term "diabetes" will refer to type 2 diabetes and the term elderly to persons aged 65 years or older unless otherwise specified.

6.1. Prevalence, Incidence, and Trends

Prevalence and Incidence

Based on the new American Diabetes Association (ADA) diagnostic criteria of fasting blood glucose 126 mg/dL or greater,[1] the Third National Health and Nutrition Examination Survey (NHANES III, 1988–1994) found that the total prevalence of diabetes (diagnosed and undiagnosed) is 17.8% among

women aged 60–74 years and 17.5% among women aged 75 years or older (Figure 6-1).[2] The percentage of older women who report that they have been diagnosed with diabetes is similar in these two age groups, 13.8% and 12.8%, respectively. The percentage with undiagnosed diabetes is 4.5% among women aged 60–74 years and 4.7% among those 75 years or older. When these estimates are applied to the 1995 U.S. population, 4.5 million women aged 60 years or older have diabetes and one-quarter of them, 1.2 million, do not know that they have the disease.

Figure 6-1. Prevalence of diagnosed and undiagnosed diabetes among U.S. adults, by age and sex- NHANES III,* 1988-94

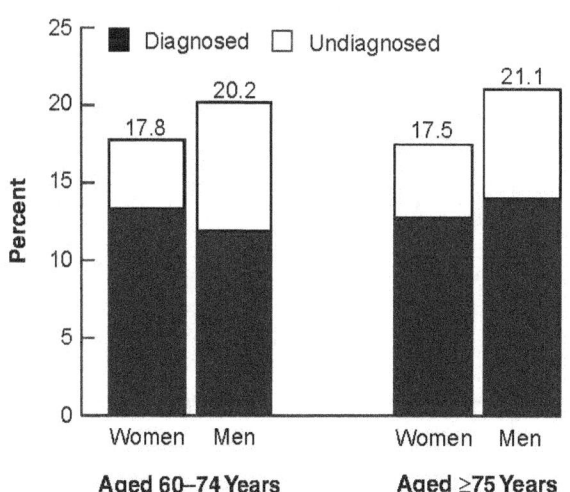

*NHANES III = Third National Health and Nutrition Examination Survey.

Source: Reference 2.

147

Recently, the number of new cases of diabetes diagnosed in the adult population increased significantly.[3] Between 1980 and 1994, data from the National Health Interview Survey (NHIS) indicate that among women aged 65 years or older, the number of new cases increased from 97,000 to 181,000 and the annual incidence rate rose 45.7% from 6.3 per 1,000 to 9.2 per 1,000.[4]

Temporal Trends

The current level of diabetes in the U.S. population reflects increasing secular trends in both the number and percentage of adults with diabetes (Figure 6-2), and the largest increase is occurring among the elderly.[3] Data from NHIS show that between 1963 and 1993, the proportion of women aged 65 years or older who reported that they had diabetes almost doubled from 5.6 per 1,000 to 10.6 per 1,000.[4,5] Similarly, the prevalence of diagnosed diabetes among older women was 50% higher in NHANES III than the prevalence found in the Second National Health and Nutrition Examination Survey (NHANES II, 1976–1980).[2,4]

These trends are not entirely explained by aging of the population.[3] Other factors that might contribute to increased prevalence of a disease include

improved identification of cases, a true increase in incidence, and declining death rates. NHIS data are based on self-reports of cases diagnosed in the previous 12 months, thus national incidence data may reflect increased case ascertainment rather than a true increase in incidence. Although, by current ADA criteria, the proportion of total diabetes that was undiagnosed did not change during 1976–1980 and 1988–1994,[2] the higher prevalence of diagnosed diabetes found suggests that case detection increased during this period.[5] However, findings from a prospective population-based study of adults in Rochester, Minnesota, indicate that true incidence of diabetes has also been increasing.[6] Overweight,[7] weight gain,[8] and lack of physical activity[9] are major risk factors for incidence of diabetes mellitus in women. These factors are very common among elderly women and increased over this time period.[10,11] Finally, a cohort study of nationally representative samples of the adult population showed that 10-year death rates among elderly women who had diabetes during 1971–1974 were not statistically different from the rates for those who had diabetes during 1982–1984.[12] Thus, the increasing prevalence of diabetes among elderly women can be attributed to the combined effects of improved case detection and an increase in the incidence of diabetes.

6.2. Sociodemographic Characteristics

Age and Sex

In the general population, the prevalence of diabetes increases with increasing age to about 75 years of age and then plateaus or decreases somewhat among persons aged 75 years or older. National surveys do not report age-specific prevalence estimates for persons older than 75 years. However, results from the Established Populations for Epidemiologic Studies in the Elderly (EPESE), a multisite prospective study of representative samples of community-dwelling adults aged 65 years or older, show that the percentages of elderly black and white women with previously diagnosed diabetes remain stable between age 65 and 85 years, then drop steeply for women aged 85 years or older.[13]

Figure 6-2. Number of new cases and incidence rate of diagnosed diabetes among women aged 65 years or older- NHIS,* 1980-94

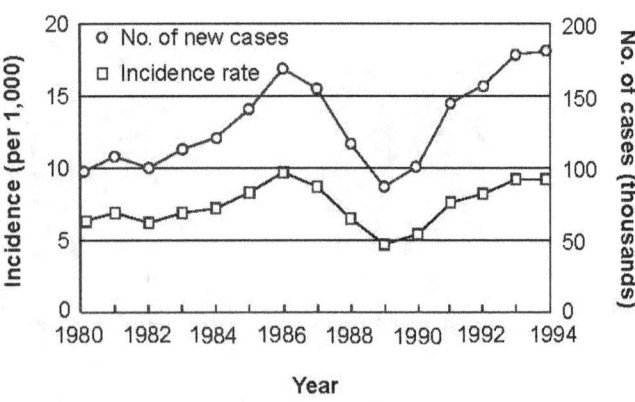

*NHIS = National Health Interview Survey.

Sources: References 4, 5.

The lower prevalence among women aged 85 years or older may result from less aggressive case ascertainment or from a survival effect. In the general population, diabetic women are older than nondiabetic women; 50% or more of all adult women with diabetes are aged 65 years or older compared with only 17.1% of women without diabetes.[14]

According to NHANES III, age-specific prevalence estimates for diagnosed diabetes are similar for both sexes (Figure 6-1). In contrast, undiagnosed diabetes was found much less frequently among elderly women than elderly men. At ages 60–74 years, prevalence of undiagnosed diabetes among women was nearly half that of men (4.5% versus 8.4%); at age 75 years or older, estimates were 4.7% and 7.3%, respectively. Nevertheless, because women make up a greater proportion of the elderly population and women with diabetes live longer than their male counterparts,[12] elderly women with diabetes outnumber elderly men with diabetes (4.5 million versus 3.7 million in 1995).

Race/Ethnicity

In the United States, type 2 diabetes is at least twice as prevalent among nonwhites of all ages as among their white counterparts.[2,13,15-21] To facilitate the discussion of comparisons among ethnic and racial groups throughout this chapter, the terms "white" and "black" will be used, regardless of Hispanic origin.

Among women aged 60–74 years, 33% of black or Mexican American women have diabetes (diagnosed and undiagnosed combined) as compared with 16% of white women; estimates are similar for women aged 75 years or older: 31%, 27%, and 17%, respectively (Figure 6-3). In each age group, black (23.9% and 19.0%) and Mexican American (29.0% and 25.0%) women were twice as likely as white women (11.7% and 12.3%) to have been previously diagnosed with diabetes (Figure 6-3). Information on the prevalence of diagnosed diabetes among older Native American women was collected in the 1987 Survey of American Indians and Alaska Natives, in which 31.8% of female respondents aged 65 years or older reported having

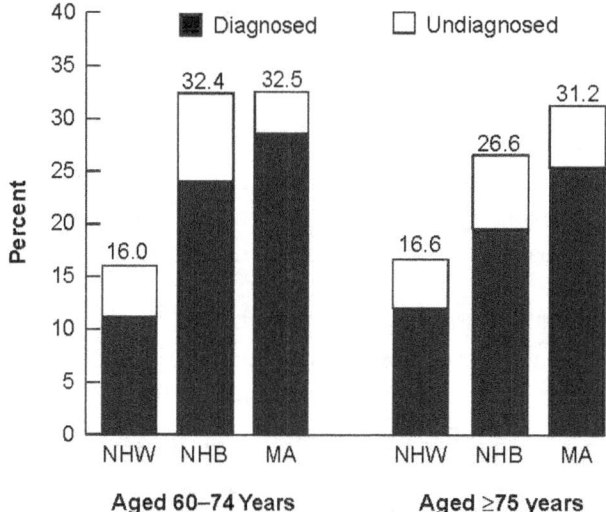

Figure 6-3. Prevalence of diagnosed and undiagnosed diabetes among U.S. women, by age and race/Hispanic origin- NHANES III,* 1988-94

*NHANES III = Third National Health and Nutrition Examination Survey; NHW = non-Hispanic white; NHB = non-Hispanic black; MA = Mexican American.

Source: Reference 2.

diabetes.[22] Additionally, among older blacks, Mexican Americans, and American Indians, diabetes is more common in women than in men.[15-22]

Data from NHANES II and the Hispanic Health and Nutrition Examination Survey (HHANES, 1982–1984)[4,21] also suggest that in the period between each of these surveys and NHANES III, the prevalence of diagnosed diabetes increased substantially among women aged 65 years or older in all ethnic and racial groups for whom findings are reported. The increase was most marked among older black (10.8% to 23.9%) and Mexican American women (21.4% to 29.0%).

Despite the higher level of diagnosed diabetes, undiagnosed diabetes is more common among black and Mexican American women than among white women.[2] However, under 75 years of age, blacks (8.5%) are twice as likely as Mexican Americans

(3.5%) and whites (4.3%) to have diabetes that is undiagnosed (Figure 6-3). At age 75 years or older, undiagnosed diabetes is present in 7.6% of blacks, 6.2% of Mexican Americans, and 4.3% of whites.

Because of their relatively small numbers, no data for older women in other ethnic and racial groups are available from national surveys. However, since the late 1970s, several surveys of diabetes among Asian Americans/Pacific Islanders and the total Hispanic population have confirmed the higher risk for diabetes among minority women at all ages compared with their white counterparts.[20,21,23]

Marital Status/Living Arrangements
Among women aged 65 years or older, women with diabetes are more likely than those without diabetes to be widowed (54.8% versus 45.4%) (Table 6-1).[14] About 4 of 10 elderly diabetic women live alone, one-third live with a spouse, and one-fifth live with some other relative. This pattern reflects the findings in the relatively larger population of white women and is different for minority women for whom national data are available. In contrast, older black women with diabetes were more likely than those without diabetes to be widowed (61.0% versus 55.8%) and less likely to be divorced or separated (5.6% versus 9.7%). Also, for this group, living arrangements did not vary by diabetic status (Table 6-1). However, black women are somewhat less likely than their white counterparts to live alone (40.0% versus 46.8%) or with a spouse (27.1% versus 35.4%), and much more likely to live with some other relative (31.0% versus 17.4%).

Education
It is well known that the level of formal education attained by older adults in the population is generally lower than that of younger adults, and elderly women have lower levels of education than elderly men. Elderly women with diabetes have even less formal education than do their counterparts without diabetes: they are more likely to have less than 9 years of education (38.0% versus 25.6%) and they are also less likely to have completed 12 or more years of education (14.4% versus 21.3%) (Table 6-1).[14] Low levels of education are especially

marked among elderly minority women with diabetes; about one-half (49.9%) of black women have fewer than 9 years of education compared with one-third (32.9%) of white women. The implications of lower levels of education among older women for diabetes management and for the design of diabetes education and health promotion programs are discussed later in this chapter.

Family Income
By age 65 years, women have half the income of men and they are twice as likely to live in poverty.[24,25] Women with diabetes are even more likely than women without diabetes to have low family incomes (Table 6-1).[14] Almost half of elderly women with diabetes (47.4%) have an annual family income less than $10,000, and for more than three-quarters (78.8%) of them this income is less than $20,000; the percentages for women without diabetes are 31.3% and 66%, respectively. The sex differential in income found among all racial and ethnic groups is amplified among persons with type 2 diabetes. Among elderly persons with diabetes, women are 2.5 times as likely as men to have an income less than $10,000. As in the general population, low income levels are considerably more common among minority women: more than 60% of elderly black women with diabetes have family incomes less than $10,000, and about 90% of them have incomes less than $20,000. Although the national data available for Mexican Americans are not specific to women aged 65 years or older, Mexican American women with diabetes are almost twice as likely as those without diabetes to have an income below $10,000.

6.3. Impact of Diabetes on Illness and Death

Risk of Death
Diabetes ranks as one of the leading underlying causes of death among women aged 65 years or older.[5] In this age group, diabetes ranks higher as an underlying cause of death among women aged 65–74 years than among those aged 75 years or older; however, the death rate for diabetes continues to increase with age. In 1992, the number of deaths

Table 6-1. Prevalence (%) of sociodemographic characteristics of women aged 65 years or older with and without type 2 diabetes, by race/Hispanic origin- United States, 1989

Characteristic	Non-Hispanic white		Non-Hispanic black		Total	
	Diabetes	No diabetes	Diabetes	No diabetes	Diabetes	No diabetes
Marital status						
Married	36.6	45.0	27.4	27.9	35.2	43.2
Widowed	54.5	44.7	61.0	55.8	54.8	45.4
Divorced or separated	4.3	5.6	5.6	9.7	5.1	6.3
Never married	4.6	4.7	6.0	6.6	4.9	5.1
Living arrangements						
Alone	46.8	42.0	40.0	40.0	44.8	41.9
Nonrelative only	0.4	1.0	1.9	0.6	0.8	0.9
Spouse	35.4	44.3	27.1	26.6	34.1	42.4
Other relative only	17.4	12.8	31.0	32.7	20.3	14.8
Household size (no. of persons)						
1	47.2	43.0	41.9	41.0	45.6	43.0
2	40.0	47.7	28.3	36.2	37.1	46.3
3	7.1	5.8	15.9	16.0	9.4	6.8
≥4	5.7	3.4	13.9	6.9	7.9	3.9
Education (years)						
<9	32.9	22.1	49.9	52.6	38.0	25.6
9–12	51.0	55.3	39.3	37.1	47.7	53.1
>12	16.1	22.6	10.8	10.3	14.4	21.3
Annual family income ($thousands)						
<10	44.4	29.1	61.4	51.6	47.4	31.3
10 – <20	32.4	34.9	28.2	35.9	31.4	34.7
20 – <40	18.9	24.4	9.3	10.4	17.3	23.4
>40	4.2	11.6	1.1	2.2	3.9	10.5
Employment status						
Employed	5.5	10.2	9.2	9.5	6.1	10.1
Unemployed	0.0	0.3	0.0	0.7	0.0	0.3
Not in labor force	94.5	89.5	90.8	89.7	93.9	89.6

Source: Reference 14.

among women aged 65 years or older with diabetes was 4.6 times the number of deaths among women aged 45–64 years with diabetes.[5] (See Figure 5-3.) The case fatality rate of 12 per 1,000 for these elderly women was 3.4 times the rate for diabetic women in midlife. However, death rates based on diabetes as an underlying cause of death are known to markedly underestimate the impact of diabetes on mortality.[26]

In the 22-year mortality follow-up study of participants in the First National Health and Nutrition Examination Survey, diabetes status was ascertained at baseline.[12,27] The data show that among persons aged 65–74 years, the overall risk of death was higher for persons with diabetes than for those without diabetes (Figure 6-4), but the effect of diabetes (rate ratio = 1.6) was less than that seen at younger ages (3.2 and 2.7 for age groups 25–34 and 45–64, respectively).[12]

Further, unlike younger women, no racial/ethnic difference in mortality was present among elderly women with diabetes (Figure 6-4). However, one study in San Antonio, Texas, found that the death rate for diabetes was almost 4 times greater among elderly Mexican American women than among elderly white women.[28]

Hospitalizations

Data from the 1989 NHIS indicate that women aged 65 years or older with diabetes were almost twice as likely as nondiabetic elderly women to report having been hospitalized in the past year (28% versus 15%).[29] At all ages, the proportion of women with diabetes who reported being hospitalized in the past year exceeded that of diabetic men, but this sex differential narrowed with age. By 65 years of age, 28% of women and 24% of men with diabetes reported a hospital stay within the past year.

National findings on hospitalization rates for older minority women with diabetes are only available for blacks.[29] In 1990, the hospitalization rate for elderly black women with diabetes (747.3 per 10,000) was 1.7 times the rate of their white counterparts (450.0 per 10,000).

Diabetes-Related Illnesses

Although elderly persons are subject to the same complications of diabetes as persons of any other age, the decreased function of major organ systems and the possible organ impairment from concurrent conditions put elderly persons at particular risk for diabetes-related illnesses.[30] Thus, in addition to being at greater risk for death from diabetes, elderly persons are also more susceptible to the complications of diabetes. Chronological age also interacts with diabetes to accelerate the chronic complications of diabetes: retinopathy, nephropathy, and neuropathy occur almost twice as quickly among elderly diabetic persons as among their younger counterparts.[31] In addition, these complications are more severe when they first occur in advanced old age.[32] Elderly women with diabetes are particularly at risk for cardiovascular disease and visual problems and may also be at greater risk for metabolic disorders and depression.

Cardiovascular and peripheral vascular diseases are the most prevalent complications among elderly

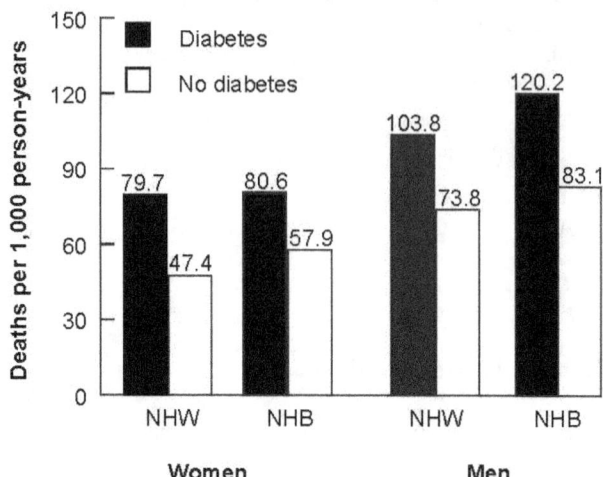

Figure 6-4. All-cause mortality rates for U.S. adults aged 65-74 years, by diabetes status, sex, and race/ Hispanic origin- 1971-93

NHW = non-Hispanic white; NHB = non-Hispanic black.

Source: Reference 12.

diabetic women, as they are among all persons with diabetes. Arthrosclerotic disease, the prevalence of which increases with age, is believed to interact with diabetes to accelerate changes in major blood vessels.[33] Epidemiologic evidence indicates that the prevalence of these macrovascular complications is greater among elderly women with diabetes than among elderly men who have the disease. For example, findings from EPESE indicated that prevalence ratios describing the association between diabetes and cardiovascular conditions (i.e., myocardial infarction, stroke, hypertension, and angina) were generally greater among elderly women than among elderly men.[14] Moreover, results from the National Hospital Discharge Survey (1979–1987) demonstrated that among patients aged 65 years or older who were discharged from the hospital with acute myocardial infarction listed as the primary diagnosis, 21.8% of women compared with 16.1% of men also had diabetes listed as a diagnosis.[34]

Most studies that have examined lower extremity arterial disease (LEAD) among elderly persons with diabetes do not present findings for elderly women specifically. However, unless otherwise noted, the findings from these are assumed to hold true for both sexes. LEAD increases with age among all persons, and among persons with diabetes, LEAD increases with the duration of the disease.[35] Diabetic neuropathy is also related to the duration of diabetes, and it may develop more rapidly in persons with diabetes diagnosed at older ages than in those with diabetes diagnosed before age 40.[36] Neuropathy and susceptibility to infection compound LEAD in persons with diabetes and contribute to LEAD progressing to foot ulcers, gangrene, and ultimately amputation.[35] The prevalence of foot ulcers increases with age, occurring in 7% of diabetic persons older than 60 years and in 14% of those aged 80 years or older.[37,38] Amputation rates also increase with age; most (64%) amputations in persons with diabetes take place in those older than age 65 years.[38] Although many of these complications associated with LEAD occur more frequently in older men than in older women,[35] the projected growth of the population of older women with diabetes[39] implies an increase in the total number of women experiencing these adverse outcomes.

Elderly persons with diabetes are also subject to metabolic complications resulting from problems with blood glucose control (e.g., hypoglycemia, hyperosmolar coma) and other clinical syndromes.[31] For example, diabetes can result in hypothermia, which is of particular concern to elderly women with diabetes as evidenced by their increased risk of being hospitalized for hypothermia compared with their male counterparts.[40]

Visual problems such as cataracts and glaucoma that are common among elderly persons are more prevalent among those who have diabetes.[41] Data from the Wisconsin Epidemiologic Study of Diabetic Retinopathy (WESDR), which examined the prevalence of ocular problems among persons with diabetes diagnosed at an older age (mean age at diagnosis, 65.4 years), showed that poorer visual acuity was associated with increasing duration of

diabetes but also that rates of legal blindness increased significantly after age 70, regardless of the duration of diabetes. In addition, a greater proportion of older women than older men had some degree of visual impairment (13.3% compared with 9.9%) and legal blindness (1.7% compared with 1.4%).

The relationship between diabetes and cognitive impairment has been equivocal in the few population-based studies of older adults that have been conducted.[42,43] However, studies of elderly patients from clinical populations with higher glycemic levels who typically have had the disease for a relatively long duration report a positive association between diabetes and cognitive dysfunction.[44,45] In these studies, elderly persons with diabetes were shown to have a greater degree of cognitive problems than did their nondiabetic age peers matched for other concurrent diseases. The effect of diabetes on cognition seems to be primarily on the ability to retain new information, and persons with diabetes may be less likely to remember changes in medication than are persons with other diseases.

Among adults, diabetes is associated with an increased risk for depression,[45] especially for those with more diabetes-related complications, and as in the general population, depression has been shown to be more common among women than men with the disease.[46,47] In persons aged 65 years or older, the incidence of depression is estimated to be about 50% greater among women than among men.[48] Thus, elderly women with diabetes may be at greater risk for depression than their male counterparts.

National estimates of diabetes-related illnesses among elderly women are not generally available for minorities. Findings from EPESE indicated stronger associations between diabetes and stroke among elderly black women than elderly white women.[14] HHANES is the only study that has examined the health and functional status of Hispanic women with diabetes, but the data are aggregated for middle-aged and elderly women (aged 45–74 years).[22] Results from this study showed that the prevalence of hypertension, kidney problems, and vision problems (i.e., cataracts, retinopathy, and glaucoma) was higher among Mexican American women with diabetes than among those without diabetes.

Disabilities

Almost one-fourth of elderly Americans have difficulty in carrying out the activities of daily living; one-fourth of women aged 65–74 years but more than half of those aged 85 years or older experience this difficulty.[49] Findings from EPESE indicated that elderly women reporting a history of diabetes were more likely than those without the disease to report a major disability (i.e., impairment in activities of daily living and physical mobility), urinary incontinence, and impairments in vision or hearing.[14] In addition, these elderly diabetic women were less likely to perceive their overall health status as excellent or good than were those without diabetes. Among a group of 2,021 participants in the Framingham Heart Study, none of whom had cardiovascular disease, diabetes was associated with physical disability in women (particularly those older than age 75) but not in men.[50] A study of self-rated health and functioning among persons with diabetes of long duration (>15 years) in the WESDR also demonstrated significantly poorer ratings of health and functional status among women than among men.[51]

As with diabetes-related illnesses, national data on disabilities associated with diabetes among elderly women are extremely limited for minority groups. In the 1989 NHIS, overall, black women with diabetes had a higher prevalence of activity limitations than did white women with diabetes, and this pattern may hold true for elderly women.[52] Data from HHANES indicated that Mexican American women aged 45–74 years with diabetes had a higher prevalence of activity limitation than did those without the disease.[53] These data also indicated that activity limitation among Mexican American women with diabetes increased with the duration of the disease. Likewise, a higher proportion of these diabetic women than nondiabetic women had a health status rated as poor by both self-evaluation and by physician assessment.

6.4. Health-Related Behaviors

Physical Inactivity

The role of health-related behaviors in the development of diabetes and its complications is well-established, and a number of these behaviors are particularly relevant to elderly women. One of the major risk factors for diabetes and its complications is physical inactivity, which increases with age among the general U.S. population.[54] In addition, contemporary elderly women tend to be less physically active than their male counterparts because they were often discouraged from active participation in exercise in their youth for a variety of cultural reasons.[55] In the 1991 NHIS, NHANES III (1988–1994), and the 1992 Behavioral Risk Factor Surveillance System, the percentages of elderly women who reported no leisure-time physical activity ranged from 32.8% to 43.4%.[56] Results from all three surveys indicate that this risk factor for diabetes and its complications is more frequent among older women than among older men.

Obesity

Total body adiposity, another recognized risk factor for diabetes and its complications, increases with age-associated decreases in metabolism. The rate of overweight among elderly women exceeds that among elderly men. Among persons aged 65 years or older with diabetes, 70.4% of women but only 38.2% of men are 20% over their desirable weight.[57] One-fourth of elderly women with diabetes, but only 5.7% of their male counterparts, are extremely obese (50% over their desirable weight).

The risk of being overweight also differentially affects older women by race and ethnicity. Among women aged 65 years or older, the prevalence of being at least 20% over the desirable body weight is 1.7 times greater among blacks (43.8%) and 1.3

times greater among Hispanics (35.5%) than among whites (25.3%).[54] Comparable national data on overweight among elderly diabetic women of other ethnic and racial groups are not available.

Smoking

Smoking is another documented risk factor for diabetes and its complications. The smoking rate among women declines with age, from 30.2% among those aged 55–64 years, to 21.5% among those aged 65–74 years, and to 8.5% among women aged 75 years or older.[58] This decline with age may be due to decreased survivorship of smokers and to rates of smoking initiation in adolescence and young adulthood becoming increasingly lower among contemporary women as age increases. Smoking rates are considerably lower among the current cohort of elderly women than among elderly men, at least in part because of social norms against smoking by women in the early 1900s. Because current younger smokers include a greater proportion of women, this risk factor for diabetes and its complications could increase significantly among elderly women in the future.

Preventive Self-Care

Effective management of diabetes depends on modifying behavioral risks and on learning appropriate diabetes management techniques and skills. Thus, the first line of therapy involves diet modification, weight control, exercise, self-monitoring of urine and blood glucose levels, and patient education.[59] Pharmacologic treatment is considered if these measures fail to produce adequate glycemic control.

Although there is little information about the prevalence of preventive self-care practices among elderly women with diabetes, more is known about preventive self-care practices for those aged 60 years or older. Among all persons who have diabetes, those aged 60 years or older have been shown to be most likely to comply with diet modifications but least likely to exercise or to test their urine for glucose levels.[60] Among persons with diabetes aged 60 years or older, women report lower levels of exercise than do men, and those who take insulin are more

likely to test their glucose levels than those who do not take insulin.[61] Barriers to and motivations for practicing preventive self-care are covered in more detail in section 6.5.[62,63]

6.5. Psychosocial Determinants of Health Behaviors and Health Outcomes

Social Environment

Social support. Social support consists of both emotional links and task-oriented assistance provided by the community, family, friends, or significant others.[64] This support, whether emotional or practical, can mitigate the negative effects of stress, including those engendered by coping with a chronic disease, and can promote healthy behaviors and self-care among older persons.[65] The type, structure, quality, and availability of social support among elderly women with diabetes will therefore affect the psychosocial resources they possess to cope with the disease.

Research on the effects of social support provided to elderly women with diabetes is negligible, and studies of adults of various ages with diabetes have had mixed findings regarding the relationship of social support, compliance with self-care practices, and glycemic control.[66,67] The most recent study investigated the role of family members in the management of diabetes in persons aged 70 years or older.[68] The types and extent of assistance provided with daily diabetes-related care tasks and participation in visits with health care providers were examined. Not unexpectedly, family involvement in the patient's diabetes care regimen increased as the patient's functional impairment increased, and patients receiving more assistance were more likely to report that they adhered to their recommended medications and diet. A modest association was also found between family assistance and glycemic control. Thus, the investigators concluded that task-oriented support provided by family members to older diabetic persons positively influences adherence to diabetes care regimens and possibly blood glucose levels.

Socioeconomic factors. As discussed above, socioeconomic factors, including income and educational attainment, have a demonstrated relationship with the prevalence of type 2 diabetes.[69] These factors influence risk factors for the development of diabetes and a person's capacity to manage this chronic disease. Evidence suggests that a high socioeconomic status is positively related to understanding a disease and negatively related to anxiety over disease symptoms and their misinterpretation.[70] The low level of education among older women thus has major implications for the design of diabetes education and health promotion programs. In addition, the economic situation of elderly women described above suggests that a high proportion of older women with diabetes may have limited access to appropriate care because their disposable income may be so low as to impose constraints on their ability, or desire, to comply with prescribed drug and diet regimens because they are unable to meet out-of-pocket costs.

Interactions with the Health Care System

Health insurance. The ability to pay for health care strongly influences an older person's use of services.[71] Older women with diabetes who have no health insurance may delay seeking medical attention for symptoms or routine preventive care. Although no research has examined the influence of health insurance on health outcomes among elderly women with diabetes, a study of adults aged 18–64 years with diabetes found that health insurance had several positive effects: persons with health insurance reported less frequent hyperglycemia and glycosuria, more frequent medical care, and more preventive self-care practices than did those who were not insured.[72]

Health care services for elderly U.S. citizens are covered by Medicare, a public health insurance program. As of 1996, 98.5% of elderly Americans had this coverage.[73,74] Medicare coverage is limited, however, to curative services; it does not pay for any primary nor for most secondary preventive services, such as periodic screening and prevention measures for hearing, dental, podiatry, and eye problems. Medicare also does not cover prescription drugs.

Many elderly Americans purchase private insurance to cover the out-of-pocket expenses and co-payments not reimbursed by Medicare. However, the proportion of elderly persons who have private insurance is lower among those who have diabetes (69.2%) than among those who do not (79.9%).[72] Medicaid is an entitlement program for low-income, disabled, and blind persons. Among persons aged 65 years or older, coverage through Medicaid is more common among those who have diabetes (15.4%) than among those who do not (6.0%). Regardless of the health insurance they have, only 52.6% of elderly Americans who have diabetes have coverage for prescription drugs.[72]

Coverage for diabetes outpatient education programs is inconsistent and is shifting throughout the private and public health insurance sectors but is generally increasing.[75] In a growing number of states, Medicare reimburses patients for participation in such education programs, but local Medicare intermediaries determine which programs meet reimbursement criteria, no self-referrals are allowed, and individual patient claims may be denied. Medicaid coverage for these programs is at the discretion of each state and is dependent on their demonstrated cost-effectiveness; currently 35 states offer this benefit.[76] Private insurance provides the most comprehensive coverage for this preventive care service for those who can afford this benefit.

Use of services. Elderly women with diabetes use health care services—both hospital care and ambulatory care—more intensively than elderly men with diabetes. According to data from the National Ambulatory Medical Care Surveys of 1991 and 1992, the average annual number of office-based physician visits in which diabetes was listed as a diagnosis was 1.5 times higher for women aged 65 years or older (7.4 million visits) than for their male counterparts (5.0 million visits).[77] Elderly women also had a higher number of physician visits specifically for diabetic complaints (4.5 million visits versus 3.2 million visits). Although these differences in use of health care services may reflect the greater propensity of women than men to report disease symptoms, the disparities may also mirror the greater burden of diabetes on elderly women than on elderly men.

Published national findings on the use of ambulatory care services by minority elders with diabetes are limited to blacks and are not sex-specific. Among elderly persons who are in poor health or who have diabetes, blacks have fewer physician contacts than do whites.[77,78] These data suggest that even though the prevalence and impact of diabetes are greater among elderly black women than among elderly white women, the former are less intensive users of ambulatory care services. Because elderly minority women are at increased risk for many diabetic complications, further characterization of their access to and use of primary medical care services is essential.

Provision of services. Because elderly persons with diabetes are more likely to have concurrent illnesses, sensory and functional deficits, and physical and financial limitations in their ability to adhere to treatment regimens, they may require more careful attention and explanation from health care providers than do younger diabetic patients. However, at least one study has found that older patients generally have shorter medical visits than do middle-aged patients despite the more impaired health status and greater number of medical problems of older patients.[79] Thus, elderly patients with diabetes may receive no more contact time with health care providers than do younger diabetic patients.

Elderly patients with diabetes may also receive less aggressive care than do their younger counterparts. In a study of adaptation to diabetes by persons in four different age groups, the oldest adults (mean age, 72 years) reported that they received the least amount of diabetes instruction.[80] In another study of persons with type 2 diabetes, those aged 65 years or older reported having been told to follow a diet, exercise, and protect and inspect their feet less often than did persons aged 45–64 years. This differential

may be due in part to clinicians being less concerned about possible long-term complications among older patients.[81] However, because elderly women have an excess risk for many of the short- and long-term complications of diabetes, active management of their diabetes is very important.

A recent national survey examined the level of preventive and monitoring services received in 1994 by fee-for-service Medicare beneficiaries (91% of whom were aged 65 years or older) who had diabetes.[82] Only 10.8% of the women received all the services recommended by the American Diabetes Association, and 10.9% received none of the preventive services recommended (Table 6-2).[82,83] (Also see Appendix E.) Receipt of preventive and monitoring services was similar among women and men, but because women account for 60% of elderly persons who have diabetes, much larger numbers of elderly women than men are likely to receive suboptimal diabetes care.

Table 6-2. Percentage of beneficiaries with diabetes who received recommended preventive and monitoring services in fee-for-service Medicare, by sex- United States, 1994

Recommended service	Women	Men
Physician visit, ≥2 per year	94.5	92.0
Dilated eye exam, ≥1 per year	43.6	39.5
Glycohemoglobin test		
≥2 per year	20.5	21.3
≥1 per year	37.5	38.7
Urinalysis, 1 per year	53.2	53.0
Serum cholesterol test, 1 per year	70.4	68.7
Influenza vaccination, 1 per fall season*	42.4	46.6

* The flu shot may be underreported in Medicare claims because people may obtain it in nonmedical settings.

Source: Reference 82.

Barriers to and Motivations for Practicing Preventive Self-Care

Among persons who have diabetes, noncompliance with preventive self-care is highest among elderly patients.[32] Noncompliance may be due to deficits in vision or hearing, arthritis, dementia, overly complicated medication regimens, lack of support from other persons, inadequate income, or the patient's beliefs and attitudes concerning the disease and the likely effects of self-care behaviors. Of the few studies that have examined the barriers to or motivations for practicing preventive self-care among elderly persons with diabetes, none present findings for elderly women specifically. However, unless otherwise noted, the findings from these are assumed to hold true for both sexes.

Although no studies have addressed exercise initiation and adherence specifically among elderly persons with diabetes, research has demonstrated that sources of motivation to exercise among the elderly include access, enjoyment, social interaction, and personal experience of the benefits, such as improved health and quality of life.[84] Tapping these motivations to exercise will be important in convincing elderly women who have diabetes to modify their existing physical activity patterns—many of which are embedded in cultural and social patterns that have been reinforced over a lifetime.[84-88]

Another study examined whether preventive self-care affected the perceived quality of life of diabetic persons aged 60–79 years who were monitoring their blood glucose.[89] The subjects did not find blood glucose monitoring to be burdensome. They also reported that modifying their diet negatively affected their quality of life more than did monitoring their blood glucose or taking diabetes medications.

The Health Belief Model, an approach to understanding the barriers to and motivations for preventive self-care, was applied in a study of diabetic persons in four age groups, including a group aged 66 years or older.[80] The study results indicated that the perceived seriousness of diabetes increased with age, yet the oldest persons were least concerned with the

potential health problems caused by the disease and were least likely to perceive the benefits of exercise and medication in controlling diabetes. Participants aged 66 years or older were most likely to try to take care of their health, try to follow medical advice as closely as possible, and feel guilty when they did things they knew were contrary to good health. However, compared with persons in other age groups, the eldest participants were not very likely to worry about their own health.

Another study expanded on the Health Belief Model to examine the associations between self-care practices and the personal constructs (i.e., beliefs about treatment effectiveness, the seriousness of the disease and its impact, and the cause of the disease) of persons aged 60 years or older with diabetes.[90] The results showed that healthy diet and physical activity among these participants were related not only to sociodemographic and medical history variables but also to personal constructs about diabetes. Belief in treatment effectiveness was the personal construct most strongly related to healthy diet. In addition, self-blame for diabetes was more likely to negatively affect adherence to diet among women than among men. Belief in treatment effectiveness was the strongest predictor of physical activity and had a stronger influence among women than among men. Feeling personally responsible for causing diabetes was also positively, but less strongly, related to physical activity among both sexes.

In addition to personal constructs, personality characteristics may influence a diabetic person's adherence to self-care practices. A study of adults aged 65–80 years with diabetes found that hardiness (defined as an adaptive personality style including the qualities of control, commitment, and challenge) was significantly associated with adherence to 24 self-care behaviors, including eating a healthy diet, regularly exercising, practicing good personal hygiene, and managing disease complications.[91]

Several researchers have investigated how elderly persons with diabetes can be motivated to practice preventive self-care. One such study examined the effects of a 4-week telephone follow-up intervention on the self-care knowledge, behaviors, and metabolic control of a group of persons aged 65 years or older who had completed an inpatient diabetes education program.[92] No significant differences in knowledge or blood glucose levels were found between participants who received the intervention and those who did not, but the former reported significantly more self-care behaviors, such as self-monitoring blood glucose and keeping records, modifying physical activities, reporting symptoms, and seeking assistance from health care professionals.

Another study examined the effect of diabetes education and peer support on weight reduction and glycemic control among older adults (mean age, 68.2 years) with diabetes.[93] Study participants received diabetes education only, diabetes education and peer support, or neither. Education focused on diabetes and its nutritional aspects and was presented in eight weekly sessions and follow-up sessions at 12 and 16 weeks. Participants who also received peer support took part in group discussions led by a trained peer support facilitator. Study participants who received diabetes education and peer support had significantly greater weight loss and glycemic control at 12 weeks than participants who received education only or no intervention. These findings suggest that diabetes education programs that are accompanied by additional support may be most effective in helping elderly women comply with preventive self-care practices.

Although there is evidence that the information and peer support provided through diabetes education programs can encourage preventive self-care, some studies indicate that older adults with diabetes may not participate in such programs as frequently as younger persons with diabetes.[62,63] Sex, duration of diabetes, type of medication, and previous experience with diabetes education programs did not affect participation rates. Apart from age, the strongest predictor of participation was how participants were recruited: those who decided independently to join the program were twice as likely to participate as those recruited by health care providers, relatives, or friends.

These studies examined factors associated with elderly adults' participation in diabetes education programs, but they do not reveal the participants' subjective perceptions of the features and processes of such programs (e.g., format, relevance of the information presented). Understanding how these perceptions translate into barriers or motivations for participation in diabetes education programs is essential to maximizing participation by and benefit to elderly women.

Traditional Beliefs

Traditional beliefs about disease causation and the nature of control over health, along with folk medical practices associated with these beliefs, may be important determinants of diabetes self-care practices among elderly women, particularly among those who live in ethnic or rural communities or who have limited access to conventional medical care. Such culturally grounded religious beliefs influence notions about the causes and care of diabetes. For example, one study of Hispanic adults with diabetes found that 78% of participants stated that they had diabetes because it was God's will, 81% said that God controlled their diabetes, and 55% said that their priests helped them control their disease.[94] Six percent of the participants—all of them older women—initially turned to God to address a diabetic problem. Other prevalent traditional beliefs among the study participants were that diabetes is caused by physiological imbalances and can be treated with herbs.[94]

In contrast, a study of the influence of age on the self-care practices of blacks with diabetes found that those aged 60–77 years were more reliant on the advice of physicians and other health professionals and less interested in alternative methods of healing than were those aged 45–59 years.[95] The older study participants used only biomedicine to control their diabetes; none supplemented standard medical care with traditional treatment, as the middle-aged persons did. The researchers speculated that this difference may be due to the greater prevalence of multiple chronic disease conditions and the perceived seriousness of these diseases among the older study participants. Nevertheless, many of these older blacks expressed traditional beliefs about the causes and management of diabetes, describing changes in blood sugar levels as "raising" and "lowering" the blood. The findings may thus also reflect the fact that the study participants were drawn from an urban diabetes clinic and thus had access to conventional medical care.

Public health practitioners need to be alert to such beliefs and practices and acknowledge their potential to influence health-related behaviors as they develop interventions and diabetes control programs targeted at older women.

6.6. Concurrent Illnesses as Determinants of Health Behaviors and Health Outcomes

Management of diabetes in elderly women is affected by changes in sensory, physical, and psychological functioning related to aging and by impairments resulting from diabetes complications (Table 6-3). These alterations directly affect the ability of elderly women who have diabetes to care for themselves.

Table 6-3. Age-associated factors affecting diabetes management in older women

Sensory changes
  Decreased vision, hearing, smell
  Altered taste perception

Difficulties in food preparation and consumption
  Impaired manual dexterity
  Impaired mobility
  Poor dentition
  Alterations in gastrointestinal function

Effects of other chronic diseases
  Increased frailty
  Increased burden of medications management

Decreased exercise and mobility

Cognitive and psychological problems
  Depression
  Cognitive impairment and dementia

Source: Reference 81.

Visual impairment can affect a person's ability to adequately inspect the feet, read markings on a syringe, or administer an insulin injection.[96] Indeed, diabetic persons who have some degree of visual impairment may have up to a 20% error rate in drawing up their insulin.[97] In addition, uncompensated hearing deficits among elderly persons can prevent patient comprehension of and interaction with health care providers who want to discuss self-care with the diabetic patient.

The ability to intervene in the diet of elderly women who have diabetes may be affected by several factors including altered perceptions of taste and smell (which may result in changes in food preferences and diet) and poor dentition. One-quarter of elderly American women are totally edentulous,[98] and many have poorly fitting partial or complete dentures that make chewing uncomfortable.[99] In addition, the decrease with age in the efficiency of peristalsis can lead to problems with digestion, absorption, and elimination that may be exacerbated in diabetic persons by autonomic neuropathy involving the gastrointestinal tract.[100] Thus, elderly diabetic women who are edentulous or who have gastrointestinal problems may substitute foods that are easily chewed and digested for those appropriate to a diabetic diet. Meal preparation (and other self-care activities necessary for diabetes management) can also be affected by chronic conditions that limit manual dexterity and mobility, such as arthritis.[101] All of these factors can put elderly persons at risk for nutritional deficiencies; frail, anorectic elderly persons who also try to follow extensive dietary restrictions for diabetes may put themselves at further risk for nutritional deficiencies.[101,102]

Self-care by elderly women who have diabetes may be affected by other comorbid conditions as well. In particular, among elderly persons with diabetes, the need to manage multiple medications for other chronic conditions is a major cause of noncompliance with preventive self-care for diabetes and its complications.[32] In addition, elderly diabetic persons who have multiple chronic conditions are at risk for problems associated with polypharmacy and for adverse drug interactions.[81]

Acute and subacute problems related to hyperglycemia can exacerbate existing chronic conditions.[30] For example, high levels of blood glucose cause increased secretion of urine and excesive urination at night, which can aggravate preexisting urinary incontinence. The estimated prevalence of urinary incontinence among noninstitutionalized adults aged 60 years or over ranges from 15% to 30%; women are twice as likely as men to have this problem.[103] Incontinence can adversely affect the quality of life for elderly women, as it is associated with pressure sores among persons who have limited mobility, urinary tract infections, and use of indwelling catheters, and it can create embarrassment and social isolation. This condition is also frequently a factor in the decision to institutionalize an elderly person. Thus, the interaction of diabetes with other commonly occurring chronic conditions can affect a woman's ability to manage diabetes as well as her physical and psychosocial functioning.

Cognitive and psychological disorders can also affect a person's ability to manage diabetes. Memory losses associated with cognitive impairment can result in overmedication or undermedication and in skipped meals,[81] and persons who are unable to retain new information may not adhere to changed medications or self-care practices.[30] Because persons with dementia may not sense hunger or thirst, they may lose weight and become dehydrated if they are not closely monitored.[81] Depression can also produce self-neglect and irregular eating patterns. Through such alterations in behavior, these cognitive and psychological disorders compromise the management and control of diabetes and its complications.

6.7. Public Health Implications

Over the next 10 years, there will be a considerable increase in the number of women aged 65 years or older among the various racial/ethnic groups. Because of the greater proportion of women in this age group, there will be significantly more women with diabetes than men. Better data and information are needed to fully assess the burden of disease in this group. Family members, friends, and community-based organizations should be involved in the process of collecting information on the elderly population because they usually play a major role in providing care and support.

Assessment
The tremendous growth projected in the number of women aged 65 years or older in the United States over the next several decades—from 19.9 million in 1990 to 29.6 million in 2020—indicates a need to collect, analyze, and disseminate timely and accurate information on elderly women. In particular, data are needed

- To better characterize diabetes among women aged 85 years or older.

- To estimate the prevalence and incidence of diabetes and its complications.

- To understand and monitor trends in racial and ethnic populations.

- To measure health-related quality of life.

- To track diabetes-related behavioral risk factors, knowledge, attitudes, and self-care practices among elderly women with diabetes.

- To evaluate the range, patterns, and adequacy of services available to elderly women, including the patient's functional and cognitive status, concurrent illnesses, the number and type of medications being used, and financial and social situation; patterns of service use, including ambulatory and inpatient care; and the views of elderly women on the adequacy and accessibility of existing programs and services.

Addressing the needs of elderly women with diabetes will help maximize the years of healthy life of older Americans by achieving a number of national health objectives for elderly adults. Achieving these objectives can substantially improve diabetes care for older women.

Policy Development

Population-based policies for elderly persons with diabetes are needed to ensure and promote

- Reimbursement for diabetes education and supplies.

- Greater coordination of services in the broader community, particularly because an increasing number of elderly women with diabetes are at risk for poverty and are more likely to live alone.

- Diabetes care that includes formal, multidimensional assessments of physical, emotional, and social functioning of each patient to determine whether barriers to self-care exist.

Assurance

Access to appropriate diabetes care and services must be assured for elderly women with diabetes. Transportation problems, insurance coverage for preventive care, and language and cultural barriers need to be considered. Diabetes care and education should be tailored to the holistic needs of elderly women.

References

1. American Diabetes Association. Report of the Expert Committee on the diagnosis and classification of diabetes mellitus. *Diabetes Care* 1997;20(7):1183–97.

2. Harris MI, Flegal KM, Cowie CC, et al. Prevalence of diabetes, impaired fasting glucose, and impaired glucose tolerance in U.S. adults. The Third National Health and Nutrition Examination Survey, 1988–1994. *Diabetes Care* 1998;21(4):518–24.

3. CDC. Trends in the prevalence and incidence of self-reported diabetes mellitus—United States, 1980–1994. *MMWR* 1997;46(43):1014–8.

4. Kenny SJ, Aubert RE, Geiss LS. Prevalence and incidence of non–insulin-dependent diabetes. In: National Diabetes Data Group, editors. *Diabetes in America.* 2nd ed. Bethesda, MD: National Institutes of Health, 1995: 47–67. (NIH Publication No. 95-1468)

5. Centers for Disease Control and Prevention. *Diabetes Surveillance, 1997.* Atlanta: U.S. Department of Health and Human Services, 1997.

6. Leibson CL, O'Brien PC, Atkinson E, Palumbo PJ, Melton LJ III. Relative contributions of incidence and survival to increasing prevalence of adult-onset diabetes mellitus: a population-based study. *Am J Epidemiol* 1997;146(1):12–22.

7. Colditz GA, Willet WC, Stampfer MJ, et al. Weight as a risk factor for clinical diabetes in women. *Am J Epidemiol* 1990;132(3):501–13.

8. Ford ES, Williamson DF, Liu S. Weight change and diabetes incidence: findings from a national cohort of U.S. adults. *Am J Epidemiol* 1997;146(3):214–22.

9. Manson JE, Rimm EB, Stampfer MJ, et al. Physical activity and incidence of non–insulin-dependent diabetes mellitus in women. *Lancet* 1991;338(8770):774–8.

10. Kuczmarski RJ, Flegal KM, Campbell SM, Johnson CL. Increasing prevalence of overweight among U.S. adults: the National Health and Nutrition Examination Surveys, 1960 to 1991. *JAMA* 1994;272(3):205–11.

11. Crespo CJ, Keteyian SJ, Heath GW, Sempos CT. Leisure-time physical activity among U.S. adults: results from the Third National Health and Nutrition Examination Survey. *Arch Intern Med* 1996;156(1):93–8.

12. Gu K, Cowie CC, Harris MI. Mortality in adults with and without diabetes in a national cohort of the U.S. population, 1971–1993. *Diabetes Care* 1998;21(7):1138–45.

13. Moritz DJ, Ostfeld AM, Blazer D, Curb D, Taylor JO, Wallace RB. The health burden of diabetes for the elderly in four communities. *Public Health Rep* 1994;109:782–90.

14. Cowie CC, Eberhardt MS. Sociodemographic characteristics of persons with diabetes. In: National Diabetes Data Group, editors. *Diabetes in America.* 2nd ed. Bethesda, MD: National Institutes of Health, 1995:85–116. (NIH Publication No. 95-1468)

15. Carter JS, Pugh JA, Monterrosa A. Non–insulin-dependent diabetes mellitus in minorities in the United States. *Ann Intern Med* 1996;125(3):221–32.

16. Ellis JL, Campos-Outcalt D. Cardiovascular disease risk factors in Native Americans: a literature review. *Am J Prev Med* 1994;10(5):295–307.

17. CDC. Prevalence of diagnosed diabetes among American Indians/Alaskan Natives—United States, 1996. *MMWR* 1998;47(42): 901–4.

18. Will JC, Strauss KF, Mendlein JM, Ballew C, White LL, Peter DG. Diabetes mellitus among Navajo Indians: findings from the Navajo Health and Nutrition Examination Survey. *J Nutr* 1997;127(10 Suppl): 2106S–2113S.

19. Lee ET, Howard BV, Savage PJ, et al. Diabetes and impaired glucose tolerance in three American Indian populations aged 45–74 years: the Strong Heart Study. *Diabetes Care* 1995;18(5):599–610.

20. Fujimoto WY. Diabetes in Asian and Pacific Islander Americans. In: National Diabetes Data Group, editors. *Diabetes in America.* 2nd ed. Bethesda, MD: National Institutes of Health, 1995:661–77. (NIH Publication No. 95-1468)

21. Flegal KM, Ezzati TM, Harris MI, et al. Prevalence of diabetes in Mexican Americans, Cubans, and Puerto Ricans from the Hispanic Health and Nutrition Examination Survey, 1982–1984. *Diabetes Care* 1991;14(7):628–38.

22. Johnson A, Taylor A. *Prevalence of Chronic Diseases: A Summary of Data from the Survey of American Indians and Alaska Natives.* Rockville, MD: Public Health Service, 1991. (AHCPR Publication No. 91-0031)

23. CDC. Self-reported prevalence of diabetes among Hispanics—United States, 1994–1997. *MMWR* 1999;48(1):8–12.

24. Costello C, Stone AJ, editors. *The American Woman 1994–95: Where We Stand.* New York: W.W. Norton & Company, Inc., 1994.

25. O'Hare WP. A new look at poverty in America. *Popul Bull* 1996;51(2):1–48.

26. Bild DE, Stevenson JM. Frequency of recording of diabetes on U.S. death certificates: analysis of the 1986 National Mortality Followback Survey. *J Clin Epidemiol* 1992;45(3):275–81.

27. Gu K, Cowie CC, Harris MI. Diabetes and decline in heart disease mortality in U.S. adults. *JAMA* 1999; 281(14):1291–7.

28. Espino DV, Parra EO, Kriehbiel R. Mortality differences between elderly Mexican Americans and non-Hispanic whites in San Antonio, Texas. *J Am Geriatr Soc* 1994; 42(6):604–8.

29. Aubert RE, Geiss LS, Ballard DJ, Cocanougher B, Herman WH. Diabetes-related hospitalization and hospital utilization. In: National Diabetes Data Group, editors. *Diabetes in America.* 2nd ed. Bethesda, MD: National Institutes of Health, 1995:553–69. (NIH Publication No. 95-1468)

30. Morley JE, Kaiser FE. Unique aspects of diabetes mellitus in the elderly. *Clin Geriatr Med* 1990;6(4):693–702.

31. Morley JE, Mooradian AD, Rosenthal MJ, Kaiser FE. Diabetes mellitus in elderly patients: is it different? *Am J Med* 1987;83(3):533–44.

32. Minaker KL. What diabetologists should know about elderly patients. *Diabetes Care* 1990;13(Suppl 2):34–46.

33. Naliboff BD, Rosenthal M. Effects of age on complications in adult-onset diabetes. *J Am Geriatr Soc* 1989; 37(9):838–42.

34. Cooper RS, Pacold IV, Ford ES. Age-related differences in case-fatality rates among diabetic patients with myocardial infarction: findings from the National Hospital Discharge Survey, 1979–1987. *Diabetes Care* 1991;14(10):903–8.

35. Palumbo PJ, Melton, LJ. Peripheral vascular disease and diabetes. In: National Diabetes Data Group, editors. *Diabetes in America.* 2nd ed. Bethesda, MD: National Institutes of Health, 1995:401–8. (NIH Publication No. 95-1468)

36. Neil HA, Thompson AV, Thorogood M, Fowler GH, Mann JI. Diabetes in the elderly: the Oxford Community Diabetes Study. *Diabet Med* 1989; 6(7):608–13.

37. Walters DP, Gatling W, Mullee MA, Hill RD. The distribution and severity of diabetic foot disease: a community study with comparison to a non-diabetic group. *Diabet Med* 1992;9(4):354–8.

38. Bild DE, Selby JV, Sinnock P, Browner WS, Bravemen P, Showstack JA. Lower-extremity amputation in people with diabetes: epidemiology and prevention. *Diabetes Care* 1989;12(1):24–31.

39. King H, Aubert RE, Herman WH. Global burden of diabetes, 1995–2025: prevalence, numerical estimates, and projections. *Diabetes Care* 1998;21(9):1414–31.

40. Neil HA, Dawson JA, Baker JE. Risk of hypothermia in elderly patients with diabetes. *Br Med J (Clin Res Ed)* 1986;293(6544):416–8.

41. Klein BE, Klein R. Ocular problems in older Americans with diabetes. *Clin Geriatr Med* 1990;6(4):827–37.

42. Robertson-Tchabo EA, Arenberg D, Tobib JD, Plotz JB. A longitudinal study of cognitive performance in non–insulin-dependent (type II) diabetic men. *Expl Gerontol* 1986;21(4–5):459–67.

43. Scott RD, Kritz-Silverstein D, Barrett-Connor E, Wiederholt WC. The association of non–insulin-dependent diabetes mellitus and cognitive function in an older cohort. *J Am Geriatr Soc* 1998;46(10):1217–22.

44. Tun PA, Nathan DM, Perlmuter LC. Cognitive and affective disorders in elderly diabetics. *Clin Geriatr Med* 1990;6(4):731–46.

45. U'Ren RC, Riddle MC, Lezak MD, Bennington-Davis M. The mental efficiency of the elderly person with type II diabetes mellitus. *J Am Geriatr Soc* 1990;38(5):505–10.

46. Gavard JA, Lustman PJ, Clouse RE. Prevalence of depression in adults with diabetes: an epidemiological evaluation. *Diabetes Care* 1993;16(8):1167–78.

47. Peyrot M, Rubin RR. Levels and risks of depression and anxiety symptomatology among diabetic adults. *Diabetes Care* 1997;20(4):585–90.

48. Anthony JC, Aboraya A. The epidemiology of selected mental disorders in later life. In: Birren JE, Sloane RB, Cohen GC, editors. *Handbook of Mental Health and Aging.* 2nd ed. San Diego, CA: Academic Press, 1992: 27–73.

49. U.S. Public Health Service. *Health Data on Older Americans: United States, 1992.* Hyattsville, MD: National Center for Health Statistics, 1993. (DHHS Publication No. PHS 93-1411)

50. Pinsky JL, Branch LG, Jette AM, et al. Framingham Disability Study: relationship of disability to cardiovascular risk factors among persons free of diagnosed cardiovascular disease. *Am J Epidemiol* 1985;122(4):644–56.

51. Klein BE, Klein R, Moss SE. Self-rated health and diabetes of long duration: the Wisconsin Epidemiologic Study of Diabetic Retinopathy. *Diabetes Care* 1998; 21(2):236–40.

52. Songer TJ. Disability in diabetes. In: National Diabetes Data Group, editors. *Diabetes in America.* 2nd ed. Bethesda, MD: National Institutes of Health, 1995: 259–82. (NIH Publication No. 95-1468)

53. Zhang J, Markides KS, Lee DJ. Health status of diabetic Mexican Americans: results from the Hispanic HANES. *Ethn Dis* 1991;1(3):273–9.

54. Schoenborn CA. *Health Promotion and Disease Prevention: United States, 1985. Vital and Health Statistics.* Hyattsville, MD: National Center for Health Statistics, U.S. Government Printing Office, 1988. Series 10, No. 163. (DHHS Publication No. PHS 88-1591)

55. O'Brien SJ, Vertinsky PA. Unfit survivors: exercise as a resource for aging women. *Gerontologist* 1991;31(3): 347–57.

56. U.S. Department of Health and Human Services. *Physical Activity and Health: A Report to the Surgeon General.* Atlanta: U.S. Department of Health and Human Services, Centers for Disease Control and Prevention, National Center for Chronic Disease Prevention and Health Promotion, 1996.

57. Harris MI. Epidemiology of diabetes mellitus among the elderly in the United States. *Clin Geriatr Med* 1990; 6(4):703–19.

58. Institute of Medicine. *The Second Fifty Years: Promoting Health and Preventing Disability.* Washington, DC: National Academy Press, 1990.

59. Fertig BJ, Simmons DA, Martin DB. Therapy for diabetes. In: National Diabetes Data Group, editors. *Diabetes in America.* 2nd ed. Bethesda, MD: National Institutes of Health, 1995:519–40. (NIH Publication No. 95-1468)

60. Glasgow RE, Toobert DJ, Hampson SE, Brown JE, Lewinsohn PM, Donnelly J. Improving self-care among older patients with type II diabetes: the "Sixty Something..." study. *Patient Educ Counsel* 1992; 19(1):61–74.

61. Rubin RR, Peyrot M, Saudek CD. Effect of diabetes education on self-care, metabolic control, and emotional well-being. *Diabetes Care* 1989;12(10):673–9.

62. Hiss RG, editor. *Diabetes in Communities.* Ann Arbor, MI: University of Michigan, Michigan Diabetes Research and Training Center, 1986.

63. Glasgow RE, Toobert DJ, Hampson SE. Participation in outpatient diabetes education programs: how many patients take part and how representative are they? *Diabetes Educ* 1991;17(5):376–80.

64. Lin N. Conceptualizing social support. In: Lin N, Dean A, Ensel W, editors. *Social Support, Life Events, and Depression.* San Diego, CA: Academic Press, 1986:17–30.

65. Ferraro KF. Widowhood and health. In: Markides KS, Cooper CL, editors. *Aging, Stress, and Health.* New York: Wiley, 1989:69–89.

66. Anderson LA, Halter JB. Diabetes care in older adults: current issues in management and research. In: Lawton MP, editor. *Annual Review of Gerontology and Geriatrics.* New York: Springer, 1989.

67. Bailey BJ, Kahn A. Apportioning illness management authority: how diabetic individuals evaluate and respond to spousal help. *Qual Health Res* 1993;3(1):55–73.

68. Silliman RA, Bhatti S, Khan A, Dukes KA, Sullivan LM. The care of older persons with diabetes mellitus: families and primary care physicians. *J Am Geriatr Soc* 1996;44(11):1314–21.

69. Rewers M, Hamman RF. Risk factors for non–insulin-dependent diabetes. In: National Diabetes Data Group, editors. *Diabetes in America.* 2nd ed. Bethesda, MD: National Institutes of Health, 1995:179–220. (NIH Publication No. 95-1468)

70. Ben-Sira Z. *Regression, Stress, and Readjustment in Aging: A Structured Bio-Psychosocial Perspective on Coping and Professional Support.* New York: Praeger, 1991.

71. Christensen S, Long SH, Rodgers J. Acute health care costs for the aged Medicare population: overview and policy options. *Milbank Q* 1987;65(3):397–425.

72. Harris MI. Health insurance and diabetes. In: National Diabetes Data Group, editors. *Diabetes in America.* 2nd ed. Bethesda, MD: National Institutes of Health, 1995:591–600. (NIH Publication No. 95-1468)

73. U.S. Bureau of the Census. *Statistical Abstract of the United States: 1997.* 117th ed. Washington, DC: U.S. Government Printing Office, 1997.

74. U.S. Department of Health and Human Services. *Health Care Financing Review: Medicare and Medicaid Statistical Supplement, 1997.* Baltimore, MD: Health Care Financing Administration, 1997. (Publication No. 03399)

75. Peddicord M, Lyons A, Tobin C, Vinicor F. Third-party reimbursement for diabetes mellitus. *Diabetes Spectrum* 1989;3:9–12.

76. American Diabetes Association. <http://www.diabetes.org/advocacy/states.asp> Last accessed January 12, 2001.

77. Janes GR. Ambulatory medical care for diabetes. In: National Diabetes Data Group, editors. *Diabetes in America.* 2nd ed. Bethesda, MD: National Institutes of Health, 1995:541–52. (NIH Publication No. 95-1468)

78. U.S. Public Health Service. *Health of Black and White Americans.* Hyattsville, MD: National Center for Health Statistics, 1990.

79. Keeler EB, Solomon DH, Beck JC, Mendenhall RC, Kane RL. Effects of patient age on duration of medical encounters with physicians. *Med Care* 1982;20(11):1101–8.

80. Jenny JL. A comparison of four age groups' adaptation to diabetes. *Can J Public Health* 1984;75(3):237–44.

81. Lipson LG. Diabetes in the elderly: diagnosis, pathogenesis, and therapy. *Am J Med* 1986;80(5A):10–21. Data used with permission from publisher.

82. U.S. Department of Health and Human Services. *Medicare Diabetes Care.* Washington, DC: Health, Education, and Human Services Division, 1997. (GAO/HEHS Publication No. 97-48)

83. American Diabetes Association. Clinical practice recommendations, 1997. *Diabetes Care* 1997;20(Suppl 1):51–70.

84. Sharon B, Hennessy CH, Brandon LJ, Boyette LW. Older adults' experiences of a strength training program. *J Nutr Health Aging* 1997;2:103–8.

85. Graham C. Exercise and aging: implications for persons with diabetes. *Diabetes Educ* 1991;17(3):189–95.

86. Hopper SV. Meeting the needs of the economically deprived diabetic. *Nurs Clin North Am* 1983;18(4):813–25.

87. Lang GC. "Making sense" about diabetes: Dakota narratives of illness. *Med Anthropol* 1989;11(3):305–27.

88. Mezitis NH, Pi-Sunyer FX. Dietary management of geriatric diabetes. *Geriatrics* 1989;44(12):70–2, 75–8.

89. Gilden JL, Casia C, Hendryx M, Singh SP. Effects of self-monitoring of blood glucose on quality of life in elderly diabetic patients. *J Am Geriatr Soc* 1990;38(5):511–5.

90. Hampson SE, Glasgow RE, Foster LS. Personal models of diabetes among older adults: relationship to self-management and other variables. *Diabetes Educ* 1995;21(4):300–7.

91. Ross ME. Hardiness and compliance in elderly patients with diabetes. *Diabetes Educ* 1991;17(5):372–5.

92. Tu KS, McDaniel G, Gay JT. Diabetes self-care knowledge, behaviors, and metabolic control of older adults—the effect of a post-educational follow-up program. *Diabetes Educ* 1993;19(1):25–30.

93. Wilson W, Pratt C. The impact of diabetes education and peer support upon weight and glycemic control of elderly persons with non–insulin-dependent diabetes mellitus (NIDDM). *Am J Public Health* 1987;77(5):634–5.

94. Zaldivar A, Smolowitz J. Perceptions of the importance placed on religion and folk medicine by non-Mexican American Hispanic adults with diabetes. *Diabetes Educ* 1994;20(4):303–6.

95. Reid BV. "It's like you're down on a bed of affliction:" Aging and diabetes among black Americans. *Soc Sci Med* 1992;34(12):1317–23.

96.   Dellasega C. Self-care for the elderly diabetic. *J Gerontol Nurs* 1990;16(1):16–20.

97.   Kesson CM, Bailie GR. Do diabetic patients inject accurate doses of insulin? *Diabetes Care* 1981;4(2):333–7.

98.   CDC. Total tooth loss in persons aged 65 years—selected states, 1995–1997. *MMWR* 1999;48(2):206–10.

99.   Ship JA, Duffy V, Jones JA, Langmore S. Geriatric oral health and its impact on eating. *J Am Geriatr Soc* 1996; 44(4):456–64.

100. Marchesseault LC. Diabetes and the elderly. *Nurs Clin North Am* 1983;18(4):791–8.

101. Palmer CF. Special issues in the management of the elderly patient with diabetes. *Mt Sinai J Med* 1991;58(4): 287–92.

102. Nickols-Richardson SM, Johnson MA, Poon LW, Martin P. Mental health and number of illnesses are predictors of nutritional risk in elderly persons. *Exp Aging Res* 1996;22(2):141–54.

103. Diokno AC, Brock BM, Brown MB, Herzog AR. Prevalence of urinary incontinence and other urological symptoms in the noninstitutionalized elderly. *J Urol* 1986;136(5):1022–5.

7

MAJOR FINDINGS, PUBLIC HEALTH IMPLICATIONS, AND CONCLUSIONS

P.E. Thompson-Reid, MAT, MPH, G.L.A. Beckles, MBBS, MSc

The findings presented in chapters 2–6 reinforce criteria put forth in a report by the U.S. Public Health Service Task Force on Women's Health Issues[1] and establish that diabetes is indeed a women's health issue. We used well-defined stages in the development of women's lives—the adolescent years, the reproductive years, the middle years, and the older years—to examine the effect of diabetes on the health of women. This approach was chosen for two reasons: first, to gain insight into the features of the social and environmental context in which women live that may constitute barriers to maintaining and improving the health status of women in general and, second, to examine whether this impact varies across the life stages of women with diabetes. Within this framework, specific and particular attention has been paid to the influence of psychosocial, socioeconomic, and environmental factors on the health behaviors and health outcomes of women with diabetes. Many of these factors are known to impair the abilities of all women, with or without diabetes, to maintain their health and to care for themselves when they are ill.

In general, we found that diabetes poses great challenges for women, and the risk factors for the disease are growing in such epidemic proportions that if we do not act soon, the problem will be even larger in the years ahead.

This final chapter presents major findings affecting all women, with particular implications for women with diabetes, and the public health implications for women with diabetes across the life stages.

7.1 Major Findings

Feminization of Old Age

There is a large proportion of women aged 65 years or older in the U.S. population and an increasing tendency for these women to be living alone when they are more likely to be frail and vulnerable. The number of women aged 65 years or older is expected to grow from approximately 20 million in 1995 to 23 million in 2010. Futhermore, the number of women aged 85 or older is projected to increase from 2.6 million in 1995 to approximately 4 million in 2010. Women live an average of 7 years longer than men, and among adults aged 75 years or older, there are nearly twice as many women as men. This difference in longevity accounts in part for the increasing tendency for women to live alone. Women with diabetes have lower life expectancy than women without diabetes; however, the median life expectancy of women with diabetes is still greater than that of men with diabetes.

Risk of Poverty

Studies have shown that indicators of social class (e.g., income, education) are associated with type 2 diabetes. In absolute terms, it is important to note that increasing numbers of women are at risk for poverty. In 1995, an estimated 13.5 million American women were living in poverty, accounting for 3 of 5 poor adults aged 18 years or older. The risk of being poor is greatest for women of childbearing age and elderly women. By age 65, women are twice as likely as men to be poor.

Trends in Employment

Approximately 3 of 5 women aged 15 years or older participate in the labor force. Many of these women experience discontinuous employment because of family responsibilities and tend to work in small companies that provide fewer benefits and lower pay than larger companies. Because the majority of women in the work force are of reproductive age, they are at risk for gestational as well as type 2 diabetes. There is also an increasing trend among women 65 years or older to remain in the labor force. Women with diabetes or other chronic conditions may work under circumstances that impede self-management and access to health care.

Inadequate Medical Insurance Coverage

Approximately 1 in 7 women are uninsured; 30% of these women are poor, and an additional 10% are nearly poor. Because of variations in eligibility for Medicaid from state to state, many of these women may not have access to health care. Medicare provides insurance for acute illness or hospitalization for persons 65 or older; however, for persons with chronic diseases such as diabetes, this type of coverage is not sufficient for recipients to gain access to quality diabetes care or to adhere to recommended preventive care practices.[2,3]

Increasing Overweight and Lack of Physical Activity

Overweight and lack of physical activity are risk factors for type 2 diabetes. In 1994, approximately 36 million female adolescents and women were overweight: 10% of adolescents aged 12–17 years, 20% of women aged 18–19 years, and 36% of women aged 20 years or older. Increasing trends in weight among women are steepest for the heaviest and youngest women. In particular, overweight adolescent girls are more likely to become overweight women than their peers who are not overweight. Three of 5 American women do not exercise regularly. School-aged female adolescents, female college students, and women are likely to engage in less physical activity as they age.

Specific Groups of Women

Issues common to specific groups of women that could potentially increase the burden of diabetes are

- The expected increase in the number of women in racial and ethnic minority populations (from 35.5 million in 1995 to 50.2 million in 2010).

- Increasing diagnosis of type 2 diabetes among adolescent black, American Indian, and Hispanic girls, which may presage a steeper rise than expected in the number of adolescent girls with diabetes in future years.

- The persisting racial and ethnic disparities in health status and access to adequate health care.

- The impact of immigration and acculturation on the diabetogenic risk profile of adolescent girls and women.

- The lack of access to adequate health care for women in rural areas, notably women of childbearing age and elderly women.

7.2 Public Health Implications

The mission of public health is to "fulfill society's interest in assuring conditions in which people can be healthy."[4] *Healthy People 2010*,[5] sets national goals to address health disparities that exist among Americans. In exercising its charge, the public health community recognizes that health disparities are expressed in a context that is influenced by social, environmental, and behavioral determinants, many of which are not clearly understood. Furthermore, in many instances, public health has no mandate to act to ameliorate some of these disparities. The health sector should acknowledge the need for research that will identify the underlying determinants of racial, ethnic, and sex disparities and should collaborate with local communities and with other sectors to develop, implement, and evaluate interventions for achieving community and national goals.

The role of public health is defined by three core functions: assessment, policy development, and assurance.[2] Public health agencies systematically collect, analyze, and disseminate information on the health status of the population. When assessment is ongoing and the data are used in the planning, implementation, and evaluation of public health activities, it is classified as surveillance. When the data collection is designed to develop or to generate new knowledge that can be applied more generally, the activity is defined as research. The data obtained from assessment activities provide the basis for the formulation of public health policy. Finally, to implement policy, it is essential that public health agencies assure that the regulations and services needed to achieve agreed upon public health goals are in place and accessible. These functions are operationally defined at the state and local levels through the work of local health departments and other public, nonprofit, and private organizations that share common goals.

The following section summarizes the public health implications of diabetes in women based on findings presented in chapters 2–6. These implications are organized by the three core public health functions: assessment, policy development, and assurance.

Assessment
Surveillance.

Population dynamics indicate that the greatest growth in the female population is expected among elderly women and among racial and ethnic minority groups at high risk for diabetes.
We need a protocol for systematic surveillance of these groups at the national and state levels. Particular emphasis should be given to analyzing and reporting data on health-related behaviors, morbidity, and mortality by the socioeconomic status of women.

The majority of the white population is dispersed relatively evenly across the United States, although racial and ethnic minority populations are concentrated in specific geographic areas, determined by their history and migration patterns.
Surveillance systems could take advantage of the regional concentrations of specific ethnic groups at risk for diabetes. In addition, the number of foreign-born women is increasing regionally. Emphasis should be given to the analysis and reporting of data on health-related behaviors, morbidity, and mortality by region, duration and generation of residence in the United States, and degree of acculturation. This approach would provide additional information to guide the development of policy and the allocation of resources for interventions targeting women in high-risk populations.

Adolescent girls, young women, and elderly women constitute high-risk groups for diabetes because of poor dietary habits, low levels of physical activity, and increasing overweight, obesity, and weight gain.
Because of the continuing increase in risks associated with diabetes in these groups, opportunities to systematically monitor diabetes-related health behaviors (e.g., eating disorders) should be undertaken. Particular attention should be paid to adolescent girls and elderly women, notably women aged 85 years or older.

Preliminary evidence suggests that the prevalence of type 2 diabetes is increasing among adolescents and reproductive-aged women, especially in minority women.
Additional surveillance information is required to confirm these initial observations and to inform programmatic activities.

Diabetes during pregnancy is a serious condition that affects not only the health of the mother but also of the unborn child. If not addressed appropriately, this condition will add to the future burden of diabetes as well as of other chronic diseases.

Surveillance systems should be developed to monitor the prevalence of gestational diabetes and differentiate between gestational and preexisting diabetes, especially in high-risk groups.

Women younger than 65 years of age who are at high risk of developing diabetes are the least likely to have adequate access to preventive health care services.

Access to and use of ambulatory diabetes-related preventive care services need to be assessed and routinely monitored, and the resulting data should be analyzed and reported for all high-risk groups of women. This information is important for the planning, promotion, and delivery of these services.

Women aged 85 years or older are the fastest growing group in the female population. They are expected to number 3.9 million in 2010 and to almost double to 7.3 million by 2020.

Because of the projected increase in the number of women in this age group, national surveillance will be needed to assess and monitor trends in behavioral risk factors for diabetes and other chronic diseases, the use of clinical preventive services, and health-related quality of life. Oversampling and special surveys may be necessary to obtain reliable estimates for these subpopulations.

Research.

The gradient of risk for diabetes and related health burden associated with socioeconomic status, geographic region, area of residence, and place of birth is often greater than the risk gradients related to the traditionally used markers of age and race/ethnicity.

We need to define and develop a consensus on valid indicators of social status and social context appropriate for use in the surveillance of the health status of various subgroups of women with or without diabetes in the United States and its territories. For example, blacks born in the South suffer poorer health than blacks born in other parts of the country. Additional information is needed to identify the determinants of excess risk for diabetes and its complications.

The role and impact of environmental factors such as availability of nutritious foods, safe neighborhoods, social policy, social context, and individual susceptibility on the development of diabetes are not well established.

We need epidemiologic and health services research to gain a better understanding of the interaction between the social and economic environment and individual characteristics to determine the effect of these variables on the incidence of diabetes.

Deterioration in the health status of immigrant females is associated with the adoption of behaviors that increase their risk for diabetes.

Research is needed to identify protective health behaviors among immigrant groups and to develop intervention strategies to preserve these behaviors. Such findings may be useful for risk reduction among other population groups.

Physical inactivity is an independent risk factor for the development of diabetes. The level of inactivity is high among all women aged 20 years or older, especially in racial and ethnic minority populations, and the level of physical activity among adolescents decreases rapidly with age.

Regular physical activity has many health benefits for female adolescents and women. Additional studies are needed to identify modifiable individual and structural barriers to physical activity among school-aged girls and to identify and assess the effectiveness of preferred types of physical activity for women in various age, cultural, and socioeconomic groups.

Overweight and obesity are major risk factors for the development of type 2 diabetes in middle-aged women.

More intensive study is needed to determine the contribution of cumulative gestational weight gain to overweight among middle-aged women and to identify the psychosocial and socioenvironmental factors that contribute to weight gain so that appropriate prevention strategies can be designed.

Women with diabetes are at greater risk for heart disease, and especially first fatal events, than men and women without diabetes.

More research is needed to gain a better understanding of the excess risk of coronary heart disease (CHD) among women with diabetes and to identify modifiable determinants of this sex differential for use in the development of effective interventions. To assess the risk-benefit ratio of aspirin treatment among diabetic women, adequate numbers of women with diabetes must be included in clinical trials of aspirin use for the primary prevention of myocardial infarction. Clinical trial data are also needed to determine the balance of benefits and risks of hormone replacement therapy (HRT) in diabetic women. Adequate numbers of women with diabetes should also be included in clinical trials of HRT because they may derive greater benefit from HRT than women at low risk for cardiovascular disease. More data are needed to determine if antioxidant or vitamin use or other potentially promising new interventions will reduce CHD in women with diabetes.

Studies document a high prevalence of depression and other mental illness among women with diabetes.

More research is needed to clarify the relationship between diabetes and depression in women. Findings from various studies are contradictory. For example, some studies show that the onset of

depression usually precedes the diagnosis of type 2 diabetes but follows the diagnosis of type 1 diabetes.

Elderly women have a higher prevalence of diabetes complications and concurrent illnesses than other women with diabetes because of the aging process and uncontrolled glycemia.

More epidemiologic research is needed to define the natural history of diabetes in elderly women. Research is needed to distinguish between outcomes resulting from aging and other comorbidities. In addition, current guidelines for diabetes control may not be appropriate for disease management among elderly persons.

Elderly women with diabetes are at high risk for poverty, are likely to live alone, and suffer disproportionately from the complications of diabetes.

The barriers to self-management of diabetes and other chronic diseases among elderly women need to be assessed at the community level, and the modifiable determinants of such barriers need to be identified to provide data for the development of appropriate interventions.

Women with diabetes use health services more often than men do.

In general, the health-seeking behaviors of women indicate more frequent office visits than men, yet women with diabetes do not fare as well with the disease as men with diabetes. Additional research is needed to elucidate the relationship between access to care, health-seeking behaviors, and hospital admission and readmission rates among women with diabetes.

Despite remarkable advances in our scientific understanding of basic disease processes, including diabetes, there is a significant gap between our knowledge base and what is actually provided to individuals for the prevention and care of diabetes.

As delineated by the Institute of Medicine,[6] the health care systems in the United States must be "redesigned" to reflect the realities and needs of chronic diseases like diabetes. Translational/effectiveness studies for diabetes prevention and control are important activities that will inform the process for improving the quality of care provided to persons with diabetes.[7]

There is a growing number of persons with diabetes in racial and ethnic minority populations, yet health care providers from these populations are underrepresented.

Studies show that members of racial and ethnic minority populations are more satisfied with health care providers of similar ethnic or cultural backgrounds. Training in cultural competency should be required for all providers, especially those serving populations with which they have little familiarity. Given the diversity of the U.S. population, health care providers should be able to communicate in the languages of the populations they serve, or suitable arrangements should be made to facilitate communication. Opportunities should also be provided to train minority health professionals, including health educators, scientists, and medical personnel. Additional research is needed to determine the effects of these strategies on the delivery of quality diabetes care.

Sex, ethnicity, socioeconomic status, and women's multiple roles are important variables that affect women's health.

As more women enter the work force and take on multiple roles, more studies are needed to elucidate the changing relationship between sex, ethnicity, socioeconomic status, social support, and the impact of these variables on health status, particularly among women with diabetes.

Policy Development

The prevalence of overweight and the incidence of obesity are increasing rapidly among adolescent girls, and these girls

appear to have an increasing risk of developing type 2 diabetes.

To make an impact on this public health issue and potential public health problem, women's health advocates and health and education agencies at the federal, state, and local levels should continue to strengthen and expand their collaboration and efforts to develop and implement programs designed to

- Ensure that foods available in schools comply with federal recommendations for healthy diets.

- Increase the incorporation of physical activity programs throughout the entire school and home life of adolescents, especially girls.

- Integrate information about the lifelong benefits of physical activity, healthy eating, and other preventive health behaviors into school curricula in all grades.

Women at high risk for diabetes are least likely to have adequate health insurance coverage.

Health insurance coverage should focus on the provision of access to optimal preventive care for women with diabetes and other chronic diseases in all age and racial/ethnic groups. Specific attention to adolescents, women less than 65 years of age, and poor and nearly poor women of all age and racial/ethnic groups should be considered. This strategy may help to reduce the growing disparities in health outcomes among persons with diabetes.

An increasing number of elderly women with diabetes are at risk for poverty and are more likely to live alone.

Access to medical care will not address all the self-management needs of elderly women with diabetes. Strategies that involve interagency collaboration should be explored because they may be helpful in the planning and delivery of community-based services that specifically target the needs of the increasing numbers of elderly women with diabetes who live alone, often in poverty.

Because of the expected growth in the elderly population, the demand for diabetes-related services will increase nationwide.

Resources need to be allocated to train health care professionals qualified in the diagnosis and management of diabetes in elderly persons.

Assurance

Sex-related differences in health communications and health-seeking behaviors should be considered in the planning and delivery of services for women with diabetes.

Protocols need to be developed to assure delivery of quality care for women to enhance the appropriate use of resources for improving health outcomes. This approach may entail designing innovative models of health care delivery that are responsive to the needs of women (e.g., extended hours, culturally competent providers, continuous access to preventive care services such as health education and self-management training). Women should have a primary health care entry point from which access can be gained to other appropriate services as needed, including enabling services such as child care and transportation.

Improving access to quality diabetes care is an important strategy for reducing the burden of diabetes in women at high risk for the disease and its complications.

Particular attention also needs to be paid to providing adequate preventive services for women younger than 65, women of childbearing age who live in nonmetropolitan areas, and elderly women who live alone. For persons with diabetes, this coverage should include access to dental and mental health services. A focused effort is needed to improve the accessibility of high-quality diabetes care for all persons with diabetes. Delivery systems such as community health centers, managed care organizations, or fee-for-service entities are important components that could be targeted for intervention.

The need will increase for health care professionals who are qualified to diagnose diabetes in women and provide comprehensive treatment.

To prepare for the future needs of persons with chronic diseases in general and those with diabetes specifically, the public health community should advocate for and facilitate the creation of incentives for training health care providers, including community health workers, who are skilled in managing health care for elderly persons with diabetes. Training for these workers should take into account that the majority of their patients will be women, many of whom will be very old.

Improved training about the risks of diabetes, its complications, and the importance of preventive care is essential for health care professionals at all levels.

Mechanisms to facilitate improved adherence to recommended standards of care, including promoting a better understanding among health care providers of the role of the family and the community, should be identified and implemented to achieve positive health outcomes for persons with diabetes. Continuing education programs addressing provider attitudes toward women, the treatment of diabetes, and the role of families and the community in the management of this disease are important topics to include in the provider curriculum. Health delivery systems should use continuous quality improvement methods to improve provider compliance with recommended standards of care.

In conclusion, it is our intent to gain the attention of the public health community, policy makers, and the general public as well. Everyone is potentially at risk for diabetes, and collaboration and the allocation of resources to reduce the burden of this disease are urgently needed. To stem the tide of the increasing societal burden of diabetes, we know there is much we can do now.

References

1. U.S. Public Health Service. *Women's Health: Report of the Public Health Service Task Force in Women's Health Issues.* Vol. 2. U.S. Department of Health and Human Services, 1987.

2. Schoeder SA. Prospects for expanding health insurance coverage. *N Engl J Med* 2001;344(11):847–52.

3. Ayanian JZ, Weissman JS, Schneider EC, Ginsburg JA, Zaslavsky KM. Unmet health needs of uninsured adults in the United States. *JAMA* 2000;284(16):2061–9.

4. Institute of Medicine. *The Future of Public Health.* Washington, DC: National Academy Press, 1988.

5. U.S. Department of Health and Human Services. *Healthy People 2010* (Conference Edition in Two Volumes). Washington, DC: U.S. Department of Health and Human Services, January 2000.

6. Institute of Medicine Committee on Quality of Health Care in America. *Crossing the Quality Chasm: A New Health System for the 21ˢᵗ Century.* Washington, DC: National Academy Press, 2001.

7. Narayan KM, Gregg EW, Engelgau MM, et al. Translation research for chronic disease: the case of diabetes. *Diabetes Care* 2000;23(12):1794–98.

When we began this project, the principal aim was to provide a reference document for public health professionals and advocates for women's health. As the work progressed, we became more acutely aware of some of the issues that affect our efforts to reduce the burden of diabetes in women. First, the challenges will soon become greater, as current trends and projections show that women will contribute greatly to the growing number of prevalent cases because of 1) the dominance of young women among those developing so-called "type 2 diabetes in youth," 2) the impact of the intrauterine environment on the subsequent development of diabetes—both in the mother following gestational diabetes and in the offspring several decades later, and 3) the fact that women live longer than men, alone and often poor, and increasingly with diabetes. Coupled with other socioeconomic and psychosocial determinants of disease, we must acknowledge this increased diabetes burden in women and begin to do something about it.

Second, it is unlikely that the traditional clinical and individual-oriented approach to disease control and prevention will, by itself, be effective. Although such approaches have been successful in eradicating and controlling certain diseases in populations throughout the world,[1] the emphasis to reduce the burden of chronic diseases has primarily focused on identifying and modifying risk *in individuals*. This 19th-century reductionist approach has persisted because many of the determinants of disease that may precede or underlie the current health status of the population (e.g., social conditions in populations) have not been studied sufficiently to influence strategies for widespread public health practice.[2-4] Throughout this document, demographic and socioeconomic disparities were recurring observations and themes at every stage of the lives of women with diabetes. As disturbing as this can

be, this focus on women also revealed the presence of structural barriers (e.g., inadequacy of insurance coverage for persons with chronic disease) in the environment that may impede efforts to reduce the burden of disease, not only for this population but for all persons with diabetes.

Third, we also found confusion in the literature in the use and understanding of the terms "gender" and "sex." In a recent report, the Institute of Medicine[5] defined sex as the classification of living things, generally as male or female according to their reproductive organs and functions assigned by the chromosomal complement, and gender as a person's self-representation as male or female, or how that person is responded to by social institutions on the basis of the individual gender presentation. Gender is shaped by environment and experience.[5] More precise use of these two terms including the development of valid indicators or measures should enhance the research agenda and inform public health practice. There are still many unanswered questions. For example, "How have the changing roles of women, work, and family responsibility affected health status?" As more women participate in the workforce, do we have policies that facilitate and support healthy lifestyles for the prevention or control of chronic diseases such as diabetes? The discordance between the traditional role expected of women and the realities of their lives may expose them to chronic psychosocial stressors that we now recognize may contribute to poor health, including the development of diabetes or other chronic diseases.

When we began this journey, there were many skeptics among our peers who voiced concern about our focus on women. Even in the literature, we found that diabetes in women was frequently discussed *only* from the perspective of "diabetes in pregnancy," and even within this limited view, protecting the child was the primary focus of practice. In other words, women's health was seen to be different solely because of their reproductive function. This particular view has framed and guided many institutional policies and has limited the scope of public health understanding and practice. The discussion of public health implications in chapter 7 addresses many of these issues and presents ideas for correcting some of these anomalies.

Finally, in using the life-stage approach to frame the body of this monograph, we hypothesized that the needs of women with diabetes would change during the various life stages, and we found this to be the case. We would like to restate this assumption, and challenge others to adopt the life-stage approach in all public health practice.

To inform health professionals and the general public in a more helpful and useful manner, there is great need for further study to understand the true burden of diabetes in women. Specifically, a major research goal could be to focus on underlying social conditions to understand how social organizations or social capital might influence the health or well-being of women. Social capital, a concept that is now being embraced by the public health community, is defined as the processes and conditions among people and organizations that lead to accomplishing a goal of mutual social benefit.[6] There is also great need for research targeting women with diabetes to translate available knowledge into effective clinical and public health practice.

To provide comprehensive care for women with diabetes and to protect and maintain the health of women throughout their lives, the medical care system and the public health system must be woven together. There are many examples of successful collaboration between these two important segments of the health sector.[7] The public and private sectors—government, universities, nongovernment organizations, and private industry—all have critical roles to play in these efforts if progress is to be made in addressing diabetes, not only in women, but in all people.

References

1. CDC. Ten great public health achievements—United States, 1900–1999. *MMWR* 1999;48(12):241–3.

2. Link BG, Phelan J. Social conditions as fundamental causes of disease. *J Health Soc Behav* 1995;Spec No: 80–94.

3. McKinlay JB, Marceau LD. To boldly go.... *Am J Public Health* 2000;90(1):25–33.

4. McKinlay JB, Marceau LD. U.S. public health in the 21st century: diabetes mellitus. Lancet 2000;356(9231): 757–61.

5. Wizemann TM, Pardue M, editors. *Exploring the Biological Contributions to Human Health: Does Sex Matter?* Committee on Understanding the Biology of Sex and Gender Differences, Board on Health Sciences Policy. Institute of Medicine. Washington, DC: The National Academy of Sciences, 2001.

6. Portes A. Social capital: its origin and application in sociology. *Annu Rev Sociol* 1998;22:1–24.

7. Lasker RD. Committee on Medicine and Public Health. *Medicine and Public Health: The Power of Collaboration.* New York: The New York Academy of Medicine, 1997.

PERCENTAGE OF U.S. ADULT POPULATION WITH
PHYSICIAN-DIAGNOSED DIABETES, BY AGE, SEX,
AND RACE/HISPANIC ORIGIN—
NHANES III,* 1988–94

Population	Age group (years)								
	20–44	45–54	55–64	65–74	≥75	45–64	≥65	≥20	≥20†
All races									
Both sexes	1.6	5.1	11.2	12.7	13.2	7.9	12.9	5.1	5.3
Women	1.7	4.5	11.0	13.3	12.8	7.6	13.1	5.4	5.2
Men	1.4	5.7	11.4	11.9	13.8	8.2	12.6	4.9	5.3
Non-Hispanic white									
Both sexes	1.4	4.5	10.2	11.5	12.6	7.1	12.0	5.0	4.8
Women	1.5	3.2	9.6	11.7	12.3	6.3	11.9	5.0	4.5
Men	1.4	5.8	10.8	11.3	13.2	8.0	12.0	5.0	5.2
Non-Hispanic black									
Both sexes	2.2	8.9	18.0	22.3	17.5	13.1	20.4	6.9	8.2
Women	2.1	10.2	19.2	26.5	19.0	14.3	23.3	7.8	9.1
Men	2.3	7.1	16.5	17.0	14.7	11.4	16.3	5.9	7.3
Mexican American									
Both sexes	1.5	12.9	17.6	27.0	21.7	14.6	25.4	5.6	9.3
Women	7.2	14.8	20.9	30.9	25.0	2.0	17.1	7.2	10.9
Men	1.0	10.9	14.2	22.2	17.8	12.1	20.8	4.2	7.7

*NHANES III = Third National Health and Nutrition Examination Survey.
†Age-standardized by direct method. Standard = 1980 U.S. population.

Sources:
Centers for Disease Control and Prevention, National Center for Chronic Disease Prevention and Health Promotion, data from the Third National Health and Nutrition Examination Survey. Data computed by the Division of Diabetes Translation.

Harris, MI, Flegal KM, Cowie CC, et al. Prevalence of diabetes, impaired fasting glucose, and impaired glucose tolerance in U.S. adults. The Third National Health and Nutrition Examination Survey, 1988–1994. *Diabetes Care* 1998;21(4)518–24.

APPENDIX B

PERCENTAGE OF U.S. ADULT POPULATION WITH UNDIAGNOSED DIABETES,* BY AGE, SEX, AND RACE/HISPANIC ORIGIN— NHANES III,[†] 1988–94

Population	Age group (years)								
	20–44	45–54	55–64	65–74	≥75	45–64	≥65	≥20	≥20[‡]
All races									
Both sexes	0.8	3.7	6.7	5.7	5.8	5.1	5.8	2.8	2.8
Women	0.6	4.4	6.0	3.6	4.9	5.2	4.2	2.5	2.5
Men	1.0	3.0	7.5	8.1	7.5	5.0	7.9	3.1	3.1
Non-Hispanic white									
Both sexes	0.5	3.0	6.0	5.9	5.0	4.4	5.6	2.5	2.5
Women	0.4	3.5	5.1	3.4	4.4	4.3	3.8	2.1	2.0
Men	0.7	2.5	6.9	8.8	6.1	4.4	7.9	3.0	2.9
Non-Hispanic black									
Both sexes	1.5	6.7	8.6	7.9	4.9	7.6	6.9	3.5	3.6
Women	1.6	7.0	11.6	9.0	7.5	9.2	8.4	4.1	4.5
Men	1.3	6.2	4.5	6.8	0.0	5.4	4.9	2.7	2.7
Mexican American									
Both sexes	2.4	3.3	12.6	3.6	8.7	6.7	5.0	3.4	4.5
Women	2.3	1.8	10.0	5.1	6.8	4.7	5.6	3.0	3.6
Men	2.6	4.8	15.2	2.0	11.1	8.7	4.3	3.8	5.4

*Based on 1997 American Diabetes Association criteria.
[†]NHANES III = Third National Health and Nutrition Examination Survey.
[‡]Age-standardized by direct method. Standard = 1980 U.S. population.

Sources:
Centers for Disease Control and Prevention, National Center for Chronic Disease Prevention and Health Promotion, data from the Third National Health and Nutrition Examination Survey. Data computed by the Division of Diabetes Translation.

Harris, MI, Flegal KM, Cowie CC, et al. Prevalence of diabetes, impaired fasting glucose, and impaired glucose tolerance in U.S. adults. The Third National Health and Nutrition Examination Survey, 1988–1994. *Diabetes Care* 1998;21(4)518–24.

AGE-STANDARDIZED PREVALENCE* OF DIAGNOSED DIABETES PER 100 ADULT FEMALE POPULATION, BY STATE— UNITED STATES, 1998–2000

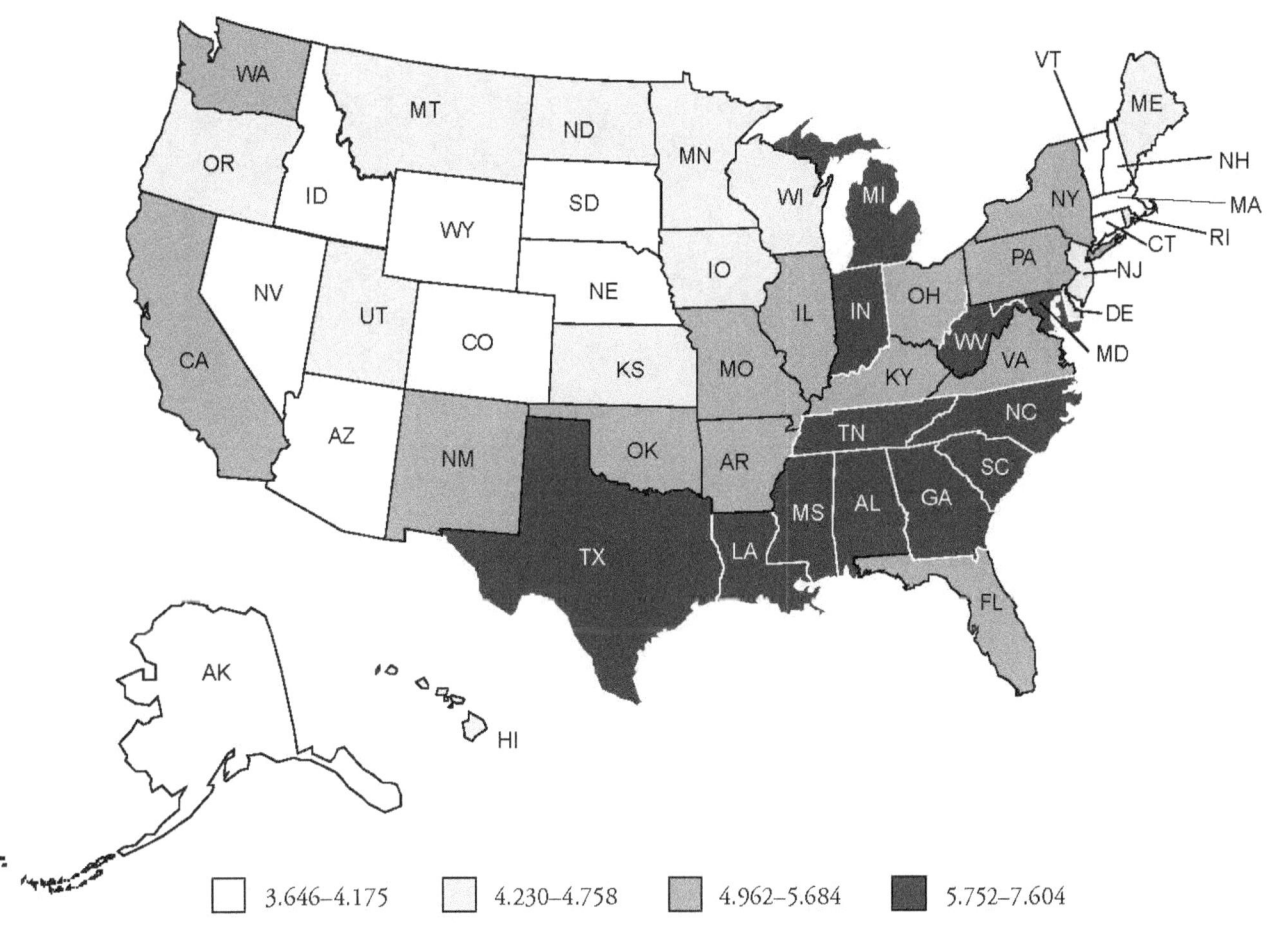

3.646–4.175   4.230–4.758   4.962–5.684   5.752–7.604

*3-year moving average.

Source: Centers for Disease Control and Prevention, National Center for Chronic Disease Prevention and Health Promotion, Division of Adult and Community Health, data from the Behavioral Risk Factor Surveillance System. Data computed by the Division of Diabetes Translation.

APPENDIX D

AGE-STANDARDIZED PREVALENCE* OF DIAGNOSED DIABETES PER 100 ADULT FEMALE POPULATION, BY STATE— UNITED STATES, 1994–96

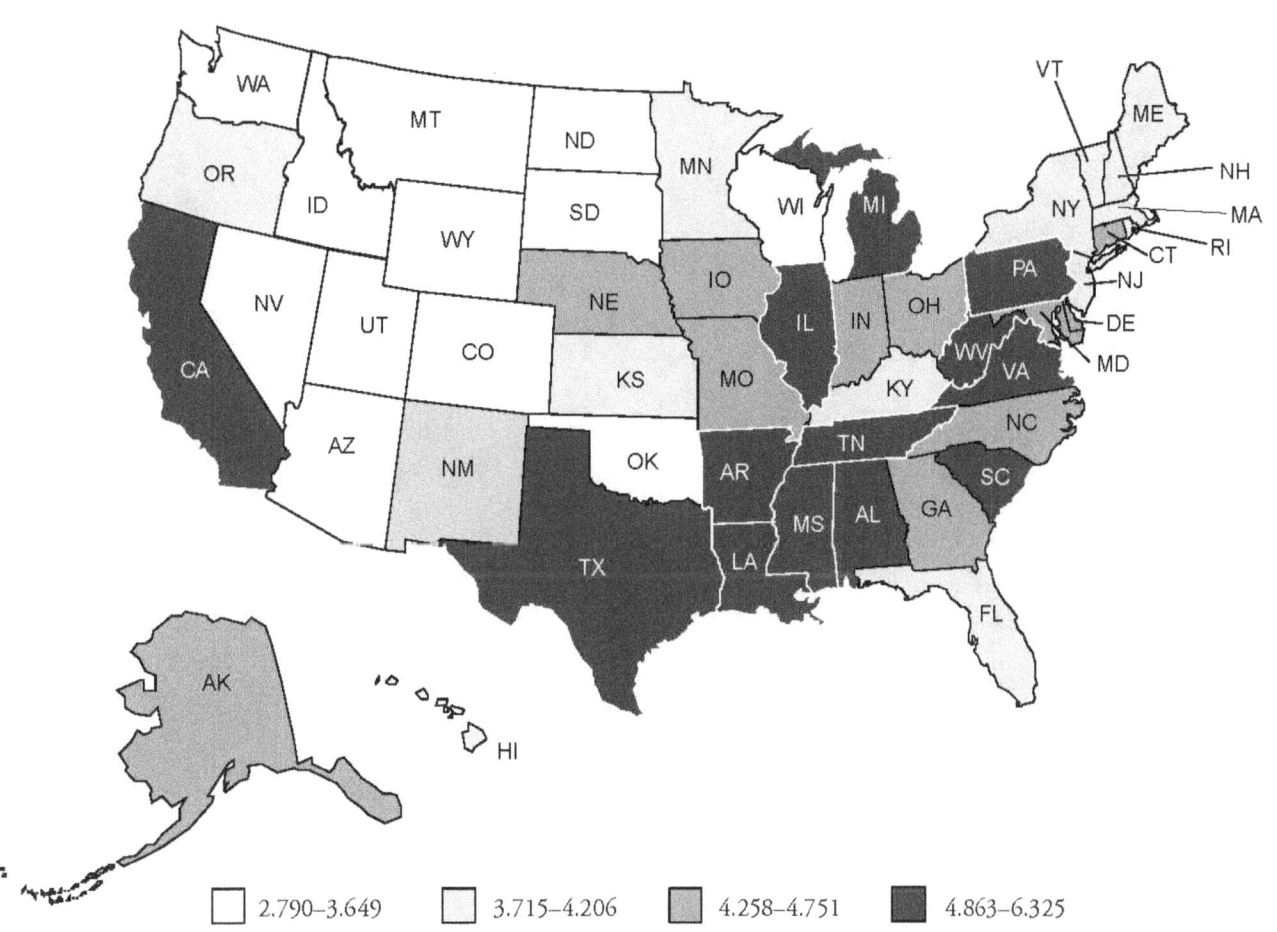

| | 2.790–3.649 | | 3.715–4.206 | | 4.258–4.751 | | 4.863–6.325 |

*3-year moving average.

Source: Centers for Disease Control and Prevention, National Center for Chronic Disease Prevention and Health Promotion, Division of Adult and Community Health, data from the Behavioral Risk Factor Surveillance System. Data computed by the Division of Diabetes Translation.

PHYSICAL ASSESSMENT

- **Visits:** Continuing care visits every six months or appropriate to meet patient's needs and treatment goals.

- **Blood Pressure:** Every continuing care visit. Goal is <130/80.**

- **Weight:** Every continuing care visit; establish growth chart for children.

- **Comprehensive Foot Exam (adults):** At least yearly (more often in patients with high-risk foot conditions).

- **Eye exam:** Yearly dilated funduscopic exam (or retinal photography); if diagnosed at age 29 or earlier, the initial eye exam should be performed within 3–5 years of diagnosis once patient is age 10 or older.

LABORATORY TESTS

- **HbA1c:** 2 times per year; more frequent if not meeting goals. Adjust goals to prevent serious hypoglycemia. Target goal is <1% above upper limit of normal (e.g., <7.0% for a HbA1c assay with an upper limit of normal of 6%). A value >2% (e.g., >8% for HbA1c) above upper limit of normal requires greater attention.**

- **Urine Protein (adults):** Microalbumin measurement annually (in the absence of previously demonstrated microalbuminuia).

- **Lipid Profile (adults):** Yearly. Target goals**: total cholesterol and triglycerides <200 mg/dL, LDL-C<100mg/dL, HDL-C>45 mg/dL in men and >55 mg/dL in women.

SELF-MANAGEMENT TRAINING

- **General Principles:** Review goals at every continuing care visit. Conduct comprehensive assessment yearly to include patient's understanding of diabetes, self-monitoring of blood glucose (SMBG), acute and chronic complications.

- **Medical Nutrition Therapy:** Review goals at every continuing care visit. Conduct comprehensive assessment yearly to include meal planning, reading food labels, weight control

- **SMBG:** Should be performed as appropriate to meet goals.

- **Physical Activity:** Review goals at every continuing care visit. Conduct comprehensive assessment yearly to include frequency and duration of activity and physical limitations.

SPECIAL SITUATIONS

- **Hypoglycemia:** Recurrent hypoglycemia calls for reassessment of treatment plan. Additional action suggested might include enhanced diabetes self-management education, comanagement with a diabetes team, referral to an endocrinologist, change in pharmacological therapy, initiation or increased SMBG, or more frequent contact with the patient.

- **Preconception Counseling:** Begin counseling at puberty; enhance counseling with adolescence; consult with high-risk perinatal programs when appropriate.

- **Pregnancy Management:** Intensify glycemic control; consult with high-risk perinatal programs when appropriate.

- **Smoking Cessation:** Emphasize and assist as much as possible.

- **Aspirin Therapy:** Enteric-coated aspirin (81mg–325mg/day) as secondary prevention for CVD. Consider for primary prevention in high-risk patients (e.g., family history, smoking, hyperlipidemia, hypertension, albuminuria).

*These guidelines have been condensed from the American Diabetes Association's Standards of Medical Care for People with Diabetes. They do not reflect all the actions that should be provided by health professionals in the medical management of diabetes. Full text of the Association's Clinical Practice Recommendations, including the Standards of Medical Care, is available at www.diabetes.org.

**If the patient is not making satisfactory progress toward treatment goals within a reasonable period (3–6 months), medical management should be enhanced. Greater attention to self-management education, comanagement with a diabetes team, referral to an endocrinologist, change in pharmacologic therapy, initiation of or increased SMBG, or more frequent contact with the patient, are examples of actions that should be considered.

Reprinted with permission from the American Diabetes Association

LIST OF ABBREVIATIONS

ADA	American Diabetes Association
ARIC	Atherosclerosis Risk in Communities Study
BRFSS	Behavioral Risk Factor Surveillance System
BMI	body mass index
CARE	Cholesterol and Recurrent Events Study
CDC	Centers for Disease Control and Prevention
CHD	coronary heart disease
CMS	Centers for Medicare and Medicaid Services (formerly HCFA)
CVD	cardiovascular disease
DCCT	Diabetes Control and Complications Trial
DERI	Diabetes Epidemiology Research International Mortality Study
DM	diabetes mellitus
DPP	Diabetes Prevention Program
DSM-IV	Diagnostic and Statistical Manual of Mental Disorders, 4th Edition
EPESE	Established Populations for Epidemiologic Studies in the Elderly
ERT	estrogen replacement therapy
ESRD	end-stage renal disease
ETDRS	Early Treatment of Diabetic Retinopathy Study
GDM	gestational diabetes mellitus
HbA_{1c}	hemoglobin A_{1c}
HDL	high-density lipoprotein
HERS	Heart and Estrogen/progestin Replacement Study
HCFA	Health Care Financing Administration (currently CMS)
HHANES	Hispanic Health and Nutrition Examination Survey (1982–84)
HOPE	Heart Outcomes Prevention and Evaluation Study
HOT	Hypertension Optimal Treatment Study
HRQOL	health-related quality of life
HRSA	Health Resources and Services Administration

HRT	hormone replacement therapy
IDDM	insulin-dependent diabetes mellitus
IGT	impaired glucose tolerance
JDRF	Juvenile Diabetes Research Foundation International
LDL	low-density lipoprotein
LEAD	lower-extremity arterial disease
NCEP	National Cholesterol Education Program
NDEP	National Diabetes Education Program
NIH	National Institutes of Health
NHANES I	First National Health and Nutrition Examination Survey (1971–75)
NHANES II	Second National Health and Nutrition Examination Survey (1976–80)
NHANES III	Third National Health and Nutrition Examination Survey (1988–94)
NHANS	Navajo Health and Nutrition Survey (1991–92)
NHDS	National Hospital Discharge Survey
NHES	National Health Examination Survey (1963–65)
NHIS	National Health Interview Survey
NHS	Nurses' Health Study
NIDDM	non–insulin-dependent diabetes mellitus
NIH	National Institutes of Health
PDR	proliferative diabetic retinopathy
Project DIRECT	Diabetes Interventions Reaching and Educating Communities Together
PVD	peripheral vascular disease
SES	socioeconomic status
UKPDS	United Kingdom Prospective Diabetes Study
WESDR	Wisconsin Epidemiology Study of Diabetic Retinopathy
WHO	World Health Organization
WHR	waist-to-hip ratio

acculturation — the process of adapting to the behaviors and norms of the majority culture. Degree of acculturation is often used to describe how much an immigrant has adopted the lifestyle of the majority culture.

acidosis — See diabetic ketoacidosis.

activities of daily living — scale developed by S. Katz and colleagues to measure personal self-maintenance ability among older adults. The activities rated are eating, toileting, dressing, bathing, transferring (e.g., getting in and out of bed), and continence.

adherence — the extent to which patients follow health care provider recommendations for disease management, including health-promoting activities. For persons with diabetes, this includes taking medications, monitoring blood glucose, and following nutrition and physical activity guidelines. Also see compliance.

adiposity — excessive fat in the body; see obesity.

age-adjusted — describes rates that have been adjusted by an established procedure to minimize the effects of differences in age composition when comparing rates for different populations.

albuminuria — more than normal amounts of the protein albumin in the urine. Albuminuria may be a sign of kidney disease.

all-cause mortality rate — an estimate of the proportion of a population that dies during a specific period due to all those diseases, morbid conditions, or injuries that either resulted in or contributed to death and the circumstances of the accident or violence that produced any such injuries.

American Diabetes Association (ADA) — non-profit national health organization that provides information, advocates policy change, and conducts research to prevent and cure diabetes and to improve the life of all people affected by diabetes. For more information, see *http://www.diabetes.org.*

angina — a condition in which the heart muscle does not receive enough blood, resulting in pain in the chest.

angiotensin converting enzyme (ACE) inhibitor — a type of drug used to lower blood pressure and to help prevent kidney disease in persons with diabetes.

anorexia — lack or loss of appetite for food.

anorexia nervosa — a serious eating disorder characterized by chronic decreased food intake that results in profound weight loss.

atherosclerosis/atherosclerotic disease — a disease in which fat builds up in the large and medium-sized arteries. This buildup of fat may slow down or stop blood flow.

atherosclerotic lesions/plaque — deposits in the arteries that result from the accumulation of cholesterol and lipids in the arteries. Persons with diabetes are at increased risk for atherosclerosis.

autonomic neuropathy — nerve damage affecting control of the internal organs, such as the bladder muscles, digestive tract, and genital organs. Autonomic neuropathy can develop as a complication of diabetes.

Behavioral Risk Factor Surveillance System (BRFSS) — an annual state-based telephone survey of the civilian, noninstitutionalized adult population conducted biannually by CDC and state health departments to assess lifestyle characteristics and risk and health-promoting behaviors. For more information, see *http://www.cdc.gov/nccdphp/brfss.*

beta cell- type of cell in the pancreas that makes and releases insulin.

body mass index (BMI) — a measure of body size that relates weight in kilograms to height in meters squared. Formula: weight in kilograms divided by height in meters squared (kg/m²). BMI correlates highly with body fat in most people.

bulemia — eating disorder characterized by binge eating and induced vomiting.

cardiovascular disease (CVD) — disease of the circulatory system, including the heart and blood vessels.

cataract — clouding of the lens of the eye. Cataracts can occur as a complication of diabetes.

central adiposity or obesity — fat deposits that form in the center of a person's body, especially around the stomach area, often assessed by measuring waist-to-hip ratio. Central adiposity increases the risk for cardiovascular complications.

cerebrovascular disease — damage to the blood vessels in the brain that can result in a stroke. (See stroke.) Cerebrovascular disease can develop as a complication of diabetes.

cholesterol — a fat-like substance in the blood, muscle, liver, brain, and other tissues. Too much cholesterol may cause fat to build up in the artery walls and cause disease that slows or stops the flow of blood.

compliance — patients' adherence to health care provider recommendations for disease management and health-promoting activities. (See adherence.)

comorbidity — the condition of having more than one illnesses at the same time (e.g., diabetes and depression, diabetes and heart disease).

continuous subcutaneous infusion of insulin (CSII) — or insulin pump, a device that delivers a continuous supply of insulin into the body. The insulin flows through the pump through a plastic tube that is connected to a needle inserted into the body and taped in place. Insulin is delivered at two rates: a low, steady rate (called basal rate) for continuous day-long coverage, and extra boosts of insulin (called bolus doses) to cover meals or when extra insulin is needed.

coronary heart disease (CHD) — a disorder that affects the heart muscle and its blood vessels. The most serious danger of coronary heart disease is a heart attack, which occurs when the supply of blood to the heart is greatly reduced or stopped due to a blockage in a coronary artery. Persons with diabetes have an increased risk for CHD.

cortisol — one of several hormones made in the adrenal glands. The primary responsibility of cortisol is to activate the immune system; it also affects the metabolism of glucose.

dementia — loss of cognitive function; a condition of deteriorated mentality.

dentition — quality and quantity of teeth, including their number, kind, and arrangement.

diabetic ketoacidosis — acute complication of diabetes characterized by a high blood glucose in the presence of ketones in the urine and bloodstream. Diabetic ketoacidocis requires emergency treatment and is often caused by illness or taking too little insulin. Symptoms include nausea and vomiting, stomach pain, and deep, rapid breathing.

Diabetes Control and Complications Trial (DCCT) — clinical study funded by the National Institutes of Health to assess the effects of intensive therapy on the long-term complications of type 1 diabetes. The study showed that intensive blood glucose control slows the onset and progression of eye, kidney, and nerve disease caused by diabetes. For more information, see *http://www.niddk.nih.gov/health/diabetes/pubs/dcct1/dcct.htm.*

Diabetes Prevention Program (DPP) — clinical trial sponsored by the National Institutes of Health that compares the effectiveness of diet/exercise with that of metformin or a placebo in reducing the risk for type 2 in high-risk persons. For more information, see *http://www.preventdiabetes.com/.*

diabetogenic risk profile — a descriptive term for a person's level of known risk factors for diabetes (e.g., body mass index, physical activity level, family history).

diabetogens — drugs or other factors that cause diabetes; some drugs cause blood glucose (sugar) to rise, resulting in diabetes.

dyslipidemia — abnormal excess of fat or lipids in the blood.

dyslipoproteinemia — abnormal concentrations of one or more lipoproteins, a combination of a lipid and a protein, used to transport cholesterol and other lipids through the bloodstream.

Early Treatment of Diabetic Retinopathy Study (ETDRS) — study that examined the effects of laser photocoagulation and aspirin on the progression of diabetic retinopathy in patients with diabetes. For more information, see *http://www.nei.nih.gov/neitrials_static/study53.htm.*

edentulous — describes the loss of teeth, especially in elderly people; toothless.

end-stage renal disease (ESRD) — the final phase of kidney disease, treated by dialysis or kidney transplantation. ESRD can be a complication of diabetes.

epinephrine — principal blood-pressure raising hormone secreted by the adrenal medulla.

estrogen replacement therapy (ERT) — refers to the use of estrogen as a prescription drug to replace the hormone estrogen that is no longer produced by the ovaries of women as a result of menopause.

excess mortality — increased rates or numbers of deaths in a specific population by age, sex, cause, and sometimes other variables.

fasting glucose — glucose concentration in a person who has not eaten recently; used to diagnose diabetes.

fatalism — a belief that events are predetermined and cannot be altered by human effort.

fibrinogen — a normal component of human plasma that functions in blood clotting.

functional impairment — damage that affects one's ability to perform daily activities.

gangrene — death of body tissue due to poor circulation. Gangrene is a serious complication of diabetes and may lead to amputation.

gestational diabetes mellitus (GDM) — type of diabetes that can occur during pregnancy; in most cases, blood sugar levels return to normal after pregnancy.

glaucoma — eye disease associated with increased pressure within the eye that can damage the optic nerve and cause impaired vision and blindness. Persons with diabetes are at increased risk for glaucoma.

glomerular filtration rate — measure of the kidney's ability to filter and remove waste products; used to diagnose kidney disease.

glucose tolerance test — test formerly used to diagnose diabetes. Blood glucose is measured before a patient has eaten that day. Blood is subsequently tested after the patient drinks a liquid containing glucose to see how the patient's body metabolizes glucose over time.

glycated hemoglobin — see HbA_{1c}.

glycemic control — maintenance of normal glucose levels.

glycosuria — high glucose in the urine, a sign of poor blood glucose control.

glycosylated hemoglobin test — see HbA_{1c}.

health-related quality of life (HRQOL) — aspects of self-perceived well-being and ability to function affected by the presence or treatment of disease. A number of instruments have been developed to assess how health affects one's functional ability.

hemoglobin A_{1c} (HbA_{1c}) — a blood test that measures a person's average blood glucose level for the 2- to 3-month period before the test.

HDL cholesterol — high-density lipoprotein cholesterol, a transport form of cholesterol in the blood. Low concentrations of HDL cholesterol are a risk factor for CVD, especially in persons with diabetes.

Hispanic Health and Nutrition Examination Survey (HHANES) — a national survey conducted during 1982–84 of approximately 16,000 Hispanic persons aged 6 months–74 years. Hispanics were included in past health and nutrition examinations but not in sufficient numbers to produce estimates of the health of Hispanics in general nor specific data for Puerto Ricans, Mexican Americans, or Cuban Americans.

hormone replacement therapy (HRT) — refers to the use of hormones as prescription drugs to replace the hormones estrogen and progesterone that women's ovaries stop producing during menopause.

hypercholesterolemia — excess of cholesterol in the blood.

hyperglycemia — too much glucose (sugar) in the blood, a sign that diabetes is out of control. Hyperglycemia can occur when the body does not have enough insulin or cannot use the insulin it does have to turn glucose into energy. Signs of hyperglycemia include a great thirst, a dry mouth, and a need to urinate often.

hyperglycemic conditions — conditions that cause an increase in the level of glucose in the blood.

hyperinsulinemia — too high a level of insulin in the blood.

hyperlipidemia — too high a level of fats (lipids) in the blood.

hyperosmolar coma — a coma related to high levels of glucose in the blood and requiring emergency treatment.

hypertension — high blood pressure, a condition that occurs when blood circulates through the arteries with too much force, increasing the risk for heart attack, stroke, and kidney problems.

hypertriglyceridemia — Too high a level of triglycerides, a type of blood fat. Triglycerides can increase when diabetes and weight are not under control.

hypoglycemia — a condition that occurs in persons with diabetes when their blood glucose levels are too low. Symptoms include feeling anxious or confused, numbness in the arms and hands, and shaking or feeling dizzy.

hypoglycemic agent — drug used to treat hyperglycemia in persons with diabetes.

impaired fasting glucose — When a person has a fasting glucose equal to or greater than 110 mg/dL and less than 126 mg/dL, they are said to have impaired fasting glucose. This result is considered a risk factor for future diabetes but, by itself, does not determine a diagnosis of diabetes.

impaired glucose tolerance (IGT) — condition diagnosed when a person is determined to have abnormal blood glucose levels, but not abnormal enough to be called diabetes. People with IGT are at increased risk of developing diabetes.

incidence — the number of new cases of a disease among a certain group of people during a certain period of time.

index pregnancy — the pregnancy in which a condition (e.g., diabetes) is first identified.

insulin — a hormone that controls the level of glucose (sugar) in the blood.

insulin resistance — abnormal metabolic pattern where body cells lose sensitivity to insulin. Insulin resistance is a risk factor for diabetes; it also increases risk for cardiovascular disease.

ischemic heart disease — See coronary heart disease.

Juvenile Diabetes Research Foundation International (JDRF) — major diabetes organization focused exclusively on diabetes research. JDRF focuses on type 1 diabetes. For more information, see *http://www.jdf.org/*.

ketoacidosis — see diabetic ketoacidosis.

LDL cholesterol — low-density lipoprotein cholesterol, a transport form of cholesterol in the blood. High concentrations of LDL cholesterol are a risk factor for cardiovascular disease, especially in persons with diabetes.

lipids — fats, including cholesterol, triglycerides, and phospolipids.

lipoprotein — component of system used to transport lipids (cholesterol, triglycerides) in the bloodstream. Major lipoproteins are LDL and HDL.

locus of control — a common measure of perceived ability to control events.

macroalbuminuria — high levels of urinary protein (albumin), a sign of kidney disease, especially in persons with diabetes.

macrovascular disease — disease of the large blood vessels caused by atherosclerosis. There are three types of macrovascular disease: coronary (heart) disease, cerebrovascular disease, and peripheral vascular disease.

metformin — a drug used to treat type 2 diabetes.

mg/dL — milligrams per deciliter. Term used to describe how much of a substance is in a specific amount of liquid (e.g., the number of milligrams of glucose in 1 deciliter of blood).

microalbuminuria — refers to albumin excretion in the urine. Microalbuminuria is a risk factor for kidney disease.

microvascular disease — disease of the small blood vessels, especially of the kidney or the eye.

myocardial infarction — also called a heart attack, results from permanent damage to an area of the heart muscle, caused by narrowed or blocked blood vessels that interrupt the blood supply to the area. A serious complication of diabetes that can cause death.

National Cholesterol Education Program (NCEP) — program begun in 1985 by the National Institutes of Health. The goal is to reduce the percentage of Americans with high blood cholesterol through educational efforts to raise awareness and understanding about high blood cholesterol as a risk factor for coronary heart disease and the benefits of lowering cholesterol levels as a means of preventing coronary heart disease. For more information, see *http://www.nhlbi.nih.gov/about/ncep/index.htm.*

National Diabetes Education Program (NDEP) — federally sponsored initiative that involves public and private partners to improve the treatment and outcomes for persons with diabetes, to promote early diagnosis, and ultimately, to prevent the onset of diabetes. For more information, see *http://www.cdc.gov/diabetes/projects/ndeps.htm.*

National Health and Nutrition Examination Survey (NHANES) — refers to the periodic National Health and Nutrition Examination Surveys that use a household interview to ascertain diagnosed diabetes and an oral glucose tolerance test to measure undiagnosed diabetes. For more information, see *http://www.cdc.gov/nchs/nhanes.htm.*

National Health Interview Survey (NHIS) — data collection program of CDC's National Center for Health Statistics that studies the health of the civilian noninstitutionalized population of the United States. Monitors trends in illness and disability and tracks progress toward national health objectives. For more information, see *http://www.cdc.gov/nchs/nhis.htm.*

nephropathy — kidney disease, a serious complication of diabetes.

neuroendocrine — pertaining to the interaction between the nervous and endocrine systems.

neuropathy — disease of the nervous system caused by damage to the nerves, a serious complication of diabetes.

oral glucose tolerance test (OGTT) — see glucose tolerance test.

parity — the state of having had children, or the number of children previously borne.

periodontal disease — disease of the gums; can be a complication of diabetes.

peripheral vascular disease (PVD) — disease of the large blood vessels of the arms, legs, and feet caused by blocking of major blood vessels.

person-years — or person-time, a measurement combining persons and time. It is the sum of individual units of time that the persons in a study population have been exposed to the condition of interest.

pharmacotherapy — the treatment of disease with medicines.

poverty — set of money income thresholds that take into account family size and composition used by the U.S. Bureau of the Census to define the official poverty level.

preeclampsia — condition characterized by high blood pressure and swelling that some women with diabetes have during the late stages of pregnancy.

prevalence — the number of people in a given group who are reported to have a disease at a certain point in time.

proliferative diabetic retinopathy (PDR) — growth of abnormal blood vessels and fibrous tissue from the optic nerve head or from the inner retinal surface elsewhere in persons with diabetes.

proteinuria — too much protein in the urine; may be a sign of kidney damage.

relative risk (RR) — the ratio of the risk of death or disease among those exposed to the risk among those unexposed.

renoprotective — describes a factor that preserves kidney function or prevents kidney disease.

reserpine — a drug used to treat hypertension.

retinopathy — a disease of the small blood vessels in the retina of the eye.

San Antonio Heart Study — a population-based study of diabetes and cardiovascular disease in Mexican Americans and non-Hispanic whites.

secular trend — change over a long period of time, generally years or decades (e.g., the rise in prevalence of diabetes in the United States in the past 20 years).

self-efficacy — one's personal judgment of one's own ability to succeed in reaching a specific goal; belief in one's ability to maintain behavioral change in the face of situational challenges.

self-management — a set of skilled behaviors that allow patients to manage their illness; for diabetes, this includes glucose management, patient education, and preventive care.

sequelae — results of a disease or injury or of complications. Sequelae of diabetes include its complications.

social network — a set of social ties that connects an individual with others.

social support — emotional or task-oriented assistance provided by the community, family, friends, or significant others.

socioeconomic status (SES) — a descriptive term for a person's position in society, using criteria such as income, educational level attained, occupation, and value of dwelling place.

standardized rate ratio (SRR) — a rate ratio in which the numerator and the denominator have been standardized to the same (standard) population distribution.

stroke — disease caused by damage to blood vessels in the brain. Depending on the part of the brain affected, stoke can cause loss of muscle function, mental function, vision, sensation, or speech. Stroke can be a complication of diabetes.

sulfonylurea — a drug used to treat type 2 diabetes that lowers the level of glucose (sugar) in the blood.

thrombosis — the formation, development, or presence of a thrombus, or blood clot, in a blood vessel. Thrombosis can develop as a complication of atherosclerosis, especially in persons with diabetes.

triglycerides — type of blood fat.

United Kingdom Prospective Diabetes Study (UKPDS) — clinical study of newly diagnosed patients with type 2 diabetes. The UKPDS demonstrated that intensive glucose control prevents complications of diabetes.

vascular — relating to the body's blood vessels (arteries, veins, capillaries). See cardiovascular disease.

vitreous hemorrhage — bleeding or leaking of the clear jelly (gel) that fills the center of the eye.

waist-to-hip ratio (WHR) — a measure of central obesity, which is related to insulin resistance and risk for diabetes. Formula: waist circumference divided by hip circumference.

Definitions for this glossary were compiled from the following sources:

National Institute of Diabetes and Digestive and Kidney Diseases. *The Diabetes Dictionary.* Bethesda, MD: U.S. Department of Health and Human Services, National Institutes of Health, NIDDK, 1994. (NIH Publication No. 98-3016)

American Heart Association. *Heart and Stroke Facts.* Dallas, Texas: American Heart Association, 1999.

Last, John M., editor. *A Dictionary of Epidemiology.* Third Edition. New York: Oxford University Press, 1995.

Merriam-Webster's Collegiate Dictionary. Tenth Edition. Springfiled, MA: Merriam-Webster, Inc., 1993.

www.ingramcontent.com/pod-product-compliance
Lightning Source LLC
Chambersburg PA
CBHW080241180526
45167CB00006B/2369